Self-Referral
Maximum Health

A New Theory Of Health and Disease

by

Dr. Michael Borger

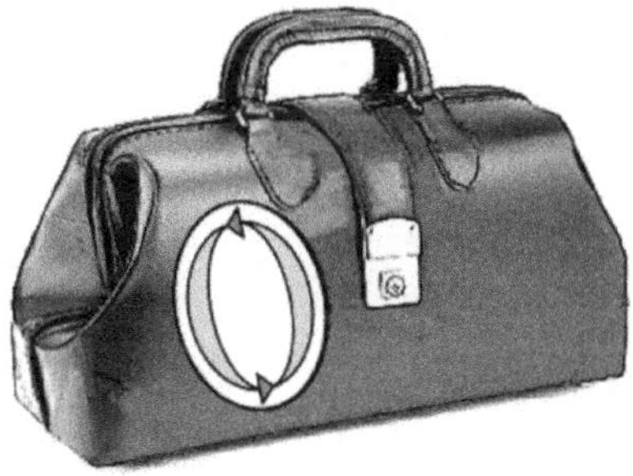

Solving the Healthcare Crisis

Published by
Northwood Enterprise Inc.

Dr. Michael Borger

ISBN 979-8-9913980-0-8

Library of Congress LCCN 2024918001

For further information:

www.MaximumHealthExpert.com

www.MaximumHealthInstitute.com

Dr. Michael Borger

www.Substack.com/@DrMichaelBorger

Northwood Enterprise Inc.
353 North Hartman Street
Nappanee, Indiana 46550
NEI@fourway.net

Photograph and Illustration Credits

Source of all historic photographs of Andrew Taylor Still MD, William Garner Sutherland, DO [Historic Collection], John Stedman Denslow, D.O. [cat # 1997.51.298], Irvin M. Korr, Ph.D. [cat # 1996.17.03], and Osteopathic Research and History courtesy of and Copyright © Museum of Osteopathic Medicine, Kirksville, Missouri, USA. The author thanks them for their kind assistance. Used by permission.

Source of photograph of R. Keith Wallace, Ph.D. Copyright © R. Keith Wallace, Ph.D. Used by permission.

Source of photograph of R. Buckminster Fuller and the Biosphere, Restored American Pavilion Expo '67 Copyright © Alamy Inc. Brooklyn, New York, USA. Used by permission.

Source of all clipart and photo images otherwise are derived from Corel Draw image collections and are Copyright © 2024 Corel Corporation, Ottawa, Canada. Used by permission. All new illustrations derived from clipart appearing in the book *Self-Referral/Maximum Health* are Copyright © Dr. Michael Borger and Northwood Enterprise Inc. All rights reserved. Used by permission. See https://www.corel.com/en/clipart-and-photos/

Dr. Michael Borger intends this book to be a tribute to all the great physicians, medical research scientists, physicists, biologists, philosophers, and spiritual thinkers mentioned in its pages. If there is any error made, it will be mine and not theirs. Thank you for your forbearance as I genuinely intend to do good through publishing this information.

Dr. Michael Borger also intends to bring information to everyone who is a patient to better work with their healthcare providers to move away from the Disease Approach and move toward the Health Approach. I urge all patients to carefully examine their lifestyle and diet habits. You are creating your own future every day of your lives. I urge you to think proactively and set a course for better health today!

Self-Referral

Maximum Health

DISCLAIMER

The advice and information in this book relates to general health care. It should be used to supplement rather than replace the advice of any doctor or trained health professional regarding your specific medical needs. All matters regarding your health require medical supervision. If you have any health concerns, please consult a trained health professional who can fully assess your needs and address them effectively.

No treatment program, including drugs, surgery, or lifestyle changes, is effective for everyone. Some people may become worse despite any treatment or lifestyle changes. Do NOT make any changes in your health care treatment without consulting your doctor or health care professional; it can be very dangerous to suddenly stop taking some medications or other treatments.

One of the purposes of this book is to teach you to participate more actively in your healthcare. You should strengthen communication between you and your doctor. You may wish to share the book *Self-Referral/Maximum Health* with your doctor. You can discuss it with your doctor so the two of you can work together more effectively to help you promote Self-Referral and achieve Maximum Health.

The author, publisher, and seller disclaim any liability for any outcomes arising directly or indirectly from the use of this book.

CONTENTS

Preface

Coronavirus COVID-19: The Wakeup Call

The Coronavirus Pandemic was a major health threat that killed multitudes of people in the United States and across the world. The pandemic also created a unique first-time medical, social, political, and financial crisis. The Coronavirus Pandemic is a wakeup call to everyone who works in the medical system – or who receives services from it.

Critical medical journal articles across the world have made a compelling case that nearly all patients admitted for hospital care due to COVID-19 had underlying comorbidities. That means if the patient had one or more chronic condition, they were far more likely to become ill enough to require hospital care. The same was true for those who died from COVID-19. The most common chronic conditions found in these patients were hypertension, obesity, and diabetes. These are all quite common health problems that – in normal times - constantly populate doctors' waiting rooms.

This underscores a fundamental problem in American medical care: we have a fixation on the Disease Approach that focuses on definable diseases found in the patient. This is not a bad thing by itself; it is generally helpful and often lifesaving. We find the disease, we treat it as effectively as possible, and get on with life. There is a downside to this bias; today's medical care spends most of the energy, attention, and money on identifying and treating Disease. Where is promoting Health in all this?

This book - *Self-Referral/Maximum Health* - teaches the Health Approach today's medical care critically needs. A vital part of this book is teaching the principle of Self-Referral as the basis of normal body operations. Through understanding how the body creates health through a vast web of interconnected feedback loops, we quickly see that Health is the natural state of the human body. Disease results from unnatural interruption of *Self-Referral*.

We must work to optimize *Self-Referral* to move toward *Maximum Health.* This brings the principle of consciousness back to the center of medical care. Everyone needs to understand this.

Three simple additions to today's medical care will bring vast improvements. The first addition is simple and effective relief from the stress of modern life – never so obvious as in our present time – and will remove the chief cause of nearly all Disease. The second addition is evidence-based natural medicine that aggressively intervenes with patients to optimize their lifestyle - including diet, exercise, stress reduction, and better synchronization with the seasons and time rhythms of nature. The third edition is a simple system of manipulative therapy – hands on care for musculoskeletal pain – that will help enormously to reduce the Opioid Crisis. The goal of all this is restoring human consciousness through restoring *Self-Referral*.

What is consciousness?

How does this idea relate to medical care?

Medical care today treats the human body as a living biomechanical device. If this or that needs removed or repaired, it is time for surgery. If blood pressure or sugar is too high, it is time for prescription medications. Granted - we do give good advice on diet, exercise, quitting smoking and so forth – but it all stays at a level of "working on" the body more than "working with" the body. Until we acknowledge that the human body is a living, self-aware organism, we will continue working at the level of mechanics doing wrench work.

When we better understand the deep workings of the human body, we quickly see the body is not a biomechanical device that needs periodic tending. Rather, the body is a self-contained, self-aware living unit that has built-in command and control settings that create Health. The body has central monitoring of all body functions and can, when necessary, take actions to self-regulate.

When external conditions change, the body capably modifies its internal environment to adapt. When the body needs to run instead of walk, the body adapts to run. The common action needed for all this to happen is *Self-Referral*. The body refers to itself, by itself, and regulates itself - and adapts to create Health.

Maximum Health is the goal of all medical care, indeed of all life. This is the absolute best health the individual can maintain given present medical conditions and all measures taken to optimize lifestyle. The way we reach *Maximum Health* is to boost the body's *Self-Referral*. How do we do this?

We do this by acknowledging that consciousness – *Self-Referral* – is the basis of creating Health. Treating Disease is critical and mandatory – but if we change the likelihood of future problems by creating Health – there will be a steady reduction in chronic conditions. And those with chronic conditions will have far better control of them.

This is how *Self-Referral/Maximum Health* provides the tools we need to rid ourselves of the chronic conditions that make us vulnerable to health challenges like COVID-19. The numbers established around the country and across the world clearly show that many people who contract COVID-19 have either no symptoms or minor symptoms. But those with chronic conditions – read poor Health Approach medical care – are those in the hospital, often in profoundly serious condition.

In the past, everyone assumed that good or bad health was beyond our control. Please take this book seriously; it turns out that this is no longer the case. We can treat existing Disease more effectively and have better outcomes. By creating Health more effectively, we will prevent chronic conditions from starting - and optimize the course of chronic conditions when they arise.

What we can accomplish together is to change the direction of time so we can avoid these problems in the future. Let us guide the destiny of medical care toward all harmony, happiness, and progress. Let us work together to learn and implement *Self-Referral/Maximum Health*.

Dr. Michael Borger
Nappanee, Indiana
August 31, 2024

The "silly question" is the first intimation
of some totally new development.

- Alfred North Whitehead

Self-Referral

Maximum Health

Introduction
Pursuit of a Theory

For too long we have tried to wrest health from our bodies as if struggling with an enemy. Let us rise to a more complete view in which everyone's normal condition is health - and let us simply restore health when disease occurs.

The Silly Question

The "silly question" I want to ask – the same question I have been asking since college days in the 1970s - is this: the focus of medicine is always on disease, or what is wrong with people. I know we must identify and correct what is wrong when people need help. That is a central function of medical care. But beyond diagnosis and treatment, how do we move people away from *disease* – what is wrong - and move people toward *health* – what is right?

Whenever we look at diagnosis, this is the process of identifying what is wrong with anyone who goes to the doctor. Disease is simply a clear definition of what is wrong. Once we diagnose the disease, the next step is determining how to treat the disease, so it no longer troubles the patient. Whether we prescribe medicine, initiate surgery, or start any other treatment, the focus is the same: we must beat the disease – we must beat what is wrong.

How do we access what is right - our health? We can easily get a to-do list of known Risk Factors to avoid and thereby prevent disease. We are advised to get enough exercise, check periodically for cancer, follow a healthy diet, and to avoid stress. But this amounts to identifying measures to simply avoid what is wrong – disease. We're back to that topic. Other than taking vitamins, exercise, and avoiding Risk Factors, we have no clear road map to health.

This undue focus on disease and its treatment has created today's *Healthcare Crisis*. That is, because nearly everyone is so focused on combating disease like an enemy in war, few are looking toward peace: achieving health. A major reason for out-of-control healthcare costs is exactly this situation: we are so busy dedicating everything to combating disease that we completely fail to seek the goal of health – which, when achieved, will make disease obsolete.

Discovering the road map to true health as opposed to simply avoiding known risk factors is a journey worth taking. This journey will require a thorough examination of health and disease, and how we can better treat disease when it raises its ugly head. Equally important is the journey of discovery to find the path to create health and completely avoid disease.

Journey with Me

This is why I want to take you on a journey with me. This journey is one of inquiry and discovery, of questions asked and answers found. We will cover a lot of ground, you and I, but do not think that it will be a journey to make you weary. Rather, this will be a journey full of the joy of discovery, of puzzle pieces found and joined, of a big picture arrived at slowly, one step at a time. And anyone who loves a good mystery, and its solution, will find lots to ponder.

This is the journey of a freshman college student - who later became a medical student. The medical student went on to become a practicing physician. That idealistic young man wondered why people get sick, and how we can make them well again. This also is the story of a practicing physician who learned over forty years how to better promote health and prevent disease.

At last, that physician found practical answers – and he now wants to share those answers to improve healthcare for everyone.

This journey covers many times and places, many cultures and philosophies, and shows the unity among them all. Our journey will find us visiting with many interesting people, in many unexpected locations. We will prowl for wisdom in ancient China with the Taoist sage Lao-Tzu and the military genius Sun Tzu. Together we will examine the India of antiquity with Maharishi Patanjali and bring Vedic knowledge into modern times with Maharishi Mahesh Yogi. We will consider the teachings of the *Bible*'s King David and Jesus and see their application to modern healthcare.

Doctors from the past and present will share their vision of the body, health, and disease with us. We will hear from doctors ancient and modern. We will travel to nineteenth century Midwest America to follow Dr. Andrew Taylor Still as he creates a uniquely American brand of medicine. Moving back to the present, we will survey the latest developments in stress and body-mind research. And – above all – we will seek practical ways for people to improve their health. Together we will seek *Self-Referral/Maximum Health.*

Pursuit of a New Theory

Most people have an outside interest that they enjoy. Perhaps they play golf, watch television, or read books. My interest blossomed into a consuming passion: the pursuit of a new theory of health and disease to improve medical practice.

Why would a busy physician spend his spare time working on such a theory? Every health professional works to relieve the suffering of sick and injured people. This theory provides one more way to meet that lofty goal. But this theory is more than just empty ideas; we will discover together many ways to create health and prevent disease before it gets started. And this is not just useless theory; practical applications of this knowledge will greatly improve medical practice. These applications will *reduce the need for medical care* – and thereby *radically reduce healthcare costs.*

Did this theory emerge all at once? No, it did not happen that way at all. It came into being a little at a time, over many years. The theory is a product of reading countless articles and books, thousands of outdoors walks, long sessions of meditation, deep thought and prayer, and discussion with many people – including medical colleagues, scientists, and patients.

When I began college in 1970, the theory was only a vague idea. I saw a single explanation of both health and disease. As I collected articles from newspapers, magazines, and scientific journals, each was a piece to the puzzle and contained ideas. Soon these ideas were cross-connecting and creating bridges, one to another. This went on through college, medical school, hospital training, and over forty years of medical practice. I now store these articles and notes in multiple file cabinets, coordinated by a computer database. The ideas have solidified at this point and this book catalogues the result of all this study.

Go East, Young Man

During my quest for knowledge, I mainly read Western textbooks and medical journals. That was driven by the demands of college, medical school, and practicing medicine. My pursuit of comprehensive literacy[1] also included the literature of the East. I concentrated on works that obviously apply to medicine. My studies have included what we in the West call Yoga and related disciplines. My interest was to find what is useful to promote health. Finally, I have included many spiritual readings, from the *Bible* to the Vedas to the *Tao te Ching* to modern writers of many faiths.

As a physician trained in the Western scientific tradition, I had to stretch my conceptual ability to learn Eastern ideas. There really is a Western and Eastern way of looking at life, the universe, and how it all works. Applying a spiritual understanding to medicine - what is to many a strictly cold, logical, and scientific subject - is equally challenging. Many of you will find yourselves scratching your heads and wondering what I am talking about while you read this book. Please bear with me; it will all come together. Your efforts will be well rewarded.

My quest for comprehensive literacy taught me a lot about Eastern traditions, and – sometimes unexpectedly - I also learned more about Western traditions in the process. We know a subject much better when we compare and contrast differing viewpoints. That is why I learned a lot about Western thought by studying Eastern ideas. Eventually, my quest taught me the philosophical unity of Eastern and Western thought. Many people quote Rudyard Kipling, saying "East is East and West is West, and never the twain shall meet."[2] I do not agree. There is more alike than different in Western science and ancient Eastern philosophy.

Unification of Western and Eastern thought will be helpful to both cultures. Western thought has solved many practical problems, but it often fails to provide inner peace for the individual. Eastern thought has solved the problem of inner peace for the individual, but often lacks practical success. It is as though each culture has gifts the other needs. If we can all simply listen and learn from each other, I believe medical care will improve enormously.

Finally, medicine is sorely in need of a renewed moral compass. Between the pressures of managed care, government regulation, and a medical system that relies more and more on technology, medicine has never had its compassion stretched so thin. Renewed attention to the spiritual basis of health and healing will vastly improve medical practice. All health professionals need to remember and practice what medicine is all about: *love and compassion for others.*

Focusing our attention on health and preventing disease through better lifestyle choices is central to this book's purpose. It is wonderful to have the miracle medications, surgery, and other aspects of Modern Medicine - when they are truly needed. Finding better ways to promote health and prevent disease will pay enormous dividends – both reducing suffering and saving money. Surely it is far better to prevent health problems before they occur than to solely rely on medication and surgery for what could easily be prevented.

Forty-Two Years in Medicine

Forty plus years in medicine have taught me a lot[3]. I mainly practice Family Medicine, but I also care for Industrial Medicine and Emergency Room patients. My patients are people of all ages - from newborn to senior citizens. My experience also includes several years as City Medical Director of our local Emergency Medical Service[4].

While my main practice is Family Medicine, I also have rendered care in patients' homes, inside rolling ambulances, at the Nursing Home, and in the Emergency Room and hospital. Because medicine is not always practiced in the daytime, I have seen patients at all hours of the day and night.

I carried out an ongoing education program for senior medical students to teach them practical skills as a part of their training. Many medical students gained instruction and experience as they rotated through my practice for clinical instruction. These young doctors in training taught me as much as I have taught them[5]. That is how, in the last forty plus years, I rendered medical care to thousands of people and taught medicine to scores of medical students in training.

All this experience has taught me a lot about people, health, and disease. As a husband and father, I know the experience of having loved ones sick or injured. As a caring human being, I have never chosen to grow calluses over my feelings. Being a physician has not made me immune to the suffering of others; it has made me more sensitive to them.

The wear and tear of life causes many physical and mental health problems. Today's fast moving, high-tech lifestyle piles on *stress* - more than any other time in history. My experience has taught me that stress is a major cause of disease. Doctors need better ways to help patients combat stress. The result will be vastly improved medical care.

Many people working in healthcare today are stressed-out. The result is they often reach and pass the burnout stage. Why does this happen? They are under pressure from government regulations, managed care, and keeping up with the Electronic Health Record in our over-regulated, hyper-technological age of medical practice.

Doctors, patients, and all health professionals desperately need to get back in touch with positive spiritual ideas, values, and practices. These are the great positive principles that have taught and inspired human beings throughout time. Healthcare personnel and patients alike will benefit from a dip in those healing spiritual waters.

Toward a New Synthesis

I have not been alone in contemplating these matters. My wife, Bonnie, is a wonderful best friend, loving wife, and excellent intellectual sparring partner. Much of this book came into being during discussions with her.

As ideas came, we winnowed them to separate the wheat from the chaff. Our most important exchange was when she told me, "Boil your ideas down. What do you have to say?" Without hesitation, I knew; I was creating a new synthesis of ideas to improve our knowledge of health and disease. My goal was to improve the practice of medicine – and all of this in a spiritual context.

The dictionary defines synthesis as "the combination of parts or elements into a whole."[6] This definition exactly captures what this book is to accomplish. Many parts of seemingly disparate knowledge must be brought together to make a new, more complete knowledge – a new whole instead of parts scattered all over the place, unconnected and without purpose.

My perspective is unique. I am a practicing physician, a scholar of the Western medical literature, and a student of Eastern knowledge. As a practicing Christian, I also am a person of faith. I believe the information that I have collected suggests a new vision of the human body, health, and disease. This unique collection of knowledge must be brought together for the good of everyone.

I have another unique perspective. I am an Osteopathic physician. Dr. Andrew Taylor Still founded Osteopathic Medicine in 1892 at Kirksville, Missouri[7]. Dr. Still founded a distinctly American reformation of medicine.[8] Today, Osteopathic physicians earn the degree DO, or Doctor of Osteopathy. DO is one of the two academic degrees one can earn in the United States to be licensed for the unlimited practice of medicine. The other degree, of course, is the more familiar MD, or Medical Doctor.

Osteopathic physicians like me practice the full range of medicine like our MD colleagues – but we also have a strong commitment to practicing Wholistic Medicine. Today, the term Wholistic (sometimes spelled as Holistic) is a popular term for widely integrated medical practice, frequently centering around a more natural approach. This is why the DO is committed to a Wholistic approach to medical care. The DO works to treat the whole person instead of just the obvious disease or symptoms. The DO also has the most effective and comprehensive system of hands-on therapy to treat medical problems of the musculoskeletal system.[9]

Modern Medicine has much to offer, but improvements are possible. Osteopathic medicine combines Modern Medicine with a wholistic approach and a sophisticated system of manipulative therapy. Both schools of medicine have much to offer, but neither has all the answers.

Eastern knowledge has seldom come to the public's attention except as a curiosity. And spiritual aspects of medicine are largely ignored except as speculation. This book is an effort to integrate these fields – and to unify them within a spiritual framework. *A major goal of this book is to harness this new synthesis of knowledge to improve medical care.*

Ideas Can Bring Change

Ideas are often the forerunners of change. This is true in politics, education, and the social sciences. It also is true in the so-called hard sciences of physics, chemistry, and medicine. This book shares ideas that are eminently useful, if not revolutionary.

R. Buckminster Fuller was a one-of-a-kind human being who, following the Great Depression, went to the library and taught himself everything he could, in every field of study he could find. Fuller is known as the inventor of the geodesic dome and originator of many other brilliant ideas and inventions. He made a career of theorizing, inventing, writing books, and lecturing in a sincere effort to help all of humanity improve itself. He taught that, by knowing as much as we can about as many subjects as we can, we can better understand and improve our world - and thereby improve the lives of all human beings.[10]

One of his central themes was this: we all need to know as much as possible about many subjects – and then integrate that knowledge to better understand our world. Fuller called the complete knowledge that he advocated *comprehensive literacy*. It is my hope that we all will emulate R. Buckminster Fuller's concept of comprehensive literacy.[11] By applying these ideas to defining health and disease, we can better understand both. We will gain a more complete vision of man's health-promoting *Self-Referral* – the way to *Maximum Health*. Combining these ideas teaches us the reality of *Self-Referral/Maximum Health*.

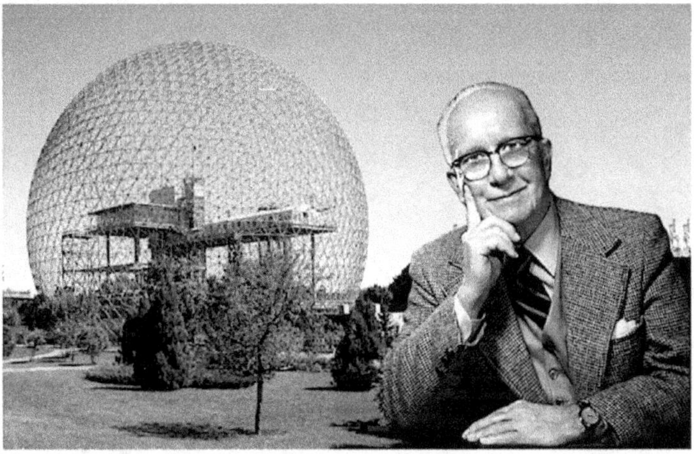

Architect-Inventor-Polymath R. Buckminster Fuller travelled the world teaching his comprehensive design science. His many inventions include the geodesic dome – a structure designed to help humanity succeed by providing a low-cost way to enclose large volumes of space for climate control. The above dome is the Biosphere constructed at the American Pavilion Expo '67, St Helen's Island, Montreal, Canada in 1967.

This book is a useful synthesis; it integrates approaches to health that were formerly thought separate and unrelated. Physicians and scientists of the world will examine these ideas and, based on their merit, will test and explore them further. The resulting knowledge will enter the mainstream of Western medical thought. This will bring a refreshing unification of many ideas, producing a clear improvement in medical care. The most important result will be a better chance for suffering people to regain their health.

For too long we have tried to wrest health from our bodies as if struggling with an enemy. Let us rise to a more complete view in which man's normal condition is health - and look to restoring health when disease occurs.

Thanks to jet planes and the electronic media, the world is fast becoming a small place where everyone knows each other. Let the West learn from the East, and the East from the West. Let all people of faith talk with and respect each other. Let us together seek *Self-Referral/Maximum Health.*

Self-Referral
Maximum Health

Chapter 1

Bringing Ideals Back to Medicine

Returning lost ideals to any field can refocus thinking and resources. Medical care can expand beyond just treating disease and work toward creating health and harmony through the *Self-Referral Paradigm*.

The Silly Question Revisited

One of the most familiar quotations from the history of science refers to a pretty basic idea. That idea is: when someone has a brand-new theory, they nearly always question what went before. This is true whether we are referring to physics, biology, chemistry, astronomy, or any other field.

Whenever someone proposes a new theory, they always have some kind of question they are working to answer. The question inspires the new theory. This is often a source of disruption to those experts of the field in question. Those who defend the old guard nearly always dismiss such questions as without merit or just plain silly. However, the question may turn out to be the start of something new and worthwhile. Alfred North Whitehead states this quite clearly:

> The "silly question" is the first intimation
> of some totally new development.

After over forty years in medicine, I have concluded we need to refocus our attention in healthcare. Yes, we need to continue combating disease as it appears, but we also need to focus on health.

This is a different point of view for many people – both in the medical field and outside of it. It is very clear to me that we desperately need to promote health – and thereby prevent disease.

When we consider pursuing the path to health - while combating disease as we encounter it - we need to examine the sweep of history that brought medical care to where we are now. How was medical care conducted in the past? Is today's medical practice the way it always was, or has it changed?

Bringing Ideals Back to Medicine

This book is about bringing ideals back to medicine. "Ideals?" you may think. "What ideals? Whose ideals? Aren't doctors, nurses and others working with ideals already? What are these ideals, anyway? Now that's a silly question. Don't we already know what the ideals of medicine are?"

Ideals are our highest possible aspirations. Some ideals include ethical behavior, universal love, and respect for all, and working for world peace. The world's great religions teach these ideals. Because such ideals usually spring from our faith, they are among the strongest beliefs we have. They are the real inner force driving our lives.

Our personal list of ideals inspires us all. Perhaps one of the best statements about ideals came from a quote by Carl Schurz on a greeting card I received:

> Ideals are like stars: you will not succeed in touching them with your hands, but like the seafaring man on the desert of waters, you choose them as your guides, and following them, you reach your destination12.

Medicine is based on the well-known ideal of the Golden Rule. "Do unto others as you would have done unto you,"[13] we have heard taught by Jesus. "Treat other people the way you want to be treated."[14] What demonstrates this ideal better than helping sick or injured people regain their health?

While helping sick people is noble, many today say that ideals are too abstract, too impractical to apply to the field of medicine. Others say that business and political concerns have driven ideals from medicine like deer before a forest fire. How can we bring ideals back to the practice of medicine?

We often learn ideals by hearing about people who are good examples. These people dedicate their lives to their profession. The quality of their work leaves an impression on our culture that inspires those who follow when they are gone. No one in the history of medicine has surpassed the excellent primary care offered by the General Practitioner doctors.

Forty years ago, the last of the fabled General Practitioner physicians were widespread. The GPs were trained in an era where all doctors learned a broad range of family medicine. Doctors who wanted to specialize had to master that formidable body of knowledge first – only then could they go on and train to become specialists. The GP focus was on families – children and adults alike.

That system of medical education and practice produced physicians who had an incredibly broad and deep skill set. They could handle anything from delivering babies to suture repairs; management of complex internal medicine problems to childhood diseases; and they practiced medicine day, night, and weekends. They often juggled an enormous office practice with concurrent care of many hospital patients.

The GPs also had a marvelous way with people. Those doctors had a magnificent personal touch. They seldom rushed anyone, and they never gave their patients less than complete respect. Those doctors made the effort to know their patients as complete human beings. Then - and only then - did they prescribe remedies. The GPs were not cold, emotionless technicians; they were members of the family.

Where Did the General Practitioners Go?

Today, the doctor who treats your soul as well as your body seems outdated, something forever gone - like poodle skirts, soda fountain Coca-Cola, or the Chevrolets with big fins on the back. Nevertheless, the GPs today – even as a memory - tell us a lot about what people want in a physician.

Do they want knowledge and technical prowess? Certainly, but there is no substitute for your family doctor who knows you and treats you like a member of their family – like the GPs truly did. Time has passed, and now the GPs have either retired or passed on. But the memory of their contribution remains, and the high standard of the care they offered is legendary.

Many miss the old Chevys and the rest, but the doctor is different. Cars and soft drinks come and go, but nearly everyone needs a doctor's care. When the doctor meets our needs, it is a wonderful healing experience, and we are deeply satisfied. Today, many people are far from satisfied; rather, they come away from medical care unhappy or even angry. What is different about today's doctors? Why are so many patients dissatisfied?

One important difference between today's doctors and those of forty years ago is specialization. Forty years ago, most doctors were broadly trained family doctors - the old GPs. They used their skills to care for everyone – any age, male or female, no matter what your health status.

The medical profession has changed since then. More doctors have specialized. Today many people complain that they cannot find a well-rounded family doctor. Instead, doctors refer patients back and forth from one specialist to another like ping-pong balls. Even with all the specialists, patients often fail to find the relief they seek.

Another difference is economics. The ongoing controversy about how to pay for medical care is one of the top hot-button issues of our time. We know that everyone needs medical care - for day-to-day problems, chronic conditions, and the major emergencies requiring hospitalization or surgery. The question of how to pay for medical care remains a Gordian knot that defies solution.

Because of economic pressures, many today see the doctor's role as anything but healing. People want the caring, healing physician like the old GPs, but feel that Ebenezer Scrooge is treating them. There is a perceived gap between what the public wants and what they see in today's doctor. Whether this is truth or propaganda, the impact on today's patient often causes disappointment and anger.

This is disconcerting - to say the least - to doctors. In previous eras the public regarded doctors as the cream of society's crop, leaders in morality, and champions of the public trust. How do we repair the damage that has occurred to the doctor-patient relationship?

Patients are equally nonplussed by changes in the healthcare system itself. Rather than getting great respect with comprehensive medical care at a leisurely pace, they are hurried through a system that often fails to respect the individual. I want to examine these issues - what is wrong? How did this situation develop? What can we do to improve things? How can we restore ideals - and dignity - to medical practice?

The Ideal of Caring

Why do people want doctors like the venerable GPs? The answer is simple: The General Practitioners of the world became personally involved with patients as people. I don't mean tending to diseases that happen to have patients attached; I mean *caring for people*.

Patients are not health statistics or dollars earned. Most especially, they are not *an interesting case*. Their needs go way past the prescription pad and the surgery table. Their needs are physical - but they also are complete human beings with emotional, psychological, social, economic, and spiritual needs. Doctors should be people-oriented servants of mercy whose mission is to relieve suffering of all kinds.

Some say doctors like this are extinct. Are there doctors like this in the world? You bet there are. Two uncles of mine[15] were real-life General Practitioners. Dr. Donald R. Hinton and Dr. Robert L. Hinton knew patients by their first names. When patients had personal problems, they dealt with them directly.

They were greeted by patients as members of the family at the hardware store, in church, or at the grocery. These were doctors to look up to, and in my practice, I try every day to follow their excellent examples.

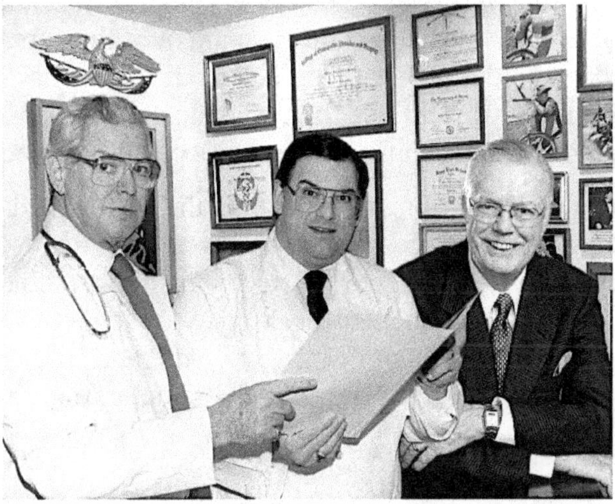

Two of the great General Practitioners: Donald R. Hinton, D.O. (left) and Robert L. Hinton, D.O. (right) – beside Michael Borger, D.O. in 1980.

Is the personal touch important? Medical experts know the personal touch can be the difference between life and death. Some newborn babies suffer from "failure to thrive:" They fail to grow and develop normally, becoming weak and sickly in spite of good nutrition and care. Some of these babies die. What causes this deadly problem? American orphanage research shows that failure to thrive results from a lack of physical cuddling and love. These babies actually die from a lack of personal love and affection.[16]

Should all doctors hug their patients? Within reason, it never hurts - and it often helps. More important is a loving, caring attitude from the doctor to the patient. People know when their doctor cares about them - through a sympathetic hand on the shoulder and an open and caring attitude. It may be difficult to measure or prove, but we all know that patients need love and concern from their doctors to recover their health. That is why one of the most important ideals of medicine is caring.

Business versus Healing

The business side of medical care is in severe disarray. Everyone needs medical care, but a solution for how to pay for it eludes us.

Patients are caught between the need for medical care and punishing medical costs. As the baby boomer segment of the population ages, the number of older people who need medical care has grown. The strain of finding ways to pay for medical care is causing a financial crisis and forces more and more emphasis on cutting medical costs.

There is nothing wrong with keeping the cost of medicine as low as possible. Cutting costs today, however, often seems more important than helping people recover their health. Insurance companies and government refuse to pay for services without rigid compliance to mountains of regulations and paperwork. The resulting conflict makes life miserable for doctors and patients alike.

Today's economic pressures threaten to make the caring doctor-patient relationship extinct. This is a tragedy because effective medical practice relies more on compassion, understanding - and, yes, love - than business concerns. When we only watch the bottom-line costs of medical care, we easily assume there is little to it other than the doctor poking around and writing prescriptions. Yes - patients need the technical knowledge and skills of the physician, but that is not all they need.

Medical care is no longer a private matter between caring people. What was once a sacred trust between doctor and patient has deteriorated into just another tough business deal. Today's medical mess results directly from doctors and patients alike turning their backs on the ideals of medicine.

Doctors are supposed to place the needs of the patient above all else. Patients are supposed to respect the doctors and take medical advice to heart. True healing requires a doctor-patient relationship based on mutual love, care, and concern. This healing relationship has more in common with family than with hard-nosed business practices. Today's healthcare system delivers just the opposite.

What can we do about this? As in all other fields, practical applications come from theories. Medicine got into the present mess by holding to the wrong theory. We need a new theory – one that will return medicine to its ideals. But whether we like it or not, we are where we are. What drives the non-caring, bottom-line approach to medicine? How can we change it?

The Scientific Tower of Babel

Bringing ideals back to medicine is important, but why do we need a new theory to change things for the better? How did we get to this point in the first place? There are thousands of doctors, nurses, and medical scientists active in the world today; why do I see a need to offer a new theory of medicine?

Several reasons come to mind. One is poor communication among physicians and research personnel. Many brilliant people simply do not know what other brilliant people are studying. The same is true for their findings. How can this happen in our age of instant communication?

Many professionals specialize in areas that hold the most interest for them. A doctor may specialize in Neurology or Internal Medicine. It is the same with researchers. One scientist may specialize in studying the lung; another may focus on the kidneys. Specialization has advanced scientific knowledge, but it also causes communication problems.

Thousands of scientists publish hundreds of articles every month. Many professionals lack the time to follow the literature outside their field. The most educated person can accidentally suffer tunnel vision. This is the case in today's world. We have a scientific Tower of Babel: many people, trying to improve medical practice, completely fail to communicate with each other. Confusion resulting from this communication snarl is preventing progress.

Let us imagine that researchers discover pieces of a large jigsaw puzzle with each article they publish. If we widely separate the pieces of the final picture, they make little sense. When we place together two pieces from different fields, they may fit together in unexpected ways, teaching us more about the big picture. They may suggest unexpected or even surprising conclusions. This is why thinking across specialty lines often yields unique perspectives. Architect-Inventor-Polymath R. Buckminster Fuller described the solution to this problem:

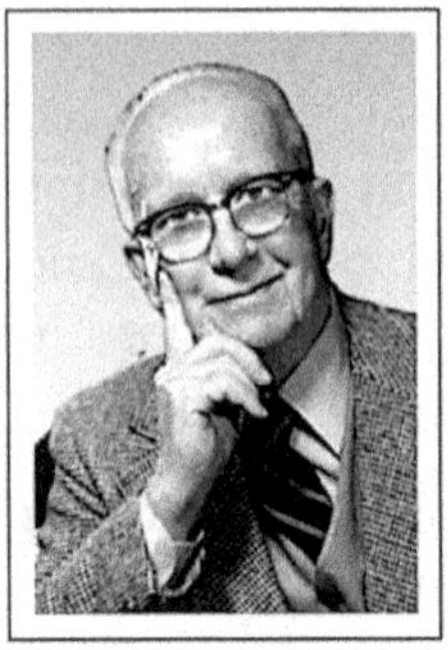

"The only way we can get somewhere is by a completely different way of seeing our world: an informational approach. You pay no attention to sovereign boundaries – you transcend them. You have to get away from any ideas of specialization and develop your comprehensive literacy. It takes a long time to know anything that way, but once you do, you know it so clearly and cleanly that anybody who'll sit down and work it out can't go wrong."[17]

I have pursued Fuller's comprehensive literacy since 1970. This book is a diligent effort to share the knowledge gained in the process. The result is a theory based on an eclectic collection of information. I also believe that it communicates clearly and cleanly what I have learned – and how all this can greatly improve medical care.

Another vital issue in improving healthcare is poor communication between medical researchers and the public. Scientists speak in precise, technical jargon. This language is often incomprehensible to the average person. The result is ongoing frustration or even anger between scientists and the lay public. Columnist Samuel Broder wrote:

> Some researchers stop trying to make their scientific goals understandable to the public. This leads to frustration on all sides . . . We must find a way to speak a common language . . . [improving] communication.[18]

Many well-known scientific geniuses of history knew the necessity of communicating well.[19] Physicist Erwin Schrödinger offered: "If you cannot – in the long run – tell everyone what you have been doing, your doing has been worthless."[20] Physicist Albert Einstein stated, "Most of the fundamental ideas of science are essentially simple, and may . . . be expressed in a language comprehensible to everyone."[21]

Doctor, We Are Not Communicating Well!

A major complaint from many is poor communication with their doctor. Some say their doctor does not take enough time with them. Others say their doctor does not seem interested in communicating with them. The result is a growing gap between doctor and patient. Most people find medical care difficult to understand. Poor communication with the doctor only amplifies fear and puts a damper on working together.

Adding to this confusion is the ubiquitous Internet. Many computer-literate people try to learn medicine online, going from one website to another. Others use the Internet to second-guess their doctor's choices on medications, surgery, or other aspects of medical care. If their doctor will not explain their health problems and treatment alternatives, who can blame people for going anywhere they can for information?

We also should remember that communication is a two-way street. Many patients refuse to communicate with their doctor. Some patients are intimidated by the doctor, or just plain nervous; they freeze up when their opportunity with the doctor comes. Others are sure they already know everything about their health status and merely need to confirm their thoughts with a quick prescription. Neither extreme is helpful.

A good doctor-patient relationship requires both parties to be willing partners. Both doctor and patient need to appreciate the need they have for each other. They must desire a positive relationship and then work together for better communication. Returning to the ideas of R. Buckminster Fuller, we see the need in medical care to communicate both clearly and cleanly.

The Need for Harmony

Considering the many sources eroding the quality of medical care, we see a common problem. I submit the problem is *a lack of harmony.*[22] Looking at business pressures, poor doctor-patient relations, overspecialization, and scientific confusion, we see little harmony. These disparate problems cause nothing but disharmony in the present healthcare system.

Harmony is something that today's medicine - and today's world - needs very badly. Critics of the medical system complain about the skyrocketing cost of medical care – and justifiably so. These concerns are driving cost reduction measures like second opinions, prior approval for hospital admissions – and healthcare reform at the national level. All these measures are, at their base, attempts at restoring harmony to the healthcare system.

Everyone seems fixated on the problem of who is going to pay for medical care. By contrast, there is little attention on *how we are practicing medicine*. This is a fundamental mistake, and I believe this error is causing everyone to miss the real problem. In fact, I suggest that the high cost of medicine is not even the root cause of medicine's problems. Rather, it is the result of *faulty assumptions about health and disease*. The fundamental lack of harmony is not caused by economics; the lack of harmony *causes* the economic problems.

This is a novel idea. Is it possible that we are fixated on the wrong problem? Could it be that economic issues are not the problem at all? Could changing our perceptions improve medicine?

Perception and Paradigms

Perception is the meaning we attach to what we see, hear, touch, taste, or smell. If we smell smoke, we assume something is hot or burning nearby. We know that someone is at the door when we hear the doorbell. When driving, our time to cross the intersection comes when the stoplight turns green. If we get cold, we know to put on a jacket. This is how perception via the five senses informs us of the world.

We rely on the senses to inform us about our surroundings, but we use our intellect to attach meaning to the information. When we have the same experience, over time, we come to assume that certain facts are true. In medicine, we assume a fever indicates an infection. Pale, cold, and clammy skin may indicate blood loss or shock. A certain rash indicates chicken pox, and a red and coated throat suggests tonsillitis.

There are many facts that nearly everyone accepts as truth. We assume that aging is inevitable. We assume we cannot avoid stress-related diseases like high blood pressure and ulcers. We assume that high cholesterol, obesity, lack of exercise, or high-risk behaviors are unavoidable. Conventional popular wisdom – and often medical wisdom - teaches that *the best we can do is cope with these problems.*

The sum of all our assumptions defines our view of the world - and how it works. We call this world view our *paradigm.* Our paradigm thus depends upon the assumptions we hold to be true. Our paradigm affects us deeply in how we think about ourselves, other people, the environment, and decisions we make every day.

If we assume that anyone we do not know is potentially dangerous, our behavior will reflect that paradigm. Someone seeing the world that way will not speak with or even look at strangers. That person will be unlikely to offer assistance to a stranger, who they see as a potential threat. If enough people adopt this paradigm, human relations will be chilly and distant.

The opposite world view or paradigm has equal implications. If we assume that other people – strangers or not - are generally trustworthy and potential friends, behavior will reflect that paradigm. Such a person will readily engage in eye contact and verbal exchange with other people. They will also be more likely to help others when needed. If enough people adopt this paradigm, human relations will be warmer and more positive.

Our paradigm thus defines how we see ourselves, other people, and how the world works. Examining the current paradigm of medical care is critical to understanding the problems we face today. Through examining today's medical paradigm, we will better understand where we are and how we got there.

Changing Paradigms for the Better

The paradigms of patients, doctors, and scientists are no different from those held by any group of people. Human beings establish paradigms slowly, over time, through the experience of people facing similar situations.

In business, industry, and medicine we often say, "there is no point in reinventing the wheel." That phrase makes it clear that people – if they are smart – learn from the experiences of others. They learn what works to achieve goals – and they learn what does not work. The application of this principle is common knowledge. Would anyone want to ride a horse coast to coast when they can take a plane and complete the trip in hours?

Breakthroughs in science, technology, or thought make big changes in our paradigm. When Thomas Edison invented the electric light bulb, it lit up the night. Suddenly we could read at night, work at night, and even attend baseball at night. When Henry Ford made the automobile available to the public, people could travel anywhere - even coast to coast. When the Wright brothers flew their airplane at Kitty Hawk, they set the stage for easy travel throughout the world. All these breakthroughs made things possible that were previously impossible. The world changed, and so did the paradigms associated with those advances.

Thomas Kuhn wrote about changes in the paradigm of scientists in his book *The Structure of Scientific Revolutions*[23]. Kuhn argues that scientists share common assumptions about the world. They agree how the world works, no matter what their area of science. The physicist, astronomer, and geologist have very different fields of study - but they share the same common knowledge about the properties of matter, energy, chemical reactions, and similar principles.

Kuhn points out fundamental changes in paradigms through the course of history. Breakthrough discoveries change basic assumptions. Before modern astronomy, the Ptolemaic view of the universe held that the sun, moon, stars, and planets revolved around the Earth. This view was the dominant paradigm of astronomy until the sixteenth century. Galileo, Kepler, and Copernicus proved that the sun was the center of the solar system. Only after a lot of religious and political struggle did the world's paradigm change. Kuhn calls this kind of radical change in thought a *paradigm shift*[24].

Changing paradigms are the foundation of Stephen Covey's best-selling book *The 7 Habits of Highly Effective People*. This book continues to revolutionize the business world.[25] Covey teaches that reexamining our most deeply held values is very important. Only by changing our way of thinking can we improve our lives, our families, our businesses, and our world. Covey shows how our paradigms define how we structure and live our lives. He writes:

> The United States today is the fruit of a paradigm shift. The traditional concept of government for centuries had been a monarchy, the divine right of kings. Then a different paradigm was developed - government of the people, by the people, and for the people. And a constitutional democracy was born, unleashing tremendous human energy and ingenuity, and creating a standard of living, of freedom and liberty, of influence and hope unequaled in the history of the world[26].

Do paradigms and paradigm shifts matter? Covey argues that paradigms are critical.

> Paradigms are powerful because they create the lens through which we see the world. The power of a paradigm shift is the essential power of quantum change, whether the shift is instantaneous or a slow and deliberate process.[27]

I suggest that the paradigm of medical practice shifted sometime between the General Practitioner era and now. The assumptions of doctors and patients alike changed, and it was not for the better. The resulting dissatisfaction continues to cause severe deterioration of the doctor-patient relationship – and degrades the medical system.

Political or economic measures will not deliver what patients really want: *doctors who meet their deepest needs*. Politics and economics will not bring what doctors want: *the ability to heal the patient*. The ineffective medical paradigm that now exists takes a terrible toll in dissatisfaction - from patients and doctors alike. This negative impact interferes with the positive emotions needed to heal. This is why patients and doctors are estranged from each other.

I suggest the problem is deeper than meeting patient and doctor expectations. The field of medicine is ripe for a paradigm shift of monumental proportions. Just as physics went through a paradigm shift from the science of Isaac Newton to that of Albert Einstein, medicine also must change. This paradigm shift will change our assumptions about the body, health, and disease – and *how we practice medicine.*

The Self-Referral Paradigm

What are today's doctors and patients about to discover? What new perceptions are on the horizon of medical progress? We may glimpse this new paradigm by reexamining the object of all medical care - the human body, and our assumptions about it.

The human body is healthy for most of the average lifetime. This hardy biological creation somehow survives a poisoned ecology, bad diet, insufficient exercise, and the stress and craziness of modern life. How does the body do it all? The body is resilient because of excellent design. The body is self-correcting and capable of adapting to any number of noxious influences – and stays mostly healthy. How does this happen?

The human body dynamically responds to challenges it encounters by adapting to the challenges. *Self-Referral* is the body's ability to regulate itself - by itself. This is how the human body maintains health throughout life.

Today's disease-focused medical care largely ignores Self-Referral, instead seeking ways to neutralize disease or irritating symptoms. By ignoring Self-Referral, today's medical care is ignoring the best road to health. Rather than ignoring Self-Referral, doctors must seek Self-Referral and work with it. The *Self-Referral Paradigm* will focus on how the human body works through Self-Referral – and restoring Self-Referral whenever possible.

Many in business now want to understand Eastern philosophy. This interest partly stems from the need to compete with Japan, China, and other Pacific Basin countries. Seekers of business wisdom have made best-sellers of formerly obscure books. These unexpected hot sellers have included Miyamoto Musashi's martial arts classic *A Book of Five Rings*,[28] an excellent source of strategy useful to business. Another example of this phenomenon is Sun Tzu's

Art of War. This venerable teaching also has sold well - in several editions – and even inspired some best-selling computer war games.[29]

Doctors and patients can glimpse the new Self-Referral Paradigm in these sources of wisdom. Thomas Cleary writes in the introduction to his translation and commentary of Sun Tzu's *Art of War*:

> According to an old story, a lord of ancient China once asked his physician, a member of a family of healers, which of them was most skilled in the art.
>
> The physician, whose reputation was such that his name became synonymous with medical science in China, replied, "My eldest brother sees the spirit of sickness and removes it before it takes shape, so his name does not get out of the house. My elder brother cures sickness when it is still extremely minute, so his name does not get out of the neighborhood. As for me, I puncture veins, prescribe potions, and massage skin, so from time to time my name gets out and is heard among the lords."[30]

Modesty is not the point here. The ancient physician tells us that prevention of disease requires much more thought, planning, and skill than treating it after the fact. Sun Tzu states the same idea in terms of the martial arts:

> To overcome others' armies without fighting is the best of skills.[31]

In today's climate of spiraling medical costs, prevention is more important than ever to doctors, patients, and budget planners. Looking for ways to defeat disease in earlier stages - or even preventing disease completely – is of great interest. *We see here that Sun Tzu's insight could be a path to both reducing patient suffering and reducing medical expenses.*

Implementing the Self-Referral Paradigm

Health care experts know that prevention of disease is far more cost-effective than treating disease after it occurs. Screening patients often identifies health problems early. When doctors treat disease in its early stages, they prevent the devastating effects of undetected long-term disease. This is why working to prevent disease prevents suffering and yields big savings.

Today's medical care does not focus on prevention; people usually see the doctor if they are sick – or after they are miserable from symptoms of advanced disease. The focus is now on disease – after it is diagnosed, often in advanced stages. Promoting health will require a reorientation of the entire medical system. *The Self-Referral Paradigm will focus on promoting health and catching disease early for effective treatment.*

Healthy lifestyle choices produce healthy patients. Everyone knows this, but a major challenge lies in changing deeply entrenched patient behavior. The constant flurry of confusing advice from media accomplishes precious little – and passing out stock pamphlets at the doctor's office seldom helps. Tailoring effective lifestyle recommendations to the individual must become a high priority. *The Self-Referral Paradigm will focus on comprehensive lifestyle intervention to optimize health.*

Considering disease prevention, we must turn to the problem of stress. Medical research shows that stress creates body wear and tear - and causes many diseases. This may be true, but how can a stressful experience translate into disease? Even if we answer this question, how can we avoid the negative effects of stress? A better understanding of stress and disease will benefit both physicians and patients. *The Self-Referral Paradigm will focus on new ways to reverse the effects of stress.*

Today, many suffer from bone and muscle pain. These health problems cost billions of dollars every year – both in lost work time and Healthcare Spending. Despite the enormous economic impact, debate is ongoing about what causes these problems – and how to treat them. *The Self-Referral Paradigm will focus on effective ways to treat painful bone and muscle problems.*

Few people live their whole lives in perfect health without need of medical assistance. Getting help when we are sick or injured is always welcome, but now we must find ways to help everyone *become as healthy as possible*. We call this *Maximum Health.*

Paradigm shifts happen because a new theory better explains known facts. We have some great ideas here, but how can we bring back ideals to medical practice? How can we refocus medical care to create Maximum Health? What is this new theory? How does this theory better explain known facts?

We have a wonderful journey ahead of us. We will travel through the world of ideas together, discovering the answers to these and many other questions. Let us explore medicine's emerging Self-Referral Paradigm. Together, we will explore *Self-Referral/Maximum Health.*

Chapter 2

Self-Referral, Health, and Disease

To discuss Self-Referral, we must know Self-Referral. To discuss medical care, we must know Health and Disease. To apply Self-Referral to medical care, we must know all three: Self-Referral, Health, and Disease.

Modern Medicine's Success

Modern Medicine has been a great success for a good reason: it works. Those served by Modern Medicine enjoy the best medical care available in known history. That is why both doctors and patients - people all over the world - accept Modern Medicine as the standard of excellence. Doctors are reluctant to change this system without strong reasons. Let us not forget; the present approach to medicine has been proven very successful.

That is why doctors are reluctant to change this system without strong reasons. Doctors scrutinize new ideas carefully before accepting them. Many today criticize Modern Medicine for being slow to adopt new ideas. I do not agree with those charges. Keeping medicine conservative serves the public well. Doctors accept new ideas slowly, but this protects the public from reckless experiments. Being conservative prevents poor or even dangerous medical care.

I want to be clear that I am not denouncing Modern Medicine. While I have some criticisms of it, they are made with deep respect for all the health professionals and institutions that make up today's medical system. I have a strong case to make advocating positive change to improve Modern Medicine, but do not mistake that for a desire to attack the medical system.

While we consider new ideas and approaches, let's not forget that we have much to be proud of in Modern Medicine. Before suggesting changes in the theory of medicine, it is good to remember how far healthcare has come. Most people today take doctors, medicine, and complete health care for granted. It was not always this way.

It is hard to believe there was no effective treatment for bacterial infections before 1935 - when a German researcher cured bacterial infection with a red dye. This was the first of the sulfa antibiotics.[32] The discovery of penicillin followed in 1946, making another major antibiotic available.[33]

Doctors now have scores of antibiotic medications for use against bacterial and even viral infection. Resistant strains of bacteria are difficult to cure - but most bacterial infection is no longer the dreaded killer that it was before 1935. To put this progress in perspective, consider this: *people used to die routinely from a strep throat.*

As medicine progressed, people have become accustomed to a higher quality of life. Quarantine and death from bacterial infection were once common. Now we consider such health problems as minor. An important result of this progress is a steadily rising definition of health. In the 1800s, living to the ripe old age of 45 was an accomplishment. People today commonly live well into their eighties, nineties, and beyond.

Medical progress since 1900 has been nothing short of astounding. Advances in immunization and medications have eliminated scores of deadly illnesses. Many disorders that used to kill thousands no longer exist. Modern Medicine has accomplished much, but the time has come to set higher goals.

Freedom from Disease is Not Enough

With improved health, the average person's thinking has changed. People now take long lives for granted. They expect to live a long time - but they also want a good quality of life.

This is in sharp contrast to even recent historical times. In the 1800s a discussion of the quality of life would have been ludicrous.

With shorter life spans, people did not live long enough to worry about the quality of life. It was enough just to stay alive - in any condition. Advanced disease crippled those who lived longer.

Medical scientists have studied the human body in great detail. As understanding of the body improved, so did medical therapy. This progressive refinement of medical knowledge has extended human life span dramatically. We now enjoy a longer life - but many older people still suffer the ravages of physical and mental disease. Those with parents or grandparents in a nursing home know longer life can be a curse as well as a blessing.

What is the *quality of life*? A healthy person has a better quality of life than someone plagued with chronic illness. Many people wonder how their retirement years will be. Will they live where they want - or will poor health force them to live in a nursing home? Will they lead an active life - or will disease confine them to a wheelchair? Given a choice, people want a higher quality of life. They want to enjoy life, and not merely endure it. This strong interest in the quality of life has caused an explosion of health information.

Modern people have a keen interest in advice on diet, exercise, and lifestyle. The news media – television, radio, and online - features some story about health nearly every day. Many people spend their online time as much at medical websites like WebMD as they do in recreational activities. Ability to participate in online discussions, subscription to email services, and blog reading also brings more health information to people.

Despite all this, Modern Medicine stays stuck in the ruts. Because of undue focus on disease, promoting health takes a long second place in doctor-patient interaction. Promoting health constantly seems to slip beyond our grasp, elusively staying out of reach.

Practice Follows Theory

Many today are frustrated with Modern Medicine. Doctors and patients are disgruntled – but this seems illogical. Why are people so critical of a system that delivers the best healthcare in history?

The reason for this dissatisfaction is a lag between what patients and doctors really want – and what Modern Medicine delivers. Patients do not want to see their doctor just when they are sick; they want to maximize their health potential – but they often do not know how to begin. Doctors know that prevention promotes health, but they can only advise against the same old list of risk factors. They have few ideas about how to promote health otherwise.

As a result, doctors feel frustrated. They simply return to what they know best: combating disease. This causes tension and frustration for doctor and patient alike. With the rising cost of healthcare, patients are paying more for what satisfies them less. This in turn creates negative public opinion and political pressure. Harassment of doctors and patients alike by government and health insurance rules and regulations is a direct result.

I believe the Disease Approach to medicine is obsolete, yet the Disease Approach still dominates medicine. Doctors and patients know, even if only subconsciously, that something is wrong. What can we do about this? We see here that we need change, but we cannot see a coherent alternative. It is not good to eliminate the Disease Approach without something better to replace it. *How can we find a better approach to medical care?*

We may find an alternative by examining the origins of the Disease Approach. An interesting question is: did it begin as a theory, and medical practice followed? Or did the Disease Approach evolve from practical considerations? Which was first: the theory or the practice? It may be impossible to say which

came first, but we might learn something useful by reviewing some medical history.

An excellent example of theory changing practice is that of operating room procedures. Today, we keep operating rooms meticulously clean. Hospital workers exhaustively scrub these areas often to maintain a germ-free environment. No one enters without first putting on sterile scrubs, cap, mask, and shoe covers. Then they extensively scrub their hands and forearms with disinfectant soap and water. Finally, they enter the surgery room – and don a sterile wraparound surgical gown and sterile gloves. In cases where extreme sterile conditions are necessary, surgeons and nurses even work in self-contained environmental suits that completely isolate them from the sterile surgery room. This is how we keep infection rates as low as possible.

It was not always that way.

The French scientist Louis Pasteur proposed his germ theory in 1864. Pasteur believed that tiny bacteria caused infection or even death. Public health officials later used his ideas to prevent disease through boiling milk; the heat kills deadly bacteria and prevents infection. Today, this is common knowledge as most people drink pasteurized milk and thereby avoid infection problems.[34]

What we take for granted today was new thinking in 1864. Doctors of Pasteur's day scoffed; they knew nothing of microscopic bacteria causing infections and death. The accepted theory of the time was spontaneous generation - a bizarre idea that infection appeared out of thin air. Few understood that tiny bacteria could cause infection and were everywhere.[35]

British Surgeon Joseph Lister challenged prevailing medical opinion in 1867. Lister put Pasteur's ideas into practice. He insisted on boiling all surgical instruments before use. He also ordered surgeons and nurses to wash thoroughly and don sterile clothing before operating.

Lister’s colleagues ridiculed him for his efforts, alleging that Lister was completely wrong and making a fool of himself. Those who kept track of numbers found quite the opposite. By using sterile procedures, Lister radically reduced his patients' rate of infection. Only then did physicians recognize Pasteur's ideas.[36] Today, all surgery takes place under strict sterile conditions.

We see that theory can influence medical practice. That is, new ideas are tested. If they improve medical practice, doctors and health professionals will adopt the new ideas. This proves that the medical system has the flexibility to accept and adopt new practices if they are found to improve medical care.

Medical schools teach the Disease Approach because it is now in vogue. We assume that a new theory, if proven true and practical, will be accepted by the medical community. Such a theory will revolutionize medicine, as did the ideas of Pasteur and Lister. The result will be a more comprehensive science of medicine. This is the basis for offering the comprehensive theory of health and disease: *Self-Referral/Maximum Health.*

The Pendulum Swings

In medicine, the pendulum of interest swings between extremes. Medicine's best minds focused on the Disease Approach in the 1930s to 1960s. This resulted in the elimination of many scourges of humanity. Medicine conquered smallpox, yellow fever, polio, and many others. Many disorders remain unconquered – such as genetic defects, cancer, and AIDS - but progress has been impressive.

Following the 1960s, the pendulum of interest swung the other way. The 1970s and 1980s focused on a Health Approach to medicine. The Health Approach also has been fruitful. Science identified risk factors for disease: smoking, overweight, high fat diet, high blood pressure, and lack of exercise.

Medical scientists showed that changing lifestyle and habits reduces the risk of future disease. This proved what many had long speculated: lowering blood pressure and positive habits like regular exercise and low-fat diet improves health. That is why people today have more control over their future quality of life than ever before.

There is a hidden error in all this. Medicine has been looking either at health *or* disease *as if each were a mutually exclusive category*. Some textbooks describe disease and how to treat it; others promote health. Medicine needs a comprehensive theory of health *and* disease. We must move people toward the best health possible – *Maximum Health.* This is the basis of *Self-Referral/Maximum Health.*

Making Things Right

Many are unhappy with today's medical system. This is because the last forty years have taken medicine in directions that doctors and patients do not like. Everyone's point of view is different, but one common theme persists. Whether you are a doctor or a patient, you doubtless feel frustration with the present system.

Politicians and bureaucrats in government and insurance try to improve the medical system. Doctors do their best with regulations and try their own ideas to improve things. Patients try to improve their health any way they can while navigating the forms and regulations thrust upon them. Throughout all this is the ongoing struggle to reduce medical costs. We thus see how the medical system is in such disarray.

It strikes me as surprising that the medical system is such a mess. Highly educated people with good intentions oversee the medical system. How did they allow things to get this bad? What happened between the era of the General Practitioner and today's medical practice that changed the healthcare system and made it worse?

One problem is *failure to see the big picture*. This is best illustrated by a story of people traveling through a forest. They became fascinated with every tree they passed. They were busy examining the bark, the branches, and the leaves of every tree - and they became lost. This is what occurs when someone cannot see the forest for the trees.

Another problem is *competing interests*. Any attempt to remedy the medical system is fraught with conflicting people and groups that make it tough for anyone to improve things.

The multitude of competing economic, political, and social interests create difficult dilemmas. Good people often quit trying to improve things because of political or economic pressures.

Adding to this is the *complexity of the medical system*. Healthcare today involves patient care – but also a myriad of interlocking economic and political concerns. All the parts interact, often affecting one another in unexpected ways. This is why fixing one part of the system often unexpectedly affects other parts of the system. The result is an endless series of failed fix attempts. Many who start to improve the system throw up their hands after poor progress with details. The whole medical system then stays the same or gets worse.

How can we deal effectively with these obstacles and make real improvements to the healthcare system? *To make things right we must reexamine our basic assumptions about medicine.* For such a reexamination to work, we must consider some new ideas.

Self-Referral Leads to Maximum Health

Most people realize that few things created by humans run well without help. If we build a bridge, it only lasts for so long and needs repaired or replaced. The same is true of a road or a building. The human body is different from manmade structures. Its normal functions create and sustain health over the typical life – these days seventy to ninety years - or even longer.

How our bodies work so well, with little assistance at all, is one of life's deepest mysteries. While science slowly uncovers how the body works, one layer at a time, the complexity seems nearly infinite. Human beings seem unable to understand the design and operation of the body. We have learned a lot, but it appears that only God can understand it all. As the *Bible*'s King David wrote in Psalm 139: -14:

For you created my inmost being;
You knit me together in my mother's womb.
I praise you because I am fearfully and wonderfully made.[37]

One thing we absolutely comprehend is that the body has excellent design, and part of that design is naturally staying healthy. To explain this natural ability to stay healthy we will use the term *Self-Referral.* Self-Referral is the natural ability of the human body to govern itself – and stay healthy. This idea seems revolutionary, yet we see evidence of it with every human being. People are born, grow to maturity, and – barring disease or an accident - usually live a long life. How does the human body do all of this?

We can best understand Self-Referral as a concept, an idea of how the human body works. As with most ideas, we cannot put Self-Referral in a test tube for scientific study. Self-Referral does not strictly refer to a person, place, or a thing. Self-Referral is an idea, a concept of how the body works.

If Self-Referral is how the body works, it is logical to find ways to improve Self-Referral – so the body works better. *It would be a major improvement in medical care if we could find ways to improve Self-Referral.* This would be a major improvement in promoting health, as well as suggesting new ways to treat diseases that doctors diagnose every day.

People throughout the medical system have varying ideas. We can all agree that we want patients to achieve the best health possible. I am calling that goal *Maximum Health*. This is a laudable goal that is worth working toward. But how can we better understand *Self-Referral* and *Maximum Health*?

Self-Referral as the Flow of the Universe

One way to explain the concept of Self-Referral is to start with the biggest, widest, and most inclusive definition. Self-Referral in its essence is an idea that describes something that we feel or experience. In Eastern philosophical terms, I think of Self-Referral as *the flow of the Universe*. In Western terms I think of Self-Referral as *the flow of God's will*.

Making all that practical is quite a chore. How can we apply such a broad term to our lives? To understand Self-Referral, try this example: We make plans to help our lives flow smoothly. Despite our plans, events beyond our control occasionally trap us. Say you have fifteen people coming over for Thanksgiving. The dog just chewed up the rug, and the children are running wild. Then your phone rings. Your aunt wants you to run an errand when you pick her up to come over.

You can deal with this situation in one of two ways. One way to handle all this is you get mad, spank the dog and children, and then tell your aunt to get lost. Thanksgiving is shot. A second way to deal with the situation is to relax, give in to it all, and cope as best you can. Thanksgiving is on, and you are working through what must be done as you go along.

The first response results in misery for you and your family; the second response is to go with the flow and is overall more effective accomplishing your goals. When we say *go with the flow of the Universe*, or *go with God's will*, we try to act harmoniously and create happiness. Go with the flow is another way to say *go with Self-Referral*. When we go with the flow, we are close to living our lives within Self-Referral.

Although he didn't call it that, the ancient Chinese philosopher Lao-Tzu taught about Self-Referral. Historians believe that Lao-Tzu lived about 500 BC. He may have been an older contemporary of Confucius. His classic work is the *Tao te Ching*, or *Book of the Way*. Lao-Tzu taught that the best way to carry out successful action is, paradoxically, to let go completely of action. He wrote in the *Tao te Ching*:

> Less and less do you need to force things, until finally you arrive at non-action. When nothing is done, nothing is left undone.[38]

This makes beautiful poetry, but many will question the practicality of these ideas. Most Western people do not think like this; we either do something - or we do not. What is non-action? What could it possibly accomplish?

Non-action can accomplish quite a lot. Stephen Mitchell writes in his excellent translation and commentary of the *Tao te Ching*:

> A good athlete can enter a state of body-awareness in which the right stroke or the right movement happens by itself, effortlessly, without any interference of the conscious will. This is . . . the purest and most effective form of action. The game plays the game; the poem writes the poem; we cannot tell the dancer from the dance.[39]

One of the best examples of an athlete performing in an effortless way is basketball great Michael Jordon when he was playing with the Chicago Bulls. Michael Jordon seemed to defy gravity as he bounded into the air, sinking shot after impossible shot, winning game after game. Commentators are at a loss to find sufficient superlatives to describe this basketball player's performance. Many sports experts name Jordon as the greatest living basketball player, perhaps the greatest basketball player of all time. The truth is that we saw someone flowing in Self-Referral every time Michael Jordon sailed through the air, winning another game.

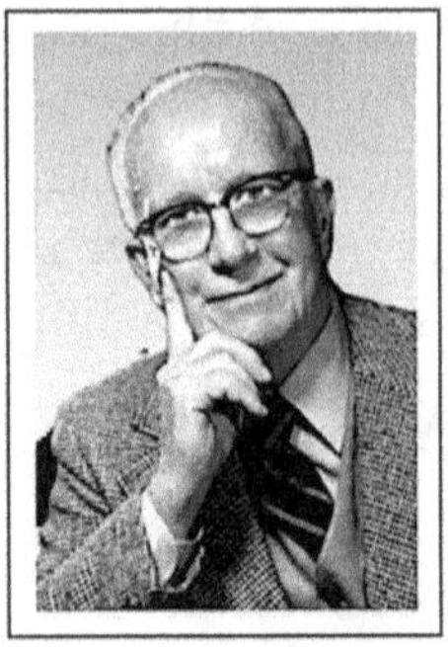

Practical application of Self-Referral is not limited to sports. We can apply it to many other fields. Architect-Inventor-Polymath R. Buckminster Fuller wrote similar ideas in his 1970 book *I Seem to Be a Verb*, Fuller wrote that humans on Earth can overcome ecological and population pressures. If we use what is already here more effectively, Fuller argued, humanity can prosper.[40]

This optimistic view contradicts doomsayers insisting the world is beyond repair - but there is a catch. Fuller challenges us to put aside our greedy ways, learn to use everything, waste nothing, and do more with less. This is a big order: it requires decision-makers to know and work with the natural flow of things. Fuller, like Michael Jordon playing basketball, was flowing with Self-Referral even as he wrote his books.

Achieving Maximum Health

Self-Referral/Maximum Health recognizes the natural flow of things and applies it to medicine. This is a great idea, but how do we work with it in a practical way? How do we find Self-Referral in the body? How can we work with *Self-Referral* to achieve *Maximum Health*?

Self-Referral implies motion, constant change, and especially balance between the pairs of opposites.[41] Motion is one definition of life. If the heart beats, the lungs breathe, blood and other fluids move through the body - this is life. Motion only stops at death.

The living person maintains the motion that sustains life through the ability to balance opposites. These opposites are physical realities that must be maintained for life to continue. Self-Referral describes the process that balances the natural flow of things to promote health.

Every person has strengths and weaknesses in their health. These arise out of genetic tendencies, injuries beyond anyone's control, and lifestyle choices that we all make every day. We cannot control accidents or what genetic tendencies we have inherited through our family - but we can do everything to make better lifestyle choices.

Many people say there is no way to achieve better health. Some health problems will always require surgery or medications - but nearly every common health problem improves with better lifestyle choices: diet, exercise, stress reduction, and related strategies. Over time, these changes can make big improvements in our health.

Many observers of life note that our culture is badly out of balance. People place too much value on material possessions and sensual experience - leaving people hostile and dissatisfied. Many want an alternative to life in the fast lane. In this context, seeking balance is a very good idea.

Today, many are suffering poor health caused by poor lifestyle choices. Examples are diabetic patients eating sugary deserts, those with high cholesterol consuming fatty foods, and heart patients living with high stress levels. All these people can improve their health greatly with aggressive lifestyle changes.

We can easily determine our current health status through medical history review, physical examination, and appropriate testing – laboratory, EKG, chest X-ray, and the like. Once we know our health strengths and weaknesses, we can better balance the physiology and improve our health. Through aggressive intervention with medications, diet, lifestyle, exercise, and stress reduction, we can move toward our best possible state of health – *Maximum Health.*

Health and Disease

Self-Referral/Maximum Health provides a new view of medicine; a view that sees health and disease as two possible outcomes in life, a choice that everyone can make. I emphasize: *we choose health OR disease*. This is truly a new way to look at medical care. By recognizing that we all can take two paths – health OR disease – we awaken to the fact that we all have a choice. This is in sharp contrast to the passive, fatalistic attitude commonly held by doctors and patients alike.

Both doctors and patients perceive health and disease as separate and unrelated conditions. When we experience health, we seldom think about it. If disease comes along, it is usually an unexpected turn of events – and often a crisis. This why people see health and disease as separate and without connection.

People want health to relish life and do what they enjoy. Disease is like a Stephen King monster; it is a bad and dangerous notion that we do not like to talk about - period. We push it out of thought, out of mind – but it is always lurking somewhere in the shadows, like the Phantom of the Opera. When we hear of disease, it is like hearing about a tornado. We know it is too bad, but what can we do about it?

Health, by contrast, is welcome to anyone. We rejoice when we get up in the morning and feel good. It is a great day when our health is perfect, and we enjoy life. We love it when we can exercise to our heart's content without obstacles. It is wonderful to have full use of our senses and enjoy the world around us. All this is automatic. This is why the average person takes their health for granted – and they simply hope that good health continues.

People seldom connect health and disease. Healthy people are too busy enjoying life to think about how their bodies stay healthy. People with disease focus on defeating their illness - and getting back to health. Today, many people wonder how they can improve their health while avoiding disease.

Health professionals like exercise experts and dietitians work to promote health. Doctors and nurses focus on combating disease. *This "either-or" situation is an illusion.* The illusion is that there are two separate human bodies: the normal body in health, the other the abnormal body in disease. *This illusion is false.*

There is only one human body: that is, all people, whether healthy or ill, have the same biological structure. Everyone has a body containing parts: the brain, heart, digestive system, and so forth. The many parts work together harmoniously to create health. When these parts fall into disharmony, they create disease. An enigma emerges. People are structurally very similar. Why does one person fall ill while another remains healthy?

It is the purpose of *Self-Referral/Maximum Health* to understand, explore, and provide solutions to promote health while preventing disease. When we understand that health and disease are merely two conditions of the same body, we better understand our options. Knowing this, we see that choices we make every day may return the body to wholeness. This wholeness produces balance that creates health.

Balance of the body's many parts and functions create harmony and health. Imbalance causes disharmony and disease. Today's medicine badly needs to find more ways to create harmony and health. We must reexamine health and disease in light of *Self-Referral/Maximum Health.*

Self-Referral is how the body usually maintains health and, by default, prevents disease. It is through Self-Referral that the healthy body keeps its many parts in balance. The heart, lungs, blood vessels and myriad other parts of the body work in harmony. This is how Self-Referral, when working normally, creates health.

Likewise, Self-Referral balances out the many pairs of opposites: hot-cold, moving-still, fast-slow - to create and maintain health. When Self-Referral fails, the pairs of opposites get out of balance. The result is a state of chaos that causes disease. Correcting this chaos and restoring the harmony that creates health is the heart of *Self-Referral/Maximum Health.*

This explains how Self-Referral creates health or disease. This is how health and disease are BOTH outcomes of Self-Referral. What is Self-Referral that it is so crucial to health? How do we know Self-Referral when we see it? How do we know when Self-Referral works or fails to work? And – most importantly – how do we restore Self-Referral when it is out of order?

Today's Disease Approach Medicine

These are good questions, but anyone who works in medical care knows that few are pondering medical theories. Medical care is intense, time-consuming, and often grueling. The pressures of medical practice force doctors to get the work done and get on to the next patient. The doctor sees the patient, hears complaints, and performs a physical examination. Then the doctor orders testing, makes a diagnosis, gives advice, and writes prescriptions. Time is up, and it is time to move on to the next patient. Has the medical system made efforts beyond this to promote health? The answer is a strong yes - medical research over many years has studied what habits promote health and what habits promote disease. The goal of such research has been to learn how we can avoid future health problems. Many studies have identified predictive elements that point to future disease. We call these elements *risk factors*.

Today's health promotion focuses on avoiding a list of risk factors. Risk factors are habits over which we presumably have some control. If we continue bad habits, we run a greater risk of disease. Likewise, if we cultivate good habits, we avoid risk factors and avoid future disease. We can literally create a future of health or disease based on the choices we make that pertain to these risk factors.

For example: tobacco smoking causes cancer, lung disease, heart disease, stroke, and many other problems. Doctors tell patients to quit smoking to avoid future disease. Other known risk factors are lack of exercise, high blood pressure, alcohol consumption, overweight, high blood sugar, high cholesterol and triglycerides, and high fat diet. Health promotion consists of pointing the patient away from harmful habits and toward healthy ones.

These efforts help people to improve their lifestyle for better health, but doctors spend only a fraction of their time giving such advice. Most day-to-day medical practice focuses on battling disease. How did medicine come to focus on disease? Let us explore a story to illustrate how this developed.

A billionaire once donated automobiles to people living on a remote tropical island. The island had plenty of gasoline and oil, and for a time the cars worked fine. Everyone was happy. However, as time went on, the cars developed mechanical problems. Some even became useless. No one knew how the cars worked, so the islanders could not repair them.

Eventually, some islanders became curious; others just wanted their cars working again. They studied automobiles needing repair. These would-be mechanics cataloged the problems they found. They often named each problem after the mechanic who first found it.

The mechanics tried various repair techniques. Little by little, by trial and error, they learned to repair the cars. Some techniques succeeded and the cars worked again. Most repairs failed, and the cars stayed the same or got worse.

Then one mechanic looked more deeply into the structure and function of the cars. He studied the engine, the drive shaft, brakes, and steering. After long study, the mechanic rediscovered the mechanisms of the automobile. People following the mechanic's methods were more successful with automobile repairs. Once the mechanics better understood the automobile's normal operation, repairs became easier and more effective. [42]

An Imbalance of Ideas

Well-meaning people can be easily confused by an imbalance of ideas. The history of medicine is quite like the automobile story. The machine - the human body - was unknown for most of recorded history. Andreas Versalius published *The Fabric of the Human Body* in 1543. The book illustrated his dissection work and was the first reliable anatomy text.[43]

Nevertheless, ignorance of human anatomy never stopped surgery. Deformed skeletons found in archaeological digs mutely testify to the efforts of prehistoric surgeons. These would-be doctors presumably employed their best guess when using the knife. We now consider such crude methods terribly risky, but we should not be too smug. Prehistoric surgeons doubtless looked upon their predecessors as primitive.

Any knowledge, no matter how accurate, is a product of its times. The common knowledge of learned physicians in 1800 is now obsolete. Since then, Modern Medicine has benefited from the dramatic upsurge in knowledge since World War II and the Space Age. Advances in physics, chemistry, computer science, and engineering have transformed medicine from a best-guess art to a profession solidly based on science. Medicine is a broad field. Textbooks used by family doctors like me easily fill four large bookshelves. These textbooks are among the largest books printed today.[44] Other books help with diagnosis, surgery, medical imaging, emergency medicine, and pediatrics. Medicine is so complex that it should be no surprise that we confuse basic ideas like health and disease.

A textbook salesperson told me that it takes five years to write and publish a medical textbook - even with today's computer-assisted publishing. The latest medical textbook thus may be five years out of date the day it is published. Even online and smart phone-based textbooks are unlikely to include the absolute latest medical knowledge.

An important factor in medical practice is the need to stay current. Changing ideas bombard physicians constantly as new knowledge rapidly replaces the old, making medicine's learning curve steeper every year. Today the field is growing at such a pace that doctors must study hard just to stay current. It thus is no surprise that broad thinking about the common origin of health and discasc is rare.

This constant shifting of the knowledge base causes confusion and disharmony. Self-Referral, by contrast, is harmony itself. Physicians need knowledge of Self-Referral to regain balance in their lives - and in their profession. The confusion created by the onslaught of changing medical knowledge creates an endless imbalance between the known and the new.

Confusion about the common origin of health and disease is such an imbalance of ideas. This is not surprising - Self-Referral is ephemeral and easy to overlook. Lao-Tzu tells us:

> Look, and it can't be seen.
> Listen, and it can't be heard.
> Reach, and it can't be grasped.
> Above, it isn't bright.
> Below, it isn't dark.
> Seamless, unnamable,
> it returns to the realm of nothing.
> Form that includes all forms,
> image without an image,
> subtle, beyond all conception.[45]

This sounds like a riddle from a Tolkien fantasy. Considering the human body, with its myriad parts and inner workings, we need a fantasy writer's imagination to comprehend it. Learning about Self-Referral requires a simpler yet more complex understanding of the human body. How does the body maintain normal operation as described in the automobile story? What process maintains health, and thus prevents disease? Where is Self-Referral in the human body, and how can we know it?

Where Is Body Self-Referral?

To find the body's Self-Referral, we must look for unity among diversity. We must find one process that is the same everywhere. Self-Referral is an idea - a principle that creates and maintains balance – and, through that balance, creates health and prevents disease.

At first glance, the human body is too complex to understand. The body's many organs and functions seem mysterious and unknowable. Suggesting a single process that unifies the body seems foolish. What could the lungs, brain, or kidneys have in common? What similarity is there between circulating blood and breathing air?

Whether we recognize it or not, the body is one unit and works as a single organism. Through many decades of life, the human body takes whatever life offers - and usually stays healthy. The idea that the body has many parts that work together is not new. The body has many organs, functions, and operations – yet somehow the body functions as a single unit. We read in the *Bible*'s Corinthians 12:12-20:

> The body is a unit, though it is made up of many parts; and though its parts are many, they form one body. If the foot should say, "Because I am not a hand, I do not belong to the body," it would not cease to be part of the body. And if the ear should say, "Because I am not an eye, I do not belong to the body," it would not cease to be part of the body. If the whole body were an eye, where would the sense of hearing be? If the whole body were an ear, where would the sense of smell be? . . . God has arranged the parts in the body, every one of them, just as he wanted them to be . . . there are many parts, but one body.[46]

All in all, it is amazing that the body works at all - let alone that it works perfectly most of the time. So many parts and processes work together to create a healthy body. How does the body accomplish the marvel of health? The human body has many natural mechanisms that maintain health. Like the clockwork of the islanders' automobiles, these mechanisms make the body's normal operation possible. We can examine these natural mechanisms and learn much about how the human body works.

One mechanism of normal operation is that of the five senses. Through the senses we see, hear, taste, touch, and smell the world around us. This is how we constantly know our surroundings - even if only subconsciously. Knowing our environment is vital to survive in an ever-changing world. If the traffic light turns red, we stop our car to avoid a collision. If we smell smoke, we look for a fire. How do these mechanisms work on a moment-to-moment basis? Can we find mechanisms of Self-Referral in the human body?

One such mechanism of Self-Referral is how our eyes respond to light. When the sun gets bright, we squint to protect our eyes. Our pupils squeeze down to a pinpoint to keep bright light out. If light becomes dim, our eyes open wider. Our pupils dilate to allow more light in dim surroundings. Here we see a glimpse of Self-Referral.

Remember - Self-Referral is the balance of opposites. When the eyes respond correctly to the opposites of light-darkness, we see balance. If they fail to adapt to sunlight, balance fails. Too much sunlight may blind a person. The other extreme is night blindness. Constant eye balance responding to light or darkness is critical for creating health and preventing disease; thus, it is one of the body's mechanisms of normal operation. This is how Self-Referral works.

Looking beyond the senses, another mechanism of normal operation is movement. Brain, bones, and muscle work together to allow us a wide variety of motion. The healthy human can walk, run, throw a baseball, or just sit still. All activities that we take for granted require constant feedback from the environment. Our bodies react to changes in position, terrain, and other conditions on a moment-to-moment basis - while we are still in motion. This is how Self-Referral works.

Many other body functions operate without conscious effort. We do not think to keep our heart beating or to breathe. We need no conscious effort to digest food or produce urine. These processes are natural and automatic. They require no effort or thinking. These body mechanisms take care of themselves. This is how Self-Referral works.

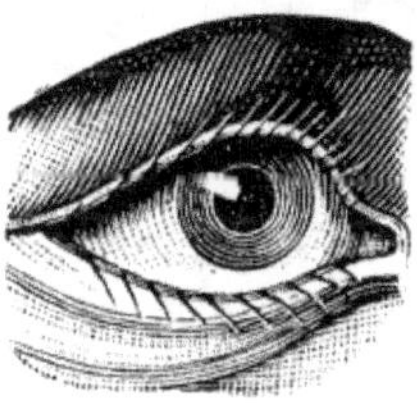

To illustrate the automatic nature of the body, consider this: how often did you blink your eyes while you read this page? Did you once have to think, "when did I last blink? Are my eyes getting dry? Should I blink to moisten them?" These mechanisms require no act of will; they are spontaneous and do not demand planning. This is how Self-Referral works.

Self-Referral of the body is its ability to balance all pairs of opposites. Some pairs of opposites are movement and rest, eating and elimination, breathing in and breathing out. The body's mechanisms seem simple, but students of the human body know that these mechanisms are far from simple. The body's normal operation requires a myriad of these mechanisms to maintain health – *through Self-Referral.*

Many Mechanisms of Self-Referral

The body's health depends on these many mechanisms of Self-Referral. These mechanisms at first seem to have little in common. How can we compare the heartbeat with sweating? Despite apparent differences, however, these mechanisms share a common underlying process. The body maintains health by a myriad of such mechanisms. Their common characteristics are:

* they refer to themselves for regulation
* they need no conscious effort.

Here we clearly see Self-Referral of the body. Through elegantly designed interlocking mechanisms, the body regulates itself. Through faultless design, the body's mechanisms have a rudimentary intelligence. Unless interfered with in some way, they are self-perpetuating as well. Listing all such mechanisms would be a formidable task. Many medical textbooks come close to precisely doing that.

The Body's Normal Operation depends on

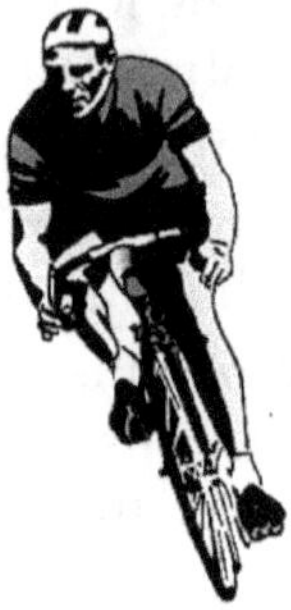

Breathing
Heart Function
Blood Pressure
Blood Oxygen
Temperature

Self-Referral allows the body to maintain constant internal conditions in an ever-changing external environment.

Even though the many individual mechanisms of self-regulation are quite different, the principle of Self-Referral is the same. The body uses this single principle of self-regulation to govern itself. This is unity from diversity. This is Self-Referral. Taking liberty with our quote from Lao-Tzu:

> We look at the body's Self-Referral and cannot see it; Listen, and it cannot be heard; Reach for it, but it cannot be grasped. *Only by inference do we know Self-Referral is there.*

Self-Referral Defined

Instead of continuously referring to the body's self-regulating mechanisms, we will use the term Self-Referral. By Self-Referral, I mean the body's natural ability of self-regulation. Through Self-Referral the body refers to itself, by itself, and regulates itself. Self-

Referral finds what changes the body needs to maintain health, and makes those changes happen.

Self-Referral

Maximum Health

Axioms Defining Self-Referral, Health, and Disease

SELF-REFERRAL is the body's process of dynamic self-regulation.

All mechanisms of SELF-REFERRAL work together to create and maintain HEALTH.

Interruption of mechanisms of SELF-REFERRAL create and maintain DISEASE.

Normal SELF-REFERRAL creates HEALTH.

Abnormal SELF-REFERRAL creates DISEASE.

HEALTH and DISEASE are functions of SELF-REFERRAL.

Self-Referral thus is the basis of health *and* disease. *The difference between health and disease is normal or abnormal functioning of Self-Referral.* And all this is as automatic as blinking our eyes.

Self-Referral and the Disease Approach

Doctors usually focus on diseases that are curable, or at least treatable. This approach is practical, but it has drawbacks. I believe this bias has produced an imbalance in medical practice.

The Disease Approach creates undue fascination with the details of disease, with apparent indifference to health. This imbalance perpetuates the myth that health and disease are separate and unrelated. Why do physicians focus on disease?

The Disease Approach organizes and simplifies medical care. Patients come to the physician with a bewildering array of complaints. Doctors need a way to sort out what ails the patient and what to do about it. The Disease Approach thus is very practical: it works. Medical knowledge has come far by first identifying disease, and then seeking treatment or cure.

The result is a cookbook approach to diagnosis and therapy. Find the correct diagnosis or disease, and the doctor proceeds with the suggested treatment. Doctors studying medicine thus learn diagnosis and treatment by rote. This has become a time-honored system because it is both effective and successful.

A second reason for the Disease Approach is medical practice's time demands. Doctors carry a heavy patient load. Consider this: in a given month, 750 of 1,000 American adults will have an illness or injury. Most will be minor problems like a cold or a stubbed toe. These people will take care of themselves. The remaining 250 will seek a physician. Nine of these will go to the hospital, but the remaining 241 will go to a doctor's office.[47] This is about one million new patients per month.[48]

Most medical problems require more than one office visit, so patients often return for care at least once. That means doctors in the United States see about three million patients every day. To understand that astonishing number, consider this: sixty-six thousand people fill the Chicago Bears football stadium for a typical Sunday game. *Doctors see 45 times that number of people every day.*[49]

When faced with the endless treadmill of medical practice, doctors must set priorities to save time and energy. This is the origin of the time-honored system of medical practice. Identify the disease, prescribe needed therapy, and move on to the next patient. This system is orderly and successful but offers little incentive to change.

A third reason for the Disease Approach is that doctors are so busy – even beyond medical practice. After a long day in the office, doctors often care for patients in the evening and on weekends. Patients constantly call with questions. Doctors go to the hospital to make rounds and perform surgery.

This lifestyle leaves little time for abstract contemplation. It does not surprise me that few physicians ponder Self-Referral or anything else beyond medical practice. Is it any wonder that doctors set their thinking and skills on the Disease Approach?

The answer to improving today's medical practice cannot be solely theoretical. A new theory alone will not solve the problems posed by the Disease Approach. Doctors and patients need practical methods to promote Self-Referral and restore the body's balance of opposites to maintain health. We also need practical methods to restore Self-Referral when the body suffers disease. What can we learn about the body's Self-Referral process? How can we improve Self-Referral?

Chapter 3

Self-Referral: The Key to Maximum Health

Self-Referral creates the body's health. If we know how to improve Self-Referral, we will know how to promote health. This is why promoting Self-Referral is the key to Maximum Health.

Finding Self-Referral

Self-Referral is the human body's capacity to govern itself. When we promote Self-Referral, we create balance. That balance creates health - and also combats disease. This is how we achieve Maximum Health. This is an interesting idea, but how do we find Self-Referral? How do we work with it?

Seeking Self-Referral is like hunting an unknown animal. Here and there we see signs of it. We can trace its activities by skillful tracking, but Self-Referral is often an elusive quarry. Like all hunters, we become discouraged. We may even doubt our quarry's reality - but, as any hunter knows, perseverance pays.

Self-Referral of the Warrior

Self-Referral is the balance of opposites, and this balance produces harmony. All physicians work to restore the body's Self-Referral, even when they do not know it. This idea seems poetic and noble, but can it be true?

Many people suffer when they are ill, and they identify disease as an enemy. They see medical care as a war against disease. This is why doctors and patients relate to the idea of the doctor as a warrior in a fight to banish disease - and restore health. If a disease is more serious, the fight to defeat it also will be more serious.

Fighting to restore health is the effort needed to restore harmony. Every doctor strives to restore harmony where there is none. The Emergency Room doctor restores harmony repairing a laceration. A specialist in Cardiology restores harmony correcting a heart-related fluid imbalance. The surgeon restores harmony removing a diseased appendix. A psychiatrist restores harmony working with troubled minds.

This is why restoring body harmony is the goal of all medical practice. An additional thought is: if we can restore harmony *before* disease becomes a serious problem, we can effectively *promote health and prevent disease*:

Restoring Harmony to Promote Health and Prevent Disease

- If disease is already present, promoting harmony will restore health - defeating disease.
- Promoting harmony has preventative effects – it can defeat disease before it exists.
- Promoting harmony creates health now and health for the future.

The philosophy of the Tao – that of seeking to establish or restore balance - greatly affected both martial arts and medical practice in ancient China. Chinese culture in Lao-Tzu's time was uniform. Most of the Chinese people shared a common philosophy. Their ideals permeated all strata of culture, from the emperor to the soldier to the physician. This commonality in thought allows us to draw parallels between the warrior and the physician.

In my practice I often feel like a general plotting strategy against disease. First, I hear reports of the enemy from the front lines as the patient describes their problem. Then I gather more information about the enemy by examining the patient. I often spy out the enemy's territory with X-ray and laboratory tests. Once I know the enemy thoroughly, I order a counterattack. I suggest behavioral or diet changes, physical therapy, exercise, medications, or surgery.

A doctor fights disease as a warrior fights an enemy in battle. When we compare physician and warrior, both must know their adversaries thoroughly. Both fields require careful strategy. Physicians and warriors resolve disharmony - an imbalance in the pairs of opposites. Both want to conquer the enemy - but with care. In war or medicine, we want to reduce complications to a minimum. And in either case - with war or medicine - the less used the better.[50]

Medications May Be Hazardous to Your Health

Just as war has unpleasant repercussions, therapeutic choices have side effects. I have on my desk the Physician's Desk Reference or PDR.[51] This massive book is a standard reference that doctors consult daily. The PDR lists medications, their common uses, and their side effects. A typical PDR entry is from one to three pages – in fine print. The prescribing information takes up about a third of this space. The rest of the entry lists every possible side effect - and there are many.[52]

Medications cure many ills, but they also can cause major problems. Medication side effects can be serious. An important scientific study found that prescription medications not only cause health problems – they also cause death. Is there proof for this in the medical literature?

A group of doctors looked at 39 major medical studies conducted over thirty years, looking for the cause of patient death. The researchers were shocked to find that adverse drug reactions were the fourth leading cause of death in the United States. Specifically, the study showed that the leading cause of death was heart disease - followed by cancer and stroke. The fourth leading cause of death – responsible for 106,000 deaths - was adverse reactions from prescribed drugs.[53]

"We were shocked," commented co-author Dr. Bruce Pomeranz, a University of Toronto researcher. Whether prescribed in the most up-to-date university center or in the local doctor's office, the threat is the same. "It doesn't matter if you're getting the drug at the Mayo Clinic or in Oshkosh, Wisconsin," Dr. Pomeranz added. "It's not a question of quality of care."[54]

It is troubling that negative side effects of prescribed medication are the fourth leading cause of death. Today's doctors and patients alike rely on medication to solve nearly any medical problem. "We are really in love with prescriptions," comments Dr. Raymond Woosley – who was chairman of the pharmacotherapy department at Washington, D.C.'s Georgetown University. He added: "We pop pills without thinking of the consequences."[55]

How is it that medications created to help people end up killing them? One reason is the too much of a good thing effect. Perhaps a blood pressure drug lowers the blood pressure too far, killing the patient. Another reason is unknown side effects.[56] Side effects are unexpected problems caused by prescribed medication.

Sometimes a beneficial medication has deadly side effects. Arthritis patients, for example, often take non-prescription drugs like aspirin, Tylenol, or ibuprofen. Because of arthritis pain, many people take too high a dose or take them too often. These medications irritate the stomach's lining. When people take these medications for a long time, ulcers can result.[57] Undetected bleeding ulcers can kill people.

Medications are usually safe when used correctly. Many side effects are a necessary tradeoff when treating serious medical problems. But - like the warrior in battle - the doctor must employ careful strategy and tactics. A doctor must do enough to restore harmony, but no more than necessary. A heavy hand on the prescription pad may make a bad situation worse.

Surgery Is Not Always Simple

Most people undergo surgery without complications - but surgery can have negative side effects. Surgery may be necessary: *the best cure for any condition that requires surgery for cure is surgery.* Surgeons who remove a badly infected gall bladder or appendix unquestionably save the patient's life.

Most operations are routine, but some patients have serious complications. Anesthesia can cause lung or heart problems. A few people die from the strain of surgery, especially those who are old or ill. Even when surgery goes well, there can be complications that later emerge.

Someone may require part of the intestine removed to save their life - but later they suffer from poor digestion and nutrition. Hip replacement for painful arthritic joints in older people is a common surgery. Hip replacement allows the person to walk, but later may interfere with the ability to drive a car or even walk normally.[58] Nevertheless, the benefits of the surgery nearly always outweigh the side effects.

Complications of surgery can be less benign – and some mistakes are positively disastrous. In one tragic case, a critically ill heart patient went to surgery for a heart transplant. Through an error, the patient received the wrong heart. The heart was of the wrong blood type, and this caused severe complications. Four days later the patient had another operation – with a correctly typed heart - that was successful, and the patient recovered.[59]

Medication and Surgery: The Less the Better

While medical care and surgery can be troublesome, we should not be unduly worried about problems. Most medications and surgery are perfectly safe, but side effects are real. Side effects are another way the art of medicine is like the art of war. We are better off without medical care or war – and if either is needed, the less used the better.

This is why prevention of illness is better than treating disease as it appears. Sun Tzu points out in *The Art of War*:

> The superior militarist foils enemies' plots; next best is to ruin their alliances; next after that is to attack their armed forces; worst is to besiege their cities.[60]

Sun Tzu's military thinking is similar to medical wisdom. "To foil the enemies' plots" is keeping patients healthy and resistant to disease; "to ruin their alliances" is avoiding contagion; "to attack their armed forces" is prescribing medicine; and "to besiege their cities" is performing surgery."[61] The modern classic *Harrison's Principles of Internal Medicine* echoes this wisdom:

> The physician who examines well individuals is not "wasting his training" when he is not constantly dealing with serious organic disease. More skill is required to recognize the early signs of ill health than to deal with what is obvious to the patient or his family. The discovery and cure of a potentially serious disease represents a far greater service to one's patient than ministrations in the course of an incurable condition.[62]

Promoting health to avoid disease is like taking measures to prevent war. By avoiding the cause of war, we may prevent war. Likewise, doctors can anticipate and prevent disease. Lao-Tzu agreed with the idea of prevention - of winning without fighting. In the *Tao te Ching* he wrote:

> Plan for what is difficult while it is easy, do what is great while it is small. The most difficult things in the world must be done while they are still easy, the greatest things in the world must be done while they are still small. For this reason, sages never do what is great; this is why they can achieve that greatness.[63]

Here we see that seeking Self-Referral is not some exotic idea. We also see that Eastern thought and Western thought is more alike than different. Wisdom is wisdom; knowledge is knowledge - no matter where or when we find it.

Self-Referral of Vital Signs

Self-Referral is the body's ability to govern itself. So far, we have only defined Self-Referral in broad terms. Do we need this idea to understand the body? What examples can we find to demonstrate Self-Referral?

Our bodies must maintain an ideal internal environment to stay alive. Doctors carefully watch what we call the vital signs - those signs that are critical to life. These are body temperature, blood gas levels, heart rate, breathing rate, and blood pressure. Disease or death is certain if any of the vital signs deviate far from normal. Why is this so?

One explanation of vital signs lies in body chemistry: many important chemical reactions only work in a narrow range of tissue acidity. This balance depends on constant blood circulation. If body cells are too acidic or not acidic enough, body chemistry fails, and cells may die in minutes. This is why the body keeps a delicate balance between nutrients and waste products.[64] The vital signs indirectly monitor delicate body chemistry. This is why doctors and nurses carefully monitor the vital signs - they are the indicators of life or death.

Doctors watch the vital signs to monitor the heart and circulation. The heart pumps blood, carrying oxygen to all body cells. If the heart stops, cell damage follows. The brain lasts only four minutes without oxygen; permanent damage occurs after that time. The heart stops if it lacks enough oxygen rich blood. Problems with breathing or blood pressure have similar deadly effects - to the brain, heart, and the rest of the body.

We see in the vital signs the balance of opposites. The heartbeat balances fast-slow. Temperature balances hot-cold. Blood pressure balances hard-soft. Breathing balances in-out. This comprehensive balance of opposites is Self-Referral.

An interesting question emerges: there is a clear balance of opposites, but how does the body maintain this balance? The body maintains Self-Referral through *mechanisms of Self-Referral*.

Self-Referral and Homeostasis

One way to understand Self-Referral is through the concept of homeostasis. The Greek root homeo means "like." Stasis means "to stand" or "to keep in place." Homeostasis thus describes the body's ability to balance all opposites and maintain normal body function.

W. B. Cannon wrote *The Wisdom of the Body* in 1932. He defined homeostasis as "the physiologic arrangements that restore the normal state once it has been disturbed."[65] Cannon described how the body responds to a changing environment. By working through its own mechanisms, the body maintains an ideal internal environment in ever-changing conditions.[66]

Today's medical textbooks define homeostasis in terms of Self-Referral, although they do not call it that. For example, *Stedman's Medical Dictionary* defines homeostasis as "the state of balance in the body" among "various functions and chemical compositions . . . of the body."[67] *Guyton's Textbook of Medical Physiology* defines homeostasis as the "maintenance of constant conditions in the internal environment."[68] *Ganong's Review of Medical Physiology* describes homeostasis as working through the principle of feedback. The body detects deviations from normal. This triggers body changes that continue until they restore the body's set point.[69]

When we look at textbook diagrams, we get an inaccurate picture. Two-dimensional drawings do not convey the moment-to-moment drama that plays out within our bodies. Homeostasis is not frozen in time; it is dynamically active every second we live.

We sweat when the weather is hot. Perspiration evaporates at the skin surface, cooling the body. We stop sweating once our body cools. Shivering is another example. When we are cold, we shiver to distribute body heat; when we warm up, shivering stops.

These experiences are common. We take them for granted – but what lies behind these experiences is not at all common. Complex mechanisms are at work below the surface. We do not think about them - they are automatic and happen so quickly. How does the body regulate itself on a moment-to-moment basis? How exactly does Self-Referral work?

Goals and Feedback Loops

We can best understand the mechanisms of Self-Referral through *Cybernetics theory*. Another important idea is the *feedback loop*. Where did these ideas originate, and what do they mean?

Norbert Wiener coined the term Cybernetics in 1948.[70] Wiener was fascinated that some self-regulated machines seemed to mimic animal behavior. Wiener noted that both animals and machines have goals. Both test the environment as they work toward meeting their goals. Once goals are met, work stops for a time.

Cybernetics is simple when applied to animal behavior. A wild animal's goal is to stay alive. It hunts for food when hungry. Once the animal eats, they accomplish their biological goal, and hunting ceases for a time. When hunger returns, the animal resumes hunting.

Cybernetics calls this process *communication* and *control*. Communication constantly checks on the changing environment, determining whether the goal is met. Control enforces work toward meeting a goal and stops work once the goal is met.[71] The idea gets more abstract when we apply it to machines. A simple machine cannot think independently, but many have self-regulating mechanisms. These machines can, in a crude way, simulate the animal model described above.

Self-regulating mechanisms use electronic or mechanical sensors to check the environment. Considering what the sensor finds, it switches other machines on or off.[72]

We can understand these ideas better by examining a common example, the thermostat. The thermostat senses a room's temperature. It can turn a central furnace on or off. If we set the thermostat at 65 degrees, it automatically turns on the furnace when the room gets cold. When room temperature rises to 65 degrees, the thermostat switches off the furnace. If thermostat and furnace are in good working order, the room will stay warm.

The thermostat and furnace form a system. This system's goal is to maintain a constant temperature of 65 degrees. The communication and control mechanisms of this system are entirely automatic. This circular system is a *Cybernetic feedback loop*.[73]

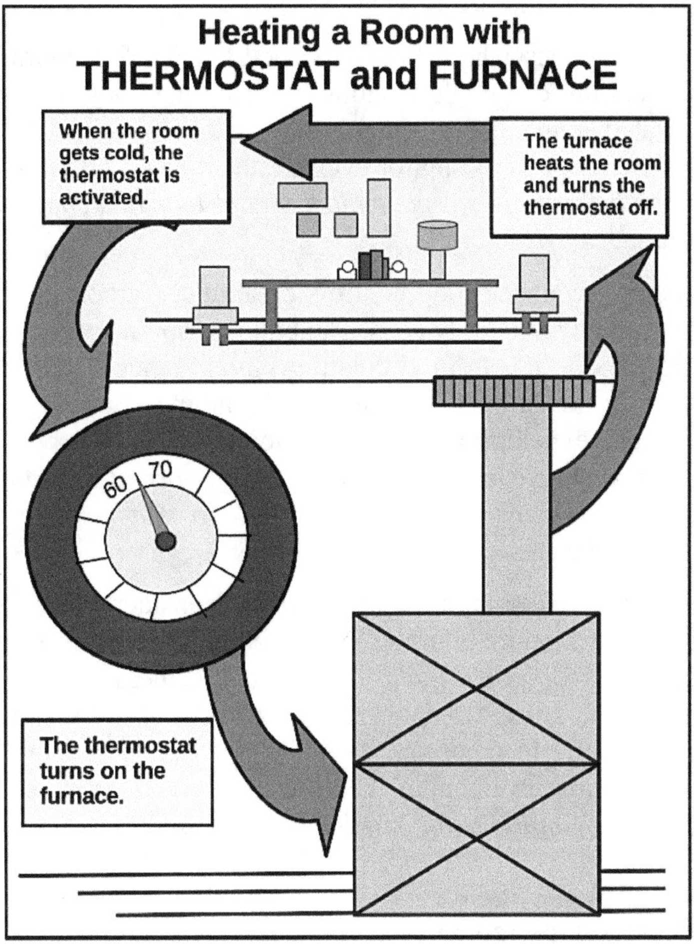

Feedback Loops in the Human Body

The body responds quickly to changing conditions - in less than a second through feedback loops. That is why feedback loops are so common throughout the body. *Feedback loops are the mechanisms of Self-Referral that make homeostasis possible.*

The body has many feedback loops. For example, one feedback loop controls blood pressure. Nerve sensors in the arteries monitor blood pressure. When blood pressure is too high, they signal the brain to decrease heart rate and relax the arteries. If blood pressure is too low, the reverse occurs: heart rate picks up and the arteries narrow to increase blood pressure.

What happens when this feedback loop fails? Abnormal high blood pressure can be devastating, wearing the body out - causing accelerated aging, heart attack, and stroke. Low blood pressure causes weakness, fainting, or even death. *Normal operation of the entire body thus depends upon the feedback loop that controls blood pressure.*[74]

Another feedback loop controls breathing. Carbon dioxide is a waste product of all body cells. The brain's respiratory center senses carbon dioxide levels in circulating blood. When carbon dioxide levels rise, the brain speeds up our breathing – pulling in more oxygen and expelling more carbon dioxide.[75] High carbon dioxide levels cause sluggish thinking or even death. *Normal operation of the entire body depends on the feedback loop that controls carbon dioxide levels.*

To better understand feedback loops, consider this. There are about 100 trillion cells in the human body. Cells form tissue, and tissue forms organs. Organs, working together, form a human being.[76] In this unfathomably complex body, all 100 trillion cells have one thing in common. Their health depends on millions of feedback loops that maintain their ideal internal environment. *Every one of these millions of feedback loops operate through Self-Referral.*

Feedback Loops and Self-Referral: Simple and Complex

Feedback loops are a natural part of the body's design. As a thermostat controls the furnace to heat a room, Self-Referral regulates the body to maintain health. Feedback loops regulate all body functions like breathing, digestion, waste disposal, and reproduction. The body accomplishes all this through millions of feedback loops.

Feedback loops are completely automatic. The body depends on them to maintain health and avoid disease. These millions of feedback loops have one purpose: they maintain an ideal internal environment by responding to external demands. *The body constantly refers to itself and changes itself - to optimize itself. This is self-regulation of the body by the body; this is Self-Referral.*

Through brilliant design the body conducts its own Self-Referral. Now we know about Self-Referral, how does the body accomplish Self-Referral? Is Self-Referral mysterious and unknowable, or does it work through familiar body structures?

Self-Referral is paradoxically simple and complex. It is simple because Self-Referral is the same everywhere in the body. It is complex because many mechanisms throughout the body make Self-Referral possible. What specific body structures make up the mechanisms of Self-Referral?

The brain and nervous system play a central role in homeostasis – and Self-Referral. They work together as the body's governor, carrying out critical communication and control functions. This is like the thermostat and wiring acting as governor to the furnace.[77] The brain and nervous system form a network of feedback loops. They are the physical correlates of Self-Referral. This is why disruption of the brain and nervous system profoundly interferes with Self-Referral.

The brain governs the body through Self-Referral. How does it do this? The brain receives information from the body, moment to moment. It compares the present situation with the ideal. The brain then sends orders through the nerves to correct imbalances. This is how the body senses the ever-changing environment - and responds to it, correcting imbalances.[78]

Environmental change is constant and unrelenting, so Self-Referral must be equally persistent. How does the human nervous system carry out this difficult task? We need more detailed knowledge of the nervous system to reveal more about Self-Referral.

A Multitude of Neurons

The human body contains about 10 billion nerve cells called neurons. Individual neurons vary in appearance according to their function, but they have a common overall structure.[79] A neuron's cell body contains the nucleus; it regulates cell function. Each neuron has two extensions: the axon and the dendrite. The axon and dendrite carry out the bulk of the nervous system's work. We can best describe that work as communication and control.[80]

A neuron works much like a telephone in its role as a communicating device. The telephone's earpiece contains a speaker to hear the caller's voice. The mouthpiece has a microphone that allows us to talk back. We must both hear and speak for a conversation to take place.

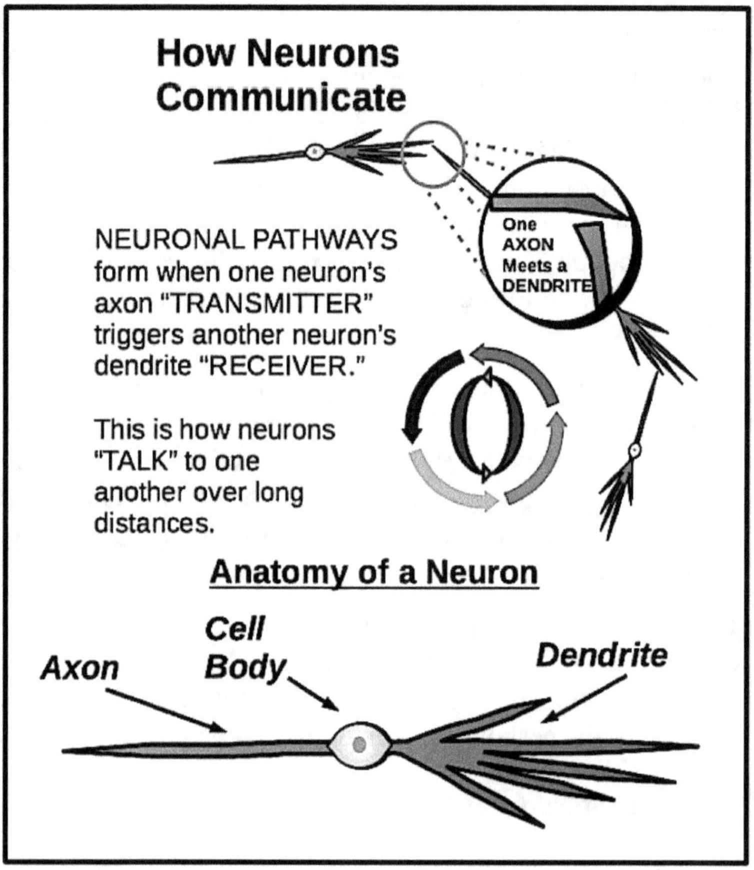

A neuron works the same way. All neurons have a dendrite acting as the telephone's speaker. The dendrite receives the incoming signal. When the dendrite receives a nerve impulse from another neuron, the axon acts as the microphone, relaying the message to the next nerve cell's dendrite. The signal is carried on this way, through long chains of neurons. This is how neurons can talk to each other, at least in a limited way.

How do neurons communicate and control the body? Let's say someone steps on your foot. A neuron in the foot senses the pain and sends the signal to another neuron. One neuron passes the pain signal to another, until it reaches the brain. The brain interprets the signal as pain. You may think "Ouch!" The brain then signals the foot to move out of the way. Finally, you move your foot and feel relief.

This is how all the many neurons communicate throughout the body. In the foot example, one neuron senses pain. Other neurons relay the signal to the brain. Brain neurons interpret the incoming signal as pain. Still other neurons signal muscles to move the toe out of the way.

This is how one neuron triggers many other neurons. The result is a complex communication and control network. *The simple neuron structure, duplicated millions of times, forms complex neuronal pathways. These are the physical correlates of Self-Referral. This is why Self-Referral is simple, yet complex.*

Neurons and Self-Referral

Each neuron is a self-contained feedback loop. It can receive a signal and pass it on to other neurons. A neuron thus is the simplest structural unit of Self-Referral. The network structure of the nervous system allows many communication pathways. Communication is not limited to a line drawn between two points. Why is this?

Neurons branch and loop to form neuronal pathways of tremendous complexity. Examining neuronal pathways one by one, the number of pathways is staggering. When we consider branching and looping, the connections are nearly infinite. This is not a system of discrete wires and cables, but something more resembling a nerve net, or even an energy field. This complexity is nearly beyond human comprehension. That is why today's scientists do not fully understand the brain and nervous system.[81]

The brain itself is a large bundle of connected complex neuronal pathways. This structure allows it to receive complex feedback from the body. Various areas of the brain test the feedback, comparing the current situation with the ideal. The brain then optimizes body function, governing the body through Self-Referral to maintain homeostasis.

When faced with such complexity, the simplicity of Self-Referral is a useful idea. Self-Referral is Self-Referral of the body – not something outside the body - but a principle defined by the body itself. Self-Referral operates through the intricate structure of the nervous system.

The nervous system is incredibly complex, but the process of Self-Referral is very simple. How can we fathom this apparently contradictory situation? We may resort to the analogy of a forest. When baffled by individual trees, we need to stand back and examine the whole forest. Lao-Tzu writes in the *Tao te Ching*:

> The Tao never does anything, yet through it all things are done.[82]

To understand the brain and nervous system, we need a better knowledge of Self-Referral. All feedback loops are mechanisms of Self-Referral. Individual feedback loops differ in structure but function identically. They are all self-regulating Cybernetic mechanisms of communication and control. *Once we know that feedback loops are mechanisms of Self-Referral, we understand all feedback loops.* We then comprehend the basis of homeostasis, and through it we see how the body maintains health and avoids disease.

We discussed individual feedback loops, like squinting the eyes to avoid harsh sunlight. Light hits the eye's optic nerve. The optic nerve passes the stimulus to the brain. The brain learns the light is too bright and signals muscles to squint the eyelids.[83] This mechanism of Self-Referral is the "light-brain-eyelids" feedback loop.

Another individual feedback loop controls stomach acid production. We might call this mechanism of Self-Referral the "food-stomach-acid" feedback loop. We chew and swallow food. The stomach senses the swallowed food and sends impulses to the brain. The brain realizes the stomach has food to digest. The brain then signals the stomach to produce acid as needed. When the food leaves the stomach, acid production stops.[84]

Self-Referral

Maximum Health

Axioms Defining Layers of Self-Referral

REMEMBER: Cells are the simplest structural unit of the body. Cells together form tissue. Tissue forms organs. Organs work together for a common purpose as organ systems. Organ systems working together form a human being.

Individual Cell SELF-REFERRAL includes all feedback loops of the individual body cells. Cells must have oxygen and nutrients. They also must dispose of waste products. This is why all body cells are layers of SELF-REFERRAL.

Body Tissue SELF-REFERRAL includes all feedback loops of body tissue. Cells combine to form tissue, and tissue forms organs. Each body tissue has specific tasks and must be healthy to fulfill its purpose. All tissue - heart, bone, lung, and all other tissue are layers of SELF-REFERRAL.

Organ System SELF-REFERRAL includes feedback loops of organ systems. Cells form tissue, tissue forms organs, and organs work together as organ systems. Each organ system has specific tasks and must be healthy to succeed. All organ systems – cardiovascular, respiratory, renal, and all other organ systems – are layers of SELF-REFERRAL.

Whole Body SELF-REFERRAL includes all the body's feedback loops. When SELF-REFERRAL works, we find health. When SELF-REFERRAL fails, we find disease.

There are a vast number of individual feedback loops throughout the body. Whole books focus on just a few of these mechanisms of Self-Referral. We should avoid becoming too fascinated with the individual feedback loops, however. The important thing is to appreciate the individual tree while maintaining the perspective of the forest.

Layers of Self-Referral

We can understand the mechanisms of Self-Referral by comparing them to an onion. The onion represents all mechanisms of Self-Referral. We inspect individual mechanisms of Self-Referral by peeling onion layers, one at a time.

Many layers of Self-Referral exist. They often operate simultaneously. How can this be? For example, human activity is often complex. A person may eat breakfast while they scan an article and still carry on a conversation. We may drive a car while listening to the radio and simultaneously think about work. Self-Referral also may have many layers – at the same time. Complex layers of activity occur in Self-Referral as follows:

We see that Self-Referral operates by layers from the whole body down to each individual cell. We also see that Self-Referral is comprehensive; it includes the macroscopic work of the body, the microscopic work of each cell, and all mechanisms of Self-Referral between the two extremes.

Self-Referral of Healing

We now have a clear understanding of Self-Referral. Self-Referral is the comprehensive, multileveled, multilayered, activity that maintains whole body health. If Self-Referral fails on any level, the body is sure to suffer. If enough disruption occurs, disease or death will certainly result.

An important question emerges: if Self-Referral is comprehensive and self-perpetuating, why doesn't everyone live forever? What goes wrong that prevents perfect health? Why do we suffer disease?

Medical textbooks and today's medical system are noncommittal on this question. Most authors simply do not address the issue, assuming it is irrelevant. Others say that disease is an expected part of life. This attitude is deeply ingrained in medicine. Like squinting in response to bright light, we don't even notice it.

Physicians constantly work to combat disease. This helps many suffering people, but is that all we can do? By limiting intervention to treating disease as we find it, we create a self-fulfilling prophecy. The Disease Approach to medicine assumes that disease is inevitable and the best we can do is treat it as it arises.

Considering the comprehensive nature of Self-Referral, we must examine new possibilities. We now know the Disease Approach to medical practice is not the only possible approach. Are we so fascinated with disease and its treatment that we cannot look beyond disease? Are we so used to looking at the trees that we cannot admit the possibility of a forest?

When we seek Self-Referral, we look for ways to work with the body's capacity for harmony. Rather than defeating diseases one at a time as enemies, we seek to restore all the body's balance. When we find this ability to restore harmony, it will revolutionize medical practice. Rather than fighting disease as a warrior, physicians can aspire to their true role: that of a facilitator of healing. *Instead of constantly being fixated on fighting disease, doctors can actively promote healing.*

Does one universal explanation of health and disease exist? Once we discover it, what new therapeutic options may we find? We have identified Self-Referral as the basis of homeostasis and the basis of health. An important question remains, however. What disrupts the body's feedback loops? *What goes wrong with Self-Referral?*

Self-Referral
Maximum Health

Chapter 4

The Rosetta Stone of Medicine

Interruption of Self-Referral creates disease. When we understand this interruption, we know what creates all disease. We quickly see this as the Rosetta Stone of Medicine

Self-Referral, Health, and Disease

We now know that Self-Referral is the body's ability to regulate itself. Self-Referral's purpose is to maintain ideal body conditions in a changing environment. At the microscopic level, Self-Referral operates within a single cell. At the macroscopic level, Self-Referral maintains homeostasis for the whole body.

There are many layers of Self-Referral throughout the body. These layers create ideal conditions from the cell, to tissue, to organs, and to the whole body. No matter what layer of Self-Referral we refer to, the principle of Self-Referral is the same. *The body regulates itself, by itself.*

Self-Referral is carried out through feedback loops. The brain, nervous system, and body work together for communication and control functions. Feedback loops are autonomous, self-perpetuating mechanisms that carry out Self-Referral. Feedback loops are automatic and usually need no outside help.

Exactly how do these feedback loops work? Remember the example of the thermostat and furnace that demonstrates the feedback loop. So long as thermostat and furnace operate normally, the room stays warm. Just as the thermostat governs the furnace, the brain governs the body. As a room stays warm with thermostat and furnace, we stay healthy through Self-Referral between brain and body.

Health and disease are two possible outcomes of Self-Referral. If all mechanisms of Self-Referral are working normally, health is the natural result. If even one of these mechanisms of Self-Referral breaks down, then disease is the equally natural outcome.

Doctors and patients work together to improve disease, working to return sick people to health. A useful question is: *how do interruptions of Self-Referral occur? What interrupts the body's elegantly designed feedback loops to create disease?*

Doctors and researchers have identified many such feedback loop interruptions. An entire sub-specialty of medicine has sprung up to deal with this problem. We can identify the cause of these interruptions with a single word: *stress*.

Stress Defined

There was once a young, ambitious research scientist named Hans Selye. The young man worked with lab rats in the 1930s, but he had a problem. It seems that Selye was clumsy, and he kept dropping the rats. He would then chase them around the room, finally capturing them by trapping them under a sink.[85]

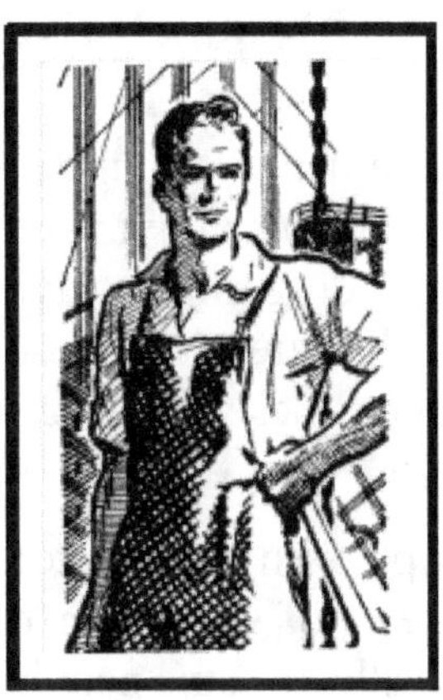

Selye became curious when he noticed the dropped rats developed ulcers and became easily infected. After testing the rats, he realized what was making the rats sick. The rats were suffering from the results of Selye's clumsy handling. Groping for a word to describe the rats' discomfort due to rough handling, Selye borrowed a word from the field of engineering: *stress*.[86]

Selye first described stress in a 1936 article titled "A Syndrome Produced by Nocuous Agents." *Selye defined* stress *as wear and tear on the body caused by the demands of life.*[87] Researchers since Selye have published over 110,000 articles and books about this important subject.[88] This research links stress with high blood pressure, ulcers, sexual problems, heart attack, stroke, kidney disorders, infections, and allergic conditions.[89] What is stress, and how can it cause so many health problems?

The stress response is a natural body reaction to demanding conditions. When we face danger, whether real or imagined, our bodies react in a unique way. Our bodies prepare to either fight or run away. *This is the classic fight or flight respon*se. Stress speeds up the heart and increases blood pressure. It causes body glands to pour stress hormones into the bloodstream.[90] This causes a sudden surge of energy and strength.

How does stress feel? Think about a time when something scared you badly without warning. Perhaps while driving you narrowly missed colliding with a car, or someone startled you unexpectedly. When this happens, you feel your heart racing. You also feel hot, flushed, and a bit shaken. Many people say they feel like they just ran a race. *The body's stress response causes all these sensations.*

The stress response thus prepares our bodies for necessary action and gives us added strength and endurance when needed. The body's stress response thus is a vital part of Self-Referral. We often need it to excel in physical activities; occasionally, we need it to survive a potentially threatening situation.

The stress response can be intense - and some situations require it. Soldiers in war, for example, often describe long periods of living on "pure adrenaline." Athletes in physically demanding competitive sports also rely on an aroused physiology. The stress response provides the alertness, strength, and endurance these situations demand.

The stress response often helps people cope with unexpected emergencies. We often hear of superhuman feats of strength and endurance during disasters. The stress response allows some people to lift a heavy tree to free a trapped loved one. It may also provide the extra physical stamina to survive airplane crashes, floods, and similar disasters.

Danger, whether real or imagined, causes stress. Noisy urban environments, job pressures, and repetitive machine operation all cause stress. Demands from other people can cause stress, particularly the demands of work and family life. The threat of failure at work or failure in the family registers to us as danger, provoking the stress response. When people say they are feeling rough from work or family problems, this is literally true – the situations are causing stress and people feel the effects.

Aggravating all this, modern life is largely sedentary. We drive to work. Then we sit at a desk or stand in a factory. We walk short distances through the day, but it does not challenge our physiology enough to be effective exercise. Then we drive home and sit down for television. *Modern life thus has many sources of stress but few opportunities for physical activity to resolve the fight or flight response.*

The stress response prepares us for action. When we have no physical outlet for it, the body works against itself. That is why people are often in a stressed state that is not appropriate, at least as a response to physical danger. Our bodies are ready to fight or run for it - but we do neither. This leaves us feeling angry and frustrated, swimming in our own metabolic waste.[91]

Stress and Future Shock

Few people have described this situation as well as Alvin Toffler in his monumental book *Future Shock.*[92] Toffler clearly points out the increased health risks associated with the stress of modern living:

> The health of the individual is intimately bound up with the adaptive demands placed on him by the environment - disease need not be the result of a germ or a virus, but a consequence of many factors, including the environment surrounding his body. Change itself - not this or that specific change but the general rate of change in a person's life - could be one of the most important environmental factors of all.[93]

Toffler illustrates these ideas with many examples from medical research.[94] In the 1960s, scientists suspected that stressful life events caused illness. What are stressful life events, and why would they cause health problems?

Alvin Toffler's book *Future Shock* Identified Increasing Stress of Modern Life Impacting Health

Futurist Alvin Toffler was among the first to recognize that modern life creates more stress than ever before. He cited the accellerating rate of change as a real danger to human health and cultural coherence. Writing in Future Shock in the late sixties, Toffler's warnings ring even more true today.

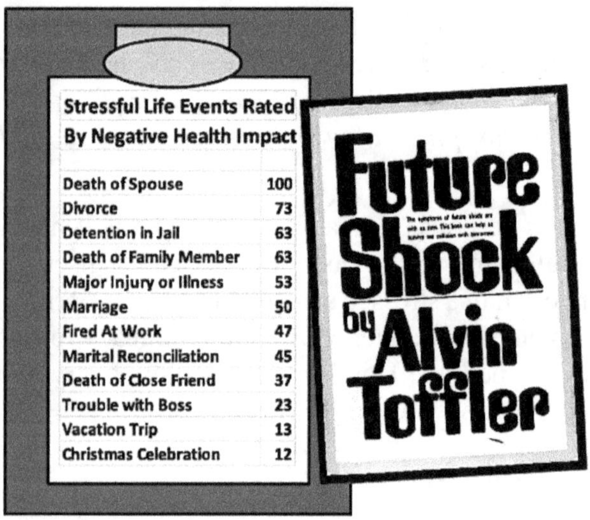
Stressful Life Events Rated
By Negative Health Impact
Death of Spouse 100
Divorce 73
Detention in Jail 63
Death of Family Member 63
Major Injury or Illness 53
Marriage 50
Fired At Work 47
Marital Reconciliation 45
Death of Close Friend 37
Trouble with Boss 23
Vacation Trip 13
Christmas Celebration 12
Future Shock
by Alvin Toffler

Stressful life events are experiences that produce stress. Some examples are the death of a spouse, changing jobs, or taking a vacation. Scientists studied stressful life events to compare people's reaction to stress.

One person, for example, might suffer the death of a parent, change jobs, and divorce a spouse within a year's time. A second person might have an uneventful year in which the biggest stressful life event is a vacation. Researchers reasoned that the first person would be much more stressed than the second, and people with more stress should have more health problems. The question was: *would differences in stress produce differences in health*?

One such study examined a large group of patients. The researchers listed the patients' stressful life events. Then they examined the patients' medical records for illness.[95] Their

conclusions were extraordinary. Without exception, *the more stressful life events in one year, the more likely patients were to fall ill the following year*.

Then the scientists rated stressful life events. The results showed that some stressful life events were more damaging to health than others. For example, the death of a spouse rated as highly stressful at 100 points. A vacation rated at 13 points, changing jobs at 20 points, and so forth.[96] Alvin Toffler pointed out the importance of this research in *Future Shock*. Toffler wrote:

> For the first time, it was possible to show . . . the rate of change in a person's life – the pace of life – is closely tied to his state of health.[97]

Good Stress and Bad Stress

Critics disagreed with these conclusions. Losing a beloved spouse would certainly cause bad stress, they argued. But would a better job cause good stress? Would bad stress cause illness, and good stress cause health?[98]

We can answer this question by defining stress more clearly. Selye defined *eustress* as stress caused by a positive event, such as changing to a better job. He defined *distress* as stress caused by a negative event, like the death of a beloved spouse.[99] Selye noted that both good stress and bad stress cause wear and tear on the body. No matter the source of stress, Selye emphasized, stress is stress and its negative health effects are the same.[100]

Much of human physiology was unknown when Hans Selye introduced the concept of stress in 1936. Selye wrote as a conceptual thinker drawing new conclusions from known facts. He worked long and hard before others accepted his new ideas - but his persistence was rewarded. *Stress is now a key part of medical thought.*

Selye wrote of this progress in the 1975 edition of his 1956 book *The Stress of Life*[101]:

> These concepts have undergone no major modifications in the course of time, and the best we can do is to polish their presentation in the light of responses to many lectures, publications, and round-table discussions . . .

Through the years Selye's conclusions have become a critical part of medical thought. Stress thus is a familiar idea that everyone in medical care – and everyone in general – knows about as common knowledge. Few health professionals now seriously question the important concept of stress.

Stress and Self-Referral

Self-Referral/Maximum Health teaches us how to improve our ability to balance the body's pairs of opposites: high blood pressure-low blood pressure, fast heart-slow heart, and so on. If stress is such a major roadblock to health, does it have a natural place in our physiology? The stress response is fundamental to biological survival, so it must be a natural part of Self-Referral - but how can we find stress or lack of stress in the body? And where is Self-Referral in all this? Answering this question requires some unusual thinking. Turning again to Lao-Tzu, as he speaks of the Tao in the *Tao te Ching*:[102]

> Listen, and it can't be heard.
> Reach, and it can't be grasped.
> Above, it isn't bright.
> Below, it isn't dark.
> Seamless, unnamable, it returns
> to the realm of nothing.
> Form that includes all forms,
> image without an image,
> subtle, beyond all conception.

Lao-Tzu tells us that the Tao – Self-Referral – requires us to stretch our thinking to find and understand it. We must seek Self-Referral by inference rather than frontal assault. The thermometer and blood pressure cuff only tell so much. We must open our mental eyes and stretch our thinking. *The stress response is yet another mechanism of Self-Referral, a useful feedback loop that provides ways to survive - in challenging and difficult situations.* How does this critical feedback loop change to work against us?

Stress causes many different diseases, so it must affect the body at a very basic level. What turns this helpful natural mechanism into a killer? How does the body turn against itself? We will examine one feedback loop at a time, discovering how stress interferes with Self-Referral. If we identify a single mechanism of interference, we can unravel the deadly relationship between stress and disease.

Our discussion of Selye's stress concept so far has been theoretical. We know that stressful life events cause increased rates of illness, but where can we find scientific proof that stress disrupts Self-Referral? *Is there specific evidence proving that disrupting Self-Referral causes disease*?

Stress and Cardiovascular Disease

Heart and blood vessel disease is the number one cause of death worldwide.[103] Doctors work hard to detect and treat it to save lives. It is interesting that *many stories from the history of medicine connect stress and heart disease*.

Doctors in history knew that stress causes disease. Emotional stress is especially a problem. The ancient Greek physician Maimonides wrote that emotional upset causes major body changes.[104] Could this emotional upset connect stress and disease?

Dr. William Harvey discovered that blood circulates through the arteries and veins. Harvey wrote in 1649 about a man who was furious after being insulted. The man began "suffering from extreme pain of the heart and breast."[105] The frightened patient described the pain as choking and terrible. This is why the symptom gained the medical name "choking chest pain" - or angina pectoris.[106] Dr. William Heberden wrote in 1768 that "any disturbance of mind" could cause angina pectoris in heart patients.[107]

Doctors through history connected several disturbances of mind with fatal heart attack. One such disturbance is *anger*. In 1776, Dr. John Fothergill described a patient who long suffered chest pain with exercise – but the patient died suddenly "in a sudden and violent transport of anger."[108]

A second disturbance of mind is *anxiety*. Dr. John Hunter wrote that his patient suffered angina pectoris whenever he had anxiety.[109] Sir William Osler commented that many famous physicians had died of angina-related illness. Osler referred here to a third disturbance of the mind:

> In a group of twenty physicians whom I know personally [who died of heart attack] the outstanding feature was the treadmill of practice . . . and *worry*.[110]

> *Anger, anxiety, and worry are common to most people*. These emotions involve the brain. We know the brain and nervous system control the heart and arteries.[111] Logically, stress must play a role in heart disease. How do these factors work together?[112] How does a fit of anger result in sudden death from heart attack?

The Mechanism of Angina Pectoris

The heart is made of muscle. Like any other muscle, it needs oxygen to work properly. The coronary arteries are small arteries that supply oxygen to heart muscle. Narrowing of the heart's arteries cuts the heart's oxygen supply – causing the terrible pain we call angina pectoris.[113] If the heart is oxygen-starved long enough, permanent damage results.[114] This is the dreaded heart attack that can cause sudden death.[115]

Autopsy of heart attack victims often reveals hardening of the arteries. Fatty deposits called plaques block blood flow inside the coronary arteries. We also find these plaques in other arteries throughout the body.[116] Plaques form in arteries during the aging process, so doctors long believed that hardening of the arteries alone caused angina pectoris and sudden death.[117] This is the *clogged pipes theory of coronary artery disease.*

By the 1970s scientists offered a more refined theory: this was coronary artery spasm. This theory suggests that wide-open coronary arteries can suddenly become narrow. The muscular wall of the artery simply goes into spasm, much like a severe cramp in the leg. This cramp was different, however; this cramp could kill. This is the *vasospasm theory of coronary artery disease.*[118]

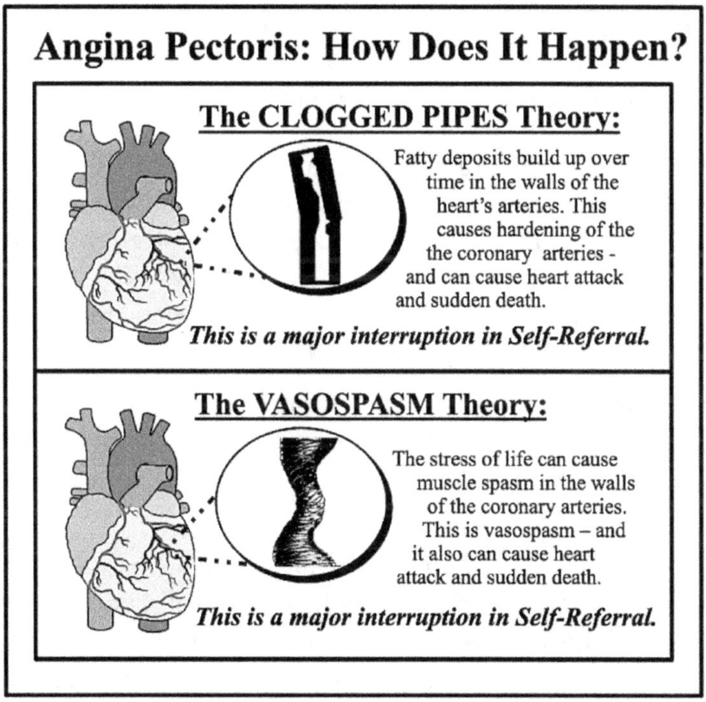

The vasospasm theory did not contradict the clogged pipes theory; it simply added deeper understanding. Where plaques were present, vasospasm worsened the condition.[119] Vasospasm also explained angina-related death in patients with no plaques.[120] Thus vasospasm alone can provoke angina pectoris or sudden death - *even with normal coronary arteries.*[121]

Now we see how abstract experience can cause physical disease.

All the Stressful Life Events referred to in Alvin Toffler's *Future Shock* contribute to the stress described by doctors in history. This is how we know that Stressful Life Events can and do cause angina pectoris. And please remember - angina pectoris is not a minor problem. Coronary artery spasm can cause angina pectoris and sudden death in short order.

Since angina pectoris and vasospasm can cause sudden death, coronary artery spasm is an extremely important disruption of Self-Referral's feedback loops. The same is true of hardening of the arteries. How do the heart and arteries maintain health through Self-Referral? By contrast, what brings about these lethal disruptions of Self-Referral?

The Cardiovascular Feedback Loop

Feedback loops are the mechanisms of Self-Referral. These elegantly designed control mechanisms usually work perfectly. Health is the natural outcome of successful Self-Referral. What work does the heart do that is so important to the body? Why is interrupting this work so devastating? We can better understand these matters by examining the *Cardiovascular Feedback Loop.*

The Cardiovascular Feedback Loop has two parts. The first is the mechanical work of the heart – pumping the blood using mechanical force. The body's blood vessels allow the blood pumped by the heart to circulate throughout the body.

The second part is the brain and nervous system doing the Cybernetic work of communication and control. They work with the heart and blood vessels to coordinate circulation. As the thermostat governs the furnace to heat a room, the brain governs the heart and blood vessels - and circulates blood throughout the body.

The reason blood circulation is so important is all cells require a constant oxygen supply – and they must dispose of waste. The cells get oxygen from circulating red blood cells. After they release oxygen, the same red cells carry away the cell's waste products.

Many chemical reactions critical to life depend on normal circulation. If oxygen is not brought to the cells, and the waste products are not carried off on time, disease or death will result. How does the body maintain circulation? Self-Referral makes this possible by coordinating the heart rate and the internal diameter of arteries.

Heart rate can change rapidly. When the heart speeds up, it pumps more blood - and circulation increases. When the heart slows down, it pumps less blood - and circulation decreases. Arteries also can change rapidly to control blood flow. When their muscular walls contract, the internal diameter narrows, and circulation increases. When arteries relax, they widen, and circulation slows.[122]

Self-Referral coordinates circulation for the whole body by controlling heart and arteries. Millions of neurons connect the brain with the heart and arteries. These sensors throughout the body provide constant feedback to the brain, updating the body's status. The brain then controls heart and arteries as conditions change. This is how the brain causes blood to flow where the body needs it most.[123]

What Disrupts the Cardiovascular Feedback Loop?

The Cardiovascular Feedback Loop is a clear example of Self-Referral, the mechanism by which the body governs itself. It is one of the body's most important feedback loops. Normal operation of this mechanism of Self-Referral produces health; disruption of it causes angina pectoris, heart attack, and high blood pressure.

Coronary vasospasm and hardening of the arteries cause angina pectoris and heart attacks. What causes these disorders? Medical scientists have long studied these problems. As they learned more, medical treatment has improved. We can better understand Self-Referral by learning more about how doctors treat heart problems.

Medicine in the 1800s was primitive by today's standards. Doctors knew nothing about hardening of the arteries or vasospasm. They found remedies by trial and error. For example, doctors found in 1867 that inhaling the chemical amyl nitrate relieves angina pectoris.[124] This medication dilates the coronary arteries, allowing more blood to reach the heart.[125] Scientists later improved amyl nitrate, producing nitroglycerin drugs. Doctors have written millions of prescriptions for these vital medications since that time.[126]

Later medical research offered better understanding of what causes angina pectoris and heart attack. Because they knew coronary artery problems caused heart attack, researchers from the 1960s forward studied how these arteries worked. Controlling coronary arteries, they reasoned, would result in fewer heart attacks.[127] What did they discover?

Part of the brain and nerves regulate automatic body functions like heart rate, blood pressure, and breathing.[128] Scientists call this the autonomic nervous system. This portion of the brain and nerves conducts Self-Referral throughout the body. By the 1970s researchers discovered drugs that work directly with the autonomic nervous system.

Beta Blocker drugs like propranolol (Inderal) lower high blood pressure[129], improve heart failure[130], and prevent the heart from beating too fast.[131] How do these medications work? The Beta receptors are local nerve control centers that regulate these functions.

In hypertension, the Beta centers are set too high, causing arteries to narrow and elevate blood pressure. Beta Blockers reduce excess Beta stimulation – causing the arteries to relax, and blood pressure drops to normal. Another benefit of these drugs is help with the heart beating too fast; Beta Blockers slow the heart to a normal rate. Finally, Beta Blocker drugs prevent coronary artery vasospasm.[132]

By the 1980s researchers produced another class of autonomic medications. These are the Calcium Channel Blocker drugs like nifedipine (Procardia).[133] They normalize artery function by blocking excess calcium activity in artery muscle. Like the Beta Blockers, these drugs cause the arteries to relax, and high blood pressure drops.[134] Calcium Channel Blockers also prevent vasospasm.[135]

A third class of autonomic medications now exists. These are the ACE Inhibitor drugs like lisinopril (Prinivil).[136] These medications block stress-related enzyme activity to control high blood pressure[137] and heart failure[138]. These medications are especially helpful in patients with weak heart muscle problems. By removing the back pressure from narrowed arteries, these medications reduce the heart's pumping load. This is why some people with enlarged hearts have seen their hearts shrink back to normal with ACE Inhibitor drugs.[139]

These three classes of drugs work through different mechanisms, but they are in one way identical. *They all reverse the effects of stress.*[140] People with high blood pressure or artery spasm are somehow locked into the fight or flight response. The heart pumps faster, arteries constrict, blood pressure rises, and the body is ready to fight or run away – translating to cardiovascular trouble. The Beta Blockers, Calcium Channel Blockers, and ACE Inhibitors are even named for what they do: *they block or inhibit the effects of stress.*

Today we also have diuretics, ACE II Inhibitors, Alpha Blockers, Alpha 2 Blockers, Aldosterone Blockers, and Renin Inhibitors. *All these medications act at similar points in the physiology to reverse the effects of stress.*[141] Another trend has been to combine these different classes of medication into one drug to have the benefits of both. It all comes down to taking the right medication to combat the effects of stress.[142] And this progress in medical care is reducing the death rate from hypertension, heart failure and heart attack.[143]

What goes wrong that causes high blood pressure? Research points to stress. When people encounter too much stress, it overwhelms their bodies. *Brain and body normally work together to maintain health, but with excess stress, the body constantly works too hard.* Just as an athlete in prime condition eventually tires, our bodies lose their ability to adapt. High blood pressure is the result. The same is true of other diseases of the heart and blood vessels. *High blood pressure, vasospasm, and heart attack are all caused by stress.*[144]

Stress and Animal Studies

Now we see that several key ideas are intimately related. The stress of life provokes the stress response – and triggers the fight or flight response. Repeated stress causes more and more stress response. This sustained state of hyper-arousal interrupts Self-Referral.[145] This in turn causes high blood pressure, angina pectoris, vasospasm - even the dreaded heart attack. But how does all this connect with modern life?

A key question is: how much of the modern environment causes enough stress to provoke these cardiovascular problems? Modern life doubtlessly causes stress, but is this enough stress to trigger these deadly diseases? *There have been some very interesting animal studies that strongly indicate modern life does in fact trigger deadly cardiovascular disease.*

One animal study connecting the stress of modern life with disease was done at the University of Miami School of Medicine. Researchers exposed Rhesus monkeys to sounds typical of modern life for an extended period. The sounds included background noise that most people assume is harmless as well as loud, obviously stressful sounds. The background noises included gargling, flushing toilets, running water, a distant motorcycle, and twenty minutes of television's Today Show. Obviously stressful sounds were loud industrial noises, alarm clock bells, and loud music.

The results were surprising. The monkeys' blood pressure rose to abnormal levels, although there was no damage to their hearing.[146] These findings suggest that human workers in noisy industry may suffer high blood pressure caused by their loud, stressful environment. Ordinary people may also suffer ill effects from the noisy urban environment or even the modern home environment.

Do these findings relate to humans and modern life? The noise of modern life is a serious problem. More than 28 million Americans suffer from a hearing impairment. The Environmental Protection Agency believes that four times that number suffer exposure to dangerously loud noise. That means about 40 percent of today's population regularly experiences noise loud enough to damage hearing.[147] And all this causes enormous levels of stress.

Drawing a relationship between stress and vasospasm makes intuitive sense, but what about the plaque formation in coronary arteries in the clogged pipes theory? *Research studies show that chronic stress causes hardening of the arteries.*

A major study at New York Medical College shows a link between stress, overstimulation of the brain, and accelerated plaque formation in rats. This suggests that stress-related chemicals in the blood may cause the plaques that block human arteries.[148]

Another study asked what caused hardening of the arteries - diet or stress? Researchers divided monkeys into two groups: one group had frequent stress by constantly introducing strange monkeys that caused crowding and increased competition for females. The other group had calm, balanced, and comfortable conditions. Both groups had the same low-fat diet.

After twenty-one months, stressed monkeys had far more hardening of the arteries than monkeys who lived in a more relaxed atmosphere. Interestingly, monkeys from both groups had normal blood levels of sugar, cholesterol, and other blood chemistry. *Stress caused plaques in stressed monkeys - even with normal laboratory blood tests.*[149]

These studies show that stress is a dangerous risk factor - and we should take stress seriously. Stress in our lives clearly can cause high blood pressure and related problems. This scientific research proves that chronic stress causes high blood pressure and hardening of the arteries.

Expanding the Cardiovascular Feedback Loop

Returning to human medicine, scientists know that high blood levels of stress chemicals cause dangerous heart rhythm problems,[150] coronary artery spasm, or even sudden death.[151] The stress chemicals also cause high blood pressure - one of the worst risk factors for heart attack and sudden death.[152]

Doctors use Beta Blockers and similar drugs to combat these problems.[153] Use of these stress-neutralizing drugs have reduced the death rate from cardiovascular disease.[154] Do these medications have other benefits?

The body controls bleeding from minor wounds through blood clotting. Platelets are blood cells that form blood clots when needed. Abnormal clots form if these cells are too sticky.

Such clots can cause heart attack, stroke, and related problems. Beta Blocker drugs reduce platelet stickiness, making abnormal clots less likely to form.[155]

Now we see the many benefits of autonomic drugs: lower blood pressure, less abnormal clot formation, fewer heart rhythm problems, less coronary artery spasm, and less hardening of the arteries. Many credit the Beta Blocker drugs for a drastic drop in death rate from heart attack[156] and stroke[157] over the last 40 years. The Calcium Channel Blockers, ACE Inhibitors, and many newer variations on these medications are also available – by themselves and in combinations. Many doctors believe these newer drugs are even more effective than the Beta Blockers.[158]

We also see that feedback loops are not theoretical fluff. Every advance in understanding these feedback loops has saved lives and produced a quantum leap in improved health. Each refinement produced a better therapeutic tool. It is like adjusting a screw - first with a baseball bat, then with a pocketknife, and finally with a screwdriver that exactly fits the screw.

Research now shows that strong links exist between coronary artery disease, migraine headache, and Raynaud's phenomenon.[159] Migraine is a type of extremely painful headache.[160] Raynaud's phenomenon is a disorder of painful circulation, often involving the hands and feet.[161] How are these apparently unrelated diseases connected with coronary artery spasm? All these disorders have a common cause: spasm of the artery, or vasospasm. It should be no surprise that these disorders respond well to Beta Blocker drugs.

Stress and Other Feedback Loops

Stress thus produces vasospasm anywhere in the body. Vasospasm results from the brain's stress response and the body changes that follow. A lead editorial of the New England Journal of Medicine asked a key question:

> If the correlation of vasospasm with these conditions is true and it seemingly is the next question may well become: "what is the mechanism of 'spontaneous' vasospasm?"[162]

Scientific research shows that spontaneous vasospasm occurs throughout the human body. The mechanism that causes this potentially deadly problem is no mystery. *The obvious mechanism for vasospasm is stress.*

We have come far in our quest for *Self-Referral/Maximum Health.* Self-Referral maintains health and, by default, prevents disease. Feedback loops are the mechanisms of Self-Referral. *Through understanding what interrupts feedback loops we have found what causes disease: stress.*

We have focused on the Cardiovascular Feedback Loop to demonstrate Self-Referral. Self-Referral, however, is not limited to brain and heart, or brain and arteries. An important question looms: is disruption of feedback loops limited to the cardiovascular system?

Since stress-mediated disruption of Self-Referral via feedback loops is universal, what do we know about stress-related disease in other organ systems? Scientists study other organ systems as they have studied the cardiovascular system. As doctors have learned more about how the body works, they have discovered better ways to treat disease. Medical therapy has improved as a direct result.

The Respiratory Feedback Loop

We breathe using the respiratory system – via the lungs and breathing passages. Because the whole body depends on oxygen, every breath we take is crucial. The respiratory system both provides oxygen – something we need constantly - and disposes of carbon dioxide - a major waste product. Oxygen enters the lungs when we breathe in, or inhale. Carbon dioxide and other gases leave the lungs when we breathe out, or exhale. How does this process work?

Red blood cells circulate through tiny blood vessels near the inner surface of the lung - where the lung meets the air. Passing this area, they release gaseous waste products like carbon dioxide, collected throughout the body. Then they absorb oxygen and carry it via the bloodstream all through the body. This is how we get the oxygen we need to live. This also disposes of gaseous waste products.[163]

The Respiratory Feedback Loop has two parts - the mechanical work of the lungs and the Cybernetics communication and control work of brain and nervous system. Chest and neck muscles work together with the diaphragm to expand the chest and allow fresh air to fill the lungs. These muscles then relax, collapsing the chest and emptying the lungs of air. This moves air in and out of the lungs.

The brain and nervous system do the Cybernetic work of communication and control. They work with the lungs and related parts to coordinate breathing. As a thermostat controls the furnace to heat a room, brain and nerves control muscles and breathing tubes to breathe. How do brain and respiratory system work together?

When we breathe faster or slower, our blood absorbs relatively more or less oxygen. This also affects whether we blow out relatively more or less gaseous waste products. The brain's respiratory center constantly monitors blood gas levels as blood circulates through it. The brain causes us to breathe faster or slower to provide ideal blood gas levels. This is how brain and body respond to a constantly changing environment.[164]

Another important task is that of controlling the lung's breathing tubes. These resemble hollow branches of a tree and allow air to pass in and out of the lungs. The largest tubes, the bronchi, must respond to changes in air temperature and humidity. To allow this, the bronchi are lined with muscle, enabling them to change their internal diameter to accommodate smooth passage of air.

How does the brain control the bronchi? In a manner strikingly similar to the artery, the Beta receptors control these muscles. The Beta receptors, in turn, are controlled by the brain.[165] This is how brain and nerves control the bronchi every moment we live.[166] The brain thus regulates the bronchi and optimizes breathing with a changing environment.

We now see the Respiratory Feedback Loop as another example of Self-Referral. Through this elegantly designed feedback loop, the body adapts to the demands of life. If Self-Referral operates normally, health is the natural result. Disruption of Self-Referral produces the equally natural result.

we call disease. This theory sounds good, but how practical are these ideas? What do we know about stress-related lung disorders?

One of the most frightening and deadly lung diseases is asthma. Asthma's underlying cause is remarkably like vasospasm of the artery: the bronchial muscle goes into spasm like a cramp in the leg.

When asthma flares up the bronchi constrict, blocking needed air exchange. Asthma attacks are both terrifying and serious. People can die of severe asthma attacks. Research has produced Beta Blocker drugs like terbutaline (Brethine)[167] and albuterol (Ventolin)[168] that reverse bronchospasm.[169] Later lung drugs build on the mechanisms these earlier medications.

We thus see that the same disruption of Self-Referral that causes high blood pressure, heart attack, stroke, and vasospasm is responsible for asthma. Stress causes overactive Beta stimulation, provoking bronchospasm in the lung. It should not be surprising to learn that bronchospasm also worsens many other lung diseases. For example, many patients with chronic lung disease and frequent lung infections suffer from underlying asthma.[170]

Self-Referral maintains health through normal operation of heart, blood vessels and lungs. Disruption of Self-Referral causes disease in these systems. When their feedback loops are disrupted, these systems can no longer maintain health. *Disease is the natural result. Stress causes these feedback loop interruptions – and we begin to see a universal connection between stress and disease.* Is this sequence of events true for other organ systems?

The G.I. Feedback Loop

Doctors use G.I. as an abbreviation for “gastrointestinal.” This refers to the organ system that includes the stomach, intestines, and related organs. The GI Feedback Loop does the work of digesting food and disposing of waste products.

How does the G.I. system do its work? We eat food via the mouth, swallowing through the esophagus. From there it enters the stomach and passes through the small and large intestines, grinding and breaking down food every step of the way. The intestines absorb water and nourishment as food moves through them. The bowel movement eliminates the rest as waste product.[171]

This Feedback Loop has two parts - the mechanical work of digesting food and the Cybernetic communication and control work of brain and nerves. Mechanical digestion breaks food down and moves it through the muscular esophagus, stomach, and intestines.

Digestion dissolves food with chemicals released on cue by various organs and glands along the way.

The brain gets constant feedback from nerve sensors located throughout the GI system. Brain and nerves control intestinal muscle movement, stomach acid production, and the release of digestive enzymes. As thermostat and furnace work together heat a room, the brain, nerves, and G.I. system work together to digest food and eliminate waste products.[172]

The G.I. Feedback Loop is another example of Self-Referral. Health naturally results when feedback loops work normally. Disease naturally results when Self-Referral is disrupted. Do we know of stress-related diseases of the G.I. system?

Stress causes the stomach to produce too much acid – and that acid erodes the lining of the esophagus, stomach, or small intestine. This causes ulcers and related disease.[173] As with other systems, research scientists have developed medications that block the effects of stress.

The H-2 Blockers cimetidine (Tagamet) and ranitidine (Zantac) block stress induced acid production in the stomach.[174] Before these drugs, patients often had their stomach's nerves surgically cut to stop ulcer disease.[175] Other drugs like omeprazole (Prilosec) work through slightly different mechanisms to reduce excess acid.[176] These drugs are effective against ulcers, GERD, and related disease - and have largely eliminated nerve-cutting surgery.[177]

Irritable bowel syndrome is a digestive disorder that causes painful cramping and diarrhea. Doctors used to dismiss it as a psychological problem,[178] but recent research has shown otherwise: it is caused by hyper-arousal of the intestines.[179] The bowel walls, regulated by the autonomic nervous system, suffer overstimulation due to stress. Like vasospasm in the artery and bronchospasm in the bronchi, stress causes muscle spasm in the intestine.

Patients with G.I. problems often have high stressful life event scores as described in *Future Shock.*[180] Many patients with irritable bowel syndrome also have poor muscle tone where the esophagus meets the stomach – allowing acid to splash up into the esophagus. This causes GERD or esophagitis.[181]

These facts confirm that stress-related disruption of intestinal muscle is universal.[182] If hyper-arousal prevents digestion, nutrition will suffer. Elimination problems will surely follow. Stress-related muscle spasm thus likely contributes to disorders like gall bladder disease or even appendicitis.[183]

We see here the same disruption of Self-Referral that causes high blood pressure, heart attack, vasospasm, stroke, and bronchospasm. Stress causes overactive H-2 stimulation, producing excess acid and ulcers. It also causes poor coordination of intestinal muscle, disrupting digestion. These interruptions in the G.I. Feedback Loop cause major diseases that often require surgery. *This is another clear connection between stress, disruption of Self-Referral, and resulting disease.*

Other Feedback Loops

We may cite many other organ systems as feedback loops of Self-Referral – and interruption of their function causes disease. The Immune Feedback Loop quickly responds to infectious agents like bacteria and viruses. When these microscopic invaders are present, white cells and other blood elements rush to the scene to fight infection. Once the infection disappears, the body returns to normal.

Disruption of the body's defenses against infection is devastating. This is the basis of the dreaded AIDS disease. The H.I.V. virus attacks the cells of the immune system, preventing them from combating infection. The result is destruction of the Immune Feedback Loop. Without frequent medications, one infection after another can gradually wear down the patient, often ending in death.[184]

The H.I.V. virus is not the only enemy of the Immune Feedback Loop. There are strong links between the nervous and immune system.[185] Research shows that stressful life events suppress the immune system.[186] These events are well within the average person's experience – including death of a spouse,[187] surgery,[188] competitive sports,[189] sleep deprivation,[190] and the general stress of life.[191] All these sources of stress inhibit the immune system. *Just like Hans Selye's roughed-up rats, stressed people develop suppressed immune systems from stress.*

Finally, the nervous system itself can fall victim to stress. Stroke has long been one of the top three causes of death.[192] The mechanism of stroke is identical to that of angina pectoris: the brain loses vital oxygen due to blocked arteries.[193] Strokes are caused by blood clots, plaques, vasospasm, or high blood pressure.[194] Research also links stress, migraine headache, and epilepsy.[195] Migraine and epilepsy both change the brain's electrical activity.[196] *This suggests that stress directly disrupts brain function.*

The Rosetta Stone of Medicine

Stress takes a terrible toll on human health. The stress of life interferes with many vital body functions. Stress affects the arteries, heart, lungs, G.I. system, immune system, and the nervous system. Disruption of brain and nerve function interferes with still other organ systems. Specific stress-related diseases include heart attack, stroke, epilepsy, high blood pressure, ulcers, infectious disease, and so on. *Can anyone doubt the importance of stress as the cause of disease*?

It is extraordinary that Beta Blockers and related drugs are effective for so many illnesses. It is also extraordinary that one type of body disruption causes so many diseases. Forty years ago, a common mechanism for angina pectoris, migraine, Raynaud's phenomenon,[197] stroke, asthma, and irritable bowel syndrome would have been preposterous. That is no longer true.[198] The very success of the Beta Blockers and other autonomic drugs proves that stress causes disease.

Sir William Osler was a highly respected physician of the early twentieth century. Osler masterfully combined compassion for patients with great medical skill. He urged his medical students to seek a single underlying disease that would explain apparently unrelated symptoms.[199] Disruption of Self-Referral by stress presents such a universal explanation for disease.[200] *This suggests that most, if not all, disease may share the same cause*. Does this not warrant closer examination - by doctors and patients alike?

Many scientists and physicians are aware of the research

described above, but they do not appreciate the full implications of it. Many just do not see the connections between these ideas. To illustrate this point, I offer a story from the history of archaeology.

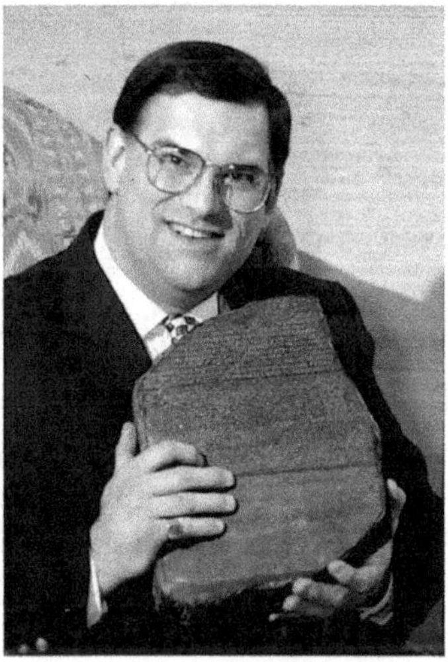

Dr. Michael Borger with a downsized replica of the Rosetta Stone in 1985.

When Napoleon invaded North Africa in 1789, he had a strong interest in ancient Egypt. He sent a group of archaeologists with the invasion force. They were to survey the conquered land and take anything of interest back to France. The French found many intriguing items, but their most important discovery was not a chest of gold or treasure. It was a simple slab of black basalt embedded in a primitive wall.

An ancient engraver had carved the same message in three languages: Greek, cursive Egyptian, and ancient Egyptian hieroglyphics. This was the Rosetta Stone. Through it, archaeologists finally deciphered the previously unknown hieroglyphic language.[201]

Archaeologists could not understand Egyptian hieroglyphics before they studied the Rosetta Stone. This made exploring the tombs and monuments of ancient Egypt very frustrating. Archaeologists found endless walls of writing they were totally unable to read.

Medical knowledge has been in a similar position for centuries. Doctors have catalogued and treated individual diseases, but they still do not understand *the common cause of disease itself*. By a new understanding of the deadly relationship between stress and disease, *we can now decipher the underlying cause of ALL diseases*. We can now formulate a new and truly comprehensive theory of health and disease.

Toward Self-Referral/Maximum Health

I submit that *Self-Referral/Maximum Health* presents such a comprehensive theory. Self-Referral maintains health, and by default prevents disease. Stress profoundly disrupts Self-Referral, interferes with homeostasis, and destroys health. The mechanism for this disruption is autonomic interference with the body's feedback loops. The body is exhausted by undue effort to maintain Self-Referral. We might state a new insight (with apologies to Lao-Tzu):

> The Tao of the Body is Self-Referral.
>
> Look, and it can't be seen.
>
> Listen, and it can't be heard.
>
> Reach, and it can't be grasped.[202]
>
> However: we ignore it at our peril.

So far, our search for *Self-Referral/Maximum Health* has been highly successful. A universal explanation for the processes of health and disease exists. Self-Referral explains health, as defined by successful homeostasis in a changing environment. Disruption of Self-Referral explains disease as well. The theory is certainly logical, but is it practical – or are we just renaming the obvious?

Self-Referral
Maximum Health

Chapter 5

One Mechanism for All Disease: Stress Syndrome

Self-Referral maintains body harmony and health. Disruption of body harmony creates disease. We must understand what disrupts the body's harmony: Stress Syndrome.

Self-Referral and Harmony

The nature of *Self-Referral/Maximum Health* is harmony. Harmony results when we balance all the body's pairs of opposites. When we seek Self-Referral, we look for the body's harmony - and this harmony creates health. How does harmony relate to health?

Harmony is a term easily applied to music. Music's pairs of opposites include loud-soft, high-low, and fast-slow. When an orchestra plays in harmony, it creates beautiful music. If the orchestra fails to keep time or plays wrong notes, we hear musical chaos. We see the same potential for harmony or chaos in the human body.

The body's many parts are startlingly different, one from another. Considering each part, we wonder how they can work together. It is a marvel that body parts as different as tongue, brain, and lung can function as a human being. The body has many parts but functions as a single unit. Like an orchestra, harmony results when all the body's parts work together. This harmony throughout the body creates health.

Self-Referral and Body Harmony

How does the body create harmony? The body's many feedback loops are mechanisms of Self-Referral and allow the body's many parts to work together. Brain works through nervous system to create body harmony.

For example, our brain balances heartbeats between too fast and too slow – and breathing between too shallow and too deep. This pattern is true for every feedback loop in the body. These feedback loops, working together, create harmony. Body harmony creates health; disruption of body harmony creates disease.

Why do we stay healthy most of the time? Asking this another way, how does the body maintain harmony? Through Self-Referral the body's many parts and processes are self-regulating. Unless something interrupts the seamless operation of Self-Referral, the body maintains health. It is as if a form of intelligence lies behind all the body's parts and processes. This is not a new observation. Lao-Tzu tells us in the *Tao te Ching*:

> The Tao is infinite, eternal.
> Why is it eternal?
> It was never born;
> Thus, it can never die.
> Why is it infinite?
> It has no desires for itself;
> Thus, it is present for all beings.[203]

Stress and Body Disharmony

Stress disrupts body harmony. The demands of life cause stress. We would like to avoid stress, but we must face it every day. Why is this? What is there about life itself that brings on stress?

From the moment we are born we face constant change. Change continues throughout our lives - until the day we die. The constant pressures of change itself create stress. We must face it; stress is part of life. To live is to be subject to stress. We can reduce stress through planning, but some stress is unavoidable.

People cope with jobs, marriage, children - many kinds of stress, pleasant and unpleasant - every day of their lives. Why do some people fall ill, while others remain healthy? How is it that some die young and others live a long life? Why do some people reach old age in good health, while others can barely function?

A dilemma emerges. We know about the negative health effects of stress.[204] Stress disrupts Self-Referral and creates disharmony. To maintain health and avoid disease, we need harmony. How can we avoid stress and the disharmony it creates?

A medieval Taoist book suggests an answer. In *The Book of Balance and Harmony* we read:

> Deep knowledge of principle knows without seeing, strong practice of the Tao accomplishes without striving.
>
> Deep knowledge is to be aware of disturbance before disturbance, to be aware of danger before danger, to be aware of destruction before destruction, to be aware of calamity before calamity.
>
> By deep knowledge of principle, one can change disturbance into order, change danger into safety, change destruction into survival, change calamity into fortune. By strong action in the Tao, one can bring the body to the realm of longevity, bring the mind to the sphere of mystery, bring the world to great peace, and bring tasks to great fulfillment.[205]

This writer knew about the body's natural harmony maintained by Self-Referral. He also knew that disharmony produces disease.

To understand disharmony in the body we need to know more about stress. Only with a deep knowledge of stress can we understand its pernicious effects on health. To gain this deep knowledge, we must examine the body's *stress response*.

Stress and Social Disharmony

Everyone knows that some people are more pleasant than others. Pleasant people are open, friendly, and usually good company. Unpleasant people are angry, full of hatred, and often carry a grudge. Pleasant people create harmony and peace through their attitudes and actions. Unpleasant people create discord or even violence. Pleasant people create the harmony of Self-Referral; unpleasant people create stress, disharmony, and strife.

Research shows that stress often produces unpleasant people.[206] The stress response provokes the urge to either fight or run away - the fight or flight rcsponsc. Strcss produces emotions of anger and fear. These negative internal sensations produce negative external attitudes and actions. Stress turns pleasant, harmonious people into unpleasant and disharmonious people.[207]

We can classify people as more or less stressed based on blood chemistry. There are many chemicals released by the body coping with stress, but studies show that *cortisol and epinephrine are key indicators of stress - the main stress chemicals produced by the human body.* A simple blood test can tell how much of these stress chemicals a person has in their circulation. Stressful life events cause more of the stress chemicals to circulate.[208]

How do these stress chemicals become elevated? The stress response begins in the brain. When a stressful event occurs, brain cells release chemicals that stimulate the pituitary gland – and it releases a hormone called ACTH into the blood stream. ACTH stimulates the adrenal glands, located above the kidneys.209 The adrenal glands then release cortisol, epinephrine, and other stress chemicals into the bloodstream.210 These stress chemicals stimulate the autonomic nervous system and cause the fight or flight response.211

The stress response occurs within seconds. When we need this natural body mechanism, as in athletics or for survival, it is beneficial. Unless there is a need for it, however, the stress response causes strain in the physiology. Too much stress response[212] causes the myriad diseases of stress: high blood pressure, ulcers, anxiety, depression, heart attack, asthma, irritable bowel problems, or vasospasm anywhere in the body.[213]

Self-Referral

Maximum Health

Axioms Defining Stress Syndrome, Disease, and the Aging Process

REMEMBER: The stress of life repeatedly triggers the stress response. When stress overwhelms the body's ability to cope, disruption of Self-Referral occurs. Local and then general breakdowns of feedback loops begin. This is Stress Syndrome.

Stress Syndrome repeatedly disrupts Self-Referral: repeated stress response causes overstimulation of the autonomic nervous system - causing high blood pressure, vasospasm, and mini-infarcts. This results in permanent tissue damage.

Stress Syndrome progressively disrupts Self-Referral throughout the body, resulting in chronic autonomic overstimulation that disrupts organs and organ systems. Disruption continues through poor organ function caused by mini-infarcts.

Stress Syndrome thus explains DISEASE and the AGING PROCESS. Feedback loops progressively break down, Self-Referral deteriorates all over the body. Feedback loops between brain and body steadily fail. Resulting disharmony creates the unpredictable results of aging, disease or death.

Vasospasm starves body tissue of oxygen and can cause tissue death. When tissue dies from lack of oxygen, we call this an *infarction*, or *infarct* for short.[214] Major vasospasm is obvious because it causes serious problems like stroke or heart attack. Minor vasospasm is not so obvious and occurs during stressful life events.

These episodes can cause *mini-infarcts* anywhere in the body.[215] This explains the gradual onset of disease and the aging process.

Stress Syndrome

This sequence of events is *Stress Syndrome* – which is what occurs when the stress of life overwhelms the body's coping abilities. Stress Syndrome disrupts Self-Referral, and the harmony and health of the body begins to fail. If this disruption continues, disease or even sudden death will result. Stress Syndrome thus accounts for most, if not all, disease *and the aging process.*

The effects of Stress Syndrome are the opposite of Self-Referral. Self-Referral creates harmony, but Stress Syndrome creates disharmony. This is important deep knowledge of principle that explains the powerful and debilitating effects of stress on human health. This is why stress is the chief cause of disease and the aging process. Feedback loops, overcome by the ruinous effects of stress, can no longer maintain Self-Referral. Harmony fails and the disharmony of disease is the logical result.

This theory is appealing in an intellectual sense. It is satisfying to link apparently unrelated facts and create a new synthesis. The symmetry between ancient and modern thought is stimulating, but how practical is this theory? Doctors and patients want to know how all this applies to real life – and how it can be used in clinical medicine.

Of Mice and Cats

One question that begs an answer is whether stress is as deadly as claimed. Many scientists since Selye have asked this question. What do we know about the effects of stress and specific diseases?

The threat of death is the most severe stressful life event. One ingenious study used the threat of death to measure the effects of stress on mice.[216] Scientists immunized two groups of mice against a type of bacteria. Ordinarily, the mice should not become infected when later exposed to these bacteria – they were already immunized against them. Would stress weaken their immune system?

Caged mice exposed to cats have no idea they are safe from the cats. They react just like they would if there was no cage at all; they fear for their lives. Their bodies thus suffer the same effects as if the imminent threat of death was absolutely real and their lives in danger.

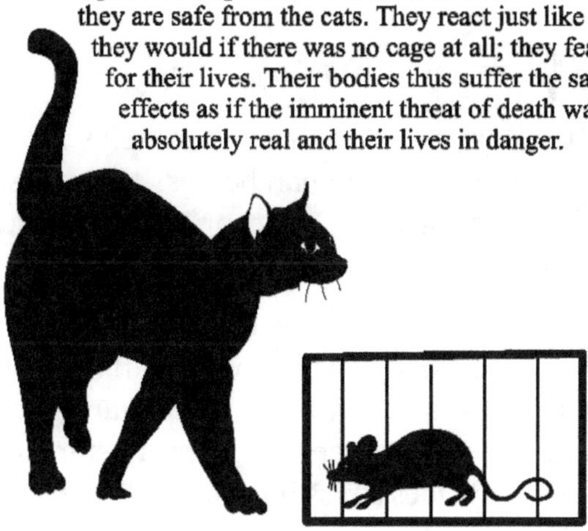

This is why mice terrorized by cats suffer severe stress. This causes strain on their immune system. This is why the stressed mice become ill more often than mice without stress.

The scientists separated the mice into two groups. Researchers threatened one group with death every day: they put the mice in a cage separated from a cat by an invisible wire wall. The mice were understandably terrified. The second group of mice received gentler treatment: the scientists simply picked the mice up and gently petted them. Both groups had stress, but the cat-terrorized mice experienced more intensely negative stress.

Then it was time to test the mice for immune system effects. The researchers repeatedly exposed all mice to the bacteria they were immunized against. The cat-terrorized mice had nearly three times more infection following the stress experiment.[217] The cat-terrorized mice thus were three times more likely to get sick - thanks to severe stress.

Our immune system promotes body harmony by defending against bacteria or viruses. Self-Referral promotes harmony; we know that stress creates disharmony. This experiment's outcome is therefore no surprise. There is no greater stress than the threat of death - and it proves that the deadly effects of stress on Self-Referral are real.

Of Mice and Men

Critics often object that animal experiments are a poor basis for drawing conclusions about human beings. The mouse experiment is interesting, but does it apply to people? Does stress weaken the human immune system?

When we encounter a virus or bacteria, the human immune system responds. The white blood cell is a critical part of the immune system. These organic soldiers attack any microorganism that invades the body's tissues. Their quick response stops most infections before we even notice them.[218] Does stress interfere with these natural agents of Self-Referral?

We know the body releases epinephrine when something triggers the stress response. In an experiment like that of the cat and mice, scientists injected epinephrine - one of the main stress chemicals - into human volunteers. The shots thus simulated intense stress.

When they compared the volunteers' white blood cells before and after the injections, the difference was striking. The patients' white cells were far less responsive to infection following epinephrine.[219] We thus see that both mice and men have similar reactions to stress.[220]

This experiment is interesting, but is it realistic? How many people routinely receive epinephrine injections? Can the body naturally produce a stress response strong enough to create these effects? The answer is shocking. It turns out that stress can make far more serious health problems than just making us sick.

Research proves that life-threatening stress can cause sudden death in humans. People subjected to physical assault or automobile accidents sometimes drop dead during the experience. Why do they die? Autopsies of these patients reveal severe heart damage. This heart damage is not an infarction; it is muscle damage caused by a huge outpouring of chemicals.[221] The facts show that these people were literally *scared to death.*[222]

We now see the effects of sudden and extreme disharmony on the body. Self-Referral promotes harmony through the balance of opposites. When stress completely overwhelms us, it causes extreme disharmony – and sometimes even death.

These facts are interesting, but critics will question the conclusions. Are the effects of stress limited to people who have terrible, life-threatening experiences? How often do average people fear for their lives? Does stress work this way in daily life?

Lives of Quiet Desperation

Stress is part of everyone's life. There are many sources of stress. No matter where we live, nearly everyone interacts with other people, doubtless creating some stress. We go to work, raise our children, and attend social events. People interact with us at a distance talking on the phone. Most people also experience frustration: the alarm clock failed to work. The car ran out of gasoline, or our bills are too high. Life itself, it seems, generates stress.

A key factor in human interaction is emotional response. Emotions are part of the human experience. In many ways, it is the most real part of real life. What connections are there between emotions and disease?

Until recently, there was little evidence to connect emotions and disease. To illustrate, doctors and patients link strong emotions with chest pain. Is there a link between stress, strong emotions, and heart disease? Can strong mental emotions caused by stress provoke a physical heart attack? Henry David Thoreau, writing over a hundred years ago in the book *Walden*, clearly described the emotional effects of stress:

> The mass of men lead lives of quiet desperation.
>
> What is called resignation is confirmed desperation.[223]

Researchers now understand this desperation because a clear link exists between stress, emotions, and heart disease. Heart disease does not always produce chest pain; researchers call this silent heart disease.[224] Vasospasm causes silent heart disease,[225] and it is just as deadly as that accompanied by chest pain.[226] Doctors call this phenomenon *silent ischemia.*

Silent ischemia is deadly because chest pain usually acts as a warning. Heart patients who experience chest pain can reduce their workload and prolong their lives. People with silent ischemia have no warning when they exceed their limits. They may cause their own death by pushing themselves far beyond their heart's abilities.[227]

When researchers identified silent ischemia, doctors wondered what activities made it worse. Some argued that *physical stress*, like riding a bicycle, was responsible. Others believed that *mental stress* was deadly. Which type of stress causes silent ischemia?

To answer these questions, scientists studied angina patients with silent ischemia. First, they tested the patients' coronary artery blood flow before, during and after a timed mental arithmetic test. Then they tested the patients before, during and after a bicycle stress test. The question was: which would cause silent ischemia - mental stress or physical stress?[228]

This study proved that *patients respond the same way to mental stress and physical stress*. They suffer silent ischemia, whether stress is mental or physical. The same areas of the heart are oxygen starved during silent ischemia - no matter what the cause. If someone takes a timed mental arithmetic test or rides a bicycle, the effect is the same. Whether stress is mental or physical, the outcome is equally real, and equally deadly.[229]

This study also proves that stress does not have to be life threatening to kill. A timed arithmetic test and bicycle riding are not unusual tasks. These activities are well within the experience of average people leading ordinary lives. We thus see that stress is part of real life - and the reality is, stress can be a killer.[230]

Life, Death, and Video Games

Today's doctors and scientists no longer question the reality of stress, disease, and sudden death. Medical professionals do not have all the answers yet, but every study reveals a little more about the monster we call stress.

Let's return for a moment to the Tao of the warrior. These researchers remind me of lonely warriors, plotting strategy for a war against disease. Thomas Cleary writes introducing his translation and commentary on Sun Tzu's *Art of War*:

> . . . the master warrior is the one who knows the psychology and mechanics of a conflict so intimately that every move of an opponent is seen through at once . . . Warriors of Asia who used Taoist or Zen arts to achieve profound calmness did not do so just to sustain the awareness of imminent death, but also to achieve the sensitivity needed to respond to situations without stopping to ponder.231

This is the deep knowledge we need to defeat stress. Many doctors and scientists throughout the world study stress. One such research warrior was Dr. Robert S. Eliot, Director of the University of Nebraska's Life Stress Simulation Laboratory. He was a world class expert on stress and the cardiovascular system.[232] Dr. Eliot established that stress is part of real life through some unusual experiments.[233]

Dr. Eliot studied the effects of stress as they happen; scientists call this studying stress in real time. How was this done? Dr. Eliot connected patients with devices that measure stress indicators like blood pressure, heart rate, and breathing. The patients carried out activities designed to provoke the stress response. Then Dr. Eliot recorded body effects while the subject performed the stress-producing activity.[234]

To illustrate, Dr. Eliot asked a heart patient to play a simple video game. He connected the patient to laboratory equipment in a quiet room. A technician explained the video game. The equipment monitored the patient while he played the game, recording his vital signs.[235]

The patient did not know it, but the computer was programmed not to let him win. The computer allowed him to almost win the first three rounds. This created the illusion that winning was possible.

Then the computer teased the patient by making the game faster and faster. Winning was then impossible because the computer was just too quick.

The researchers watched the patient react to the stress of frustration. His physical changes were like those of an athlete in action. Blood pressure rose from 140/80 to 183/125. Heart rate increased from 80 beats per minute to 109. The body's circulation clamped down because of autonomic overstimulation.[236]

After a while, Dr. Eliot stopped the experiment. He told the patient it was "like drag racing a car with the brakes on. The engine was overheating and starting to fail." The patient, caught up in the thrill of the game, replied "I'm just getting the hang of it. Give me a few more minutes and I'll get the best of the bloody machine." Dr. Eliot explained "You will never beat the computer. The question is: *is this effort worth dying for*?"[237]

Self-Referral, Personality, and Stress

Many doctors in history connect strong emotions like anger and fear with death from heart attack. Observers of human nature often note that personalities are not alike. Some people easily adapt to changing conditions with limited stress. Other people can tolerate little change without slipping into fear or anger. Do personality traits – often matters of emotion – impact how we cope with stress?

Self-Referral promotes harmony, and harmony creates health. Stress causes disharmony through negative emotions like anger, worry, and fear. We might look at personality to learn more about stress. This is not a new idea. Lao-Tzu tells us in the *Tao te Ching*:

> Knowing others is intelligence; knowing yourself is true wisdom.
>
> Mastering others is strength; mastering yourself is true power.[238]

Doctors and patients often connect strong emotions like anger, fear, and worry with angina pectoris. This is why researchers look for a coronary-prone personality. Some classify people as stress seekers

– those who consider stress a positive experience - or as stress avoiders, who regard stress as unpleasant and try to avoid it.[239]

Another classification of personality calls the stress seekers racehorse types. They are like racehorses, barely under control and constantly straining to break into a run. They call the opposite people – the stress avoiders - the turtle types. They are like turtles, going into their shell whenever they see stress coming.[240]

A third way to classify personality is Type A or Type B. Type A subjects have intense ambition and strong competitive drive. They are always in a hurry, fidget a lot, focus unduly on deadlines, and speak in short, curt phrases. Type B subjects are more easygoing.[241]

Type A subjects have a more intense stress response than Type B subjects. They also have higher levels of stress chemicals in their urine. This suggests that Type A people have high levels of stress chemicals in their blood stream. This proves that Type A people are more stressed.[242]

Lately the idea of Type A and Type B personality has come under attack. Some researchers question the relationship between Type A personality and heart disease.[243] Others suggest that Type A people may be a subset of all people at risk for heart attack.[244] This larger group may have an underlying disorder unrelated to personality.[245]

The Worst Stress: Hot Reactors

Dr. Robert Eliot believed such a group exists, based on his research. He divided people into two groups: those who tolerate the stressful video game he called normal. Those who responded with increased heart rate and blood pressure he called abnormal.[246]

Dr. Eliot called the abnormal subjects *Hot Reactors*. He characterized Hot Reactors as hostile, impatient, and unnecessarily competitive. Hot Reactors will suffer dangerous reaction to stress, simulated or otherwise. *Dr. Eliot believed at least half the American population may be Hot Reactors.*[247]

Once again, we see that stress does not have to be life threatening to cause coronary problems. Ordinary activities like playing a video game can cause a Hot Reactor response. "We recognize that the central nervous system can provide a powerful cardiovascular response," Dr. Eliot stated. "What nature intended to be helpful can be a killer.

"Let's put this in perspective. During one year, coronary heart disease killed about one million Americans. Half of them - about twelve hundred per day - died suddenly within the day," Dr. Eliot says. "*Stress outweighs the other standard risk factors in these deaths*."[248]

The research of Dr. Eliot and others teaches us that stress is a clear and present danger. Stress is no longer an esoteric topic limited to academic circles. People know they are in trouble, and the cause of it is stress.[249]

Stress Syndrome is not an abstract idea; most people these days know what is happening. I recently repaired a laceration on a factory worker. This man complained bitterly about his job. He said that no matter how hard they worked, there was more pressure to work harder. He wore an interesting T-shirt. Written in large letters across it was the following message:

> Just when you thought you were winning the rat race, along came *faster rats*.

Stress Syndrome is The Enemy

We know that stress causes Stress Syndrome. Through repeated triggering of the stress response, the harmony of Self-Referral breaks down. Little by little, Stress Syndrome erodes the many feedback loops the body depends on to maintain health.

The impact of ongoing attacks on Self-Referral by Stress Syndrome is real. As the stress of life strains the body's natural ability to maintain health, disease is the natural result. Likewise, the ongoing strain of Stress Syndrome drives the aging process, steadily wearing us down year after year.

All the research we have reviewed points in one direction: *stress is the enemy that destroys health and creates disease*. We now know that the stress of life overcomes the harmony of Self-Referral. We must answer an important question: why is stress such a problem now, today? What is going on in the modern world that is creating so much stress? Answering this question will give all of us a better chance for a long life through Maximum Health.

Self-Referral

Maximum Health

Chapter 6

The Adaptation Crisis

Self-Referral creates harmony in the body, and harmony creates health. Stress Syndrome disrupts Self-Referral and creates disease. Why do so many today suffer the disharmony of stress?

Self-Referral and Adaptation

When we seek *Self-Referral/Maximum Health*, we look for ways to help the body govern itself. The body governs itself through elegantly designed feedback loops. These feedback loops are the mechanisms of Self-Referral. They maintain health and, by default, prevent disease.

We have traveled far in our search for *Self-Referral/Maximum Health*. When we began our search, Self-Referral was totally unknown to us. What is Self-Referral, we asked? We learned that Self-Referral is the balance of opposites. We see Self-Referral in the body's many feedback loops. How can the harmony of the Tao – the balance of opposites – help us understand human health? Lao-Tzu helps us to understand in the *Tao te Ching*:

> The Tao is nowhere to be found. Yet it nourishes and completes all things.[250]

We again confront a Tolkien-like riddle. The Tao-like harmony of the body is Self-Referral. We know that Self-Referral exists after thoroughly examining its role in the body. Despite this detailed examination, we likely still have some questions about it. Exactly how it is that Self-Referral keeps us healthy?

Adaptation is the body's ability to successfully adjust to changing conditions. Exercise, for example, causes our bodies to adapt. We can see this when we walk and run. Walking is usually an easy, effortless experience – but when we run, our bodies must adapt to a greater workload. Our heart speeds up, breathing becomes deeper, blood pressure rises, and our muscles work harder – we can only run so far, and we must stop to rest.

In health, Self-Referral easily responds to changing conditions and adapts the body to succeed. In disease, the body is out of balance and cannot respond dynamically to changing conditions. Such a person may be unable to run, or even walk. In that case the body simply cannot meet challenges when they arise. This is *failure of adaptation* – the body simply cannot muster what is needed to carry out the desired action.

We know that disease is not limited to obvious problems like heart attack, stroke, or other major and dramatic health crises. Most disease is silent and the person developing the problem is not even aware of it. Aging itself falls into this category, silently taking its toll until one day people realize they cannot do things they used to take for granted.

Stress disrupts Self-Referral, and we know that modern life causes more stress than ever before. Many sources of stress today converge on peoples' lives, disrupting Self-Referral. The result is a crisis in the ability to cope with stress. Alvin Toffler called this *Future Shock.*

We know from Dr. Robert Eliot's research that half of all Americans may be Hot Reactors. These people routinely overreact to mental or physical stress. The Hot Reactor suffers a basic inability to adapt to stressful conditions. That is why Hot Reactors are more prone to stress disorders like high blood pressure, angina pectoris, and sudden death.

Modern life sets the stage for people to become Hot Reactors. This is the basis of the Adaptation Crisis causing today's explosion in stress-related disease. The term Adaptation Crisis suggests a true emergency. Some, however, will ask if this is an overstatement. What evidence can we find of an authentic Adaptation Crisis?

Stress and Modern Life

By way of historical perspective, medicine only learned about stress recently. Selye's stress research was first published in the 1930s. In the ninety plus years since Hans Selye's articles, research proved that stress is the basis of disease. Researchers then developed drugs to treat the effects of stress.

Many ask why stress is such an important issue at this time in history. Is modern life truly more stressful, or are we just noticing stress for the first time? Did stress cause the same health problems in earlier times? People have always endured the death of a spouse, moving one's home, or changing jobs. Today's lifestyle is different, however; it adds new stress to that which has always been with us.

One unique aspect of modern life is technology. *Our many electronic and mechanical devices help us – but they also stress us.* We rely on these devices – but they also drive us hard and irritate us.

Today's unnatural pace of living accelerates the rate of stress. It also makes the negative effects of stress stronger. Why is this so? A hundred years ago there were no buzzing clock radios or buzzing cell phones. There were no banging air hammers or roaring jet planes. Life was slower and more predictable. People worked hard, but they had more peace and quiet. Compared to driving today's car, riding a carriage was slow and the horse did most of the decision making.

In today's world people often find it difficult to finish a conversation without cell phones interrupting. Automobiles, computers, and machine-based jobs force people to think and work at a frantic pace. Every day we contend with rush hour traffic, meet the demands of our jobs, and keep going nearly any time of the day and night. Cable, satellite, and streaming television and video players allow us to watch what we want, 24 hours a day. This electronic cacophony converges to create more stress than ever – piling on stress, stress, and more stress.

What can we do to counteract these multiple sources of stress? One problem is that people can't make a living in today's world without technology. An additional factor is that technology is very enjoyable, for entertainment purposes and otherwise. Nowhere is this problem more obvious than the management of something at the center of everyone's life: television.

Violence in Entertainment

Experts who study children and the family express concern about television's negative effects. Many children spend eleven hours a day bleary-eyed in front of the television: parents find it easier to place a child in front of the television than to interact meaningfully with the kids. Leaving the television on is also cheaper than hiring a baby-sitter.

Violence has become more and more a part of television fare. By age 18, a child will have seen 200,000 acts of violence on television. Social researchers believe this exposure to violence increases aggression in children. Research shows that young children who watch television many hours per week are more likely to behave badly or even fight. One study shows that children who frequently watch TV violence are more likely to commit violent crime by age 30, including beating their own children.[251]

Video and computer games are more violent. First there was Mortal Kombat, a martial arts video game that showed the loser's head flying off, complete with blood spewing from the neck. Then came Night Trap, the computer game that featured vampires using an electric drill on a teenage girl's jugular vein. Game gore then advanced via the first-person shooter games that started with DOOM.[252] Computer columnist John C. Dvorak of *PC Magazine* wrote about DOOM:

> In many ways, DOOM may be the most violent computer game ever written. The people and things you kill make a sickening groan as blood splashes all over the place. You can even use a chain saw to ravage the enemy, chopping him into a mess of blood and guts.[253]

Since DOOM, more violent computer games have entered our lives. Adding to their impact is more and more realistic graphics and sound as computer hardware and software improved over the years. The result of games like DOOM and its descendants is a growing realization that these are not innocent games like the old Pac Man or Mario Brothers.

Many claim these games are nothing more than harmless cartoons, but critics argue otherwise. Angry parents, educators, and family experts across the country demanded action from Congress. The resulting furor caused the introduction of a U.S. Senate bill to develop a voluntary rating system within the video game industry. The ratings warn parents about violence, foul language, and sexual content in computer and video games.[254]

While the ratings system is helpful, creative children can still access violent games anyway. Five kids aged 9 to 15 years old had no problem purchasing gory computer games that were too strong for them according to the rating system.[255] Kids also can easily rent games, regardless whether they are suitable for children. And now streaming game services make unlimited game access for children easy.

Dr. Robert Eliot's work with video games makes a clear case that today's electronic environment aggravates the Hot Reactor in all of us. Violent video games, television shows, and movies will surely trigger Hot Reactors.[256] The tremendous upsurge in game machines, Internet streaming video shows, and movies – whether on television or on notebook computers or smart phones – brings more and more R-rated violent material into people's lives.

War on the Home Front

Television news coverage brings crime, violence, and war into our homes. *TIME* magazine columnist Lance Morrow wrote about the electronic news coverage of Operation Desert Storm:

> Television brought the Vietnam War into America's living rooms only when the fighting was underway. [During Operation Desert Storm]
>
> Americans are watching the preparations in the sand on television every night. . . Time gets dismantled somehow; slaughter gets projected

> into the hypothetical. The adrenaline rushes prematurely; the cost gets reckoned before the deployment. So much anticipation overworks the nerves. The process causes hallucinations and jitters. Normally war begins without such neurotic projections.[257]

Witnessing war, natural disasters, and violent crime without being affected by them changes us. Newspaper columnist Vaughn Moreno wrote:

> My experience in Vietnam showed how constant exposure to violence makes a person less aware of it and less sensitive to it. Violence that shocked me at the beginning of my tour of duty seemed not even worthy of notice at the end. I believe the same dynamic is at work on our collective consciousness. Television could very well be renamed tele violence.[258]

Does all this matter? Many who fight crime argue that all this does matter. Detective Joe Fox is a homicide detective in crime-ridden Washington, D.C. He has a job few would envy – he investigates the crime scenes of recent murders. Like the characters in television shows like The X Files, Bones, Cold Case Files, and NCIS he carefully studies dead and often mangled bodies to find clues to these crimes.

Detective Fox reports there has been a change in his homicide cases. Thirty years ago, Fox reports, most murders resulted from domestic or family quarrels that got out of hand. He says that murders are now more likely to be acts of random violence, or even bizarre cases with dark psychological overtones.[259] These are the notorious serial killer cases, where people murder not as part of committing another crime, but purely for the enjoyment of killing.

Because serial murder cases lack many clues, statistics on them are often unreliable. Nevertheless, criminologist Marc Ridel of Southern Illinois University thinks they may account for as much as 25% to 35% of the national murders. This is a threefold increase from just twenty years previously. Other crimes like robbery, assault, and carjacking also have increased in frequency.[260] Is this upswing in violence coincidental with increased violence in the electronic media?

Television exposes millions of people to mass trauma through news stories focused on violence, disasters, or warfare. Televised events like the 9-11 attack expose millions of television viewers to levels of violence and destruction they ordinarily would never encounter in day-to-day life. Streaming documentary and reality shows feature such disturbing content every day. Mental health experts express concern that people watching television violence suffer trauma from witnessing such events.[261]

Television, Television, and Television

There are well over 93 million television sets in the United States – and when you include computers and smart phones, it may be impossible to measure how many screens exist. Children aged 2 to 5 years old typically watch 22 hours of television per week. The number of viewing hours per week increases with age: people aged 35 or more watch between 25 and 37 hours of television per week. By the time today's teenagers reach age 70, they will have watched 7 years' worth of television – and with more screens to watch, this number will climb substantially.[262]

Of the homes with television, 75 percent own at least one video player – DVD, Blu-Ray, or digital video recording machines. Those who record television typically watch an average of two hours delayed television per day. There are 6 million movies rented daily – online or otherwise. By contrast, people check out daily only 3 million items from the public library. Television in its various forms thus dominates people's leisure time.[263]

What are the effects of all this television viewing? While everyone who watches TV does not become a serial killer, it has other negative effects. One effect is that of creating a jittery, nervous mind set. In an interview, Jurassic Park author Michael Crichton offered:

> When I'm working hard, I go for six weeks without TV, and I feel different. One of the most interesting things about experiencing television is its ever-accelerating pace. I realize that when I take a walk in the woods, or make the bed or cook a meal, our everyday rhythms are much slower than television. That's a reason I'm drawn to watch slow political discussions on CSPAN. It puts you back in human time.[264]

Hyperactivity is a widespread problem among children. This behavior disorder causes kids to constantly move about, unable to stay in one place. They also have attention problems that interfere with learning. Their behavior is so disruptive that teachers cannot conduct class work around them. These children suffer from attention deficit hyperactivity disorder, or ADHD. Doctors treat these children with medications like Ritalin, Adderall, or Vyvanse.

Recent research shows that ADHD has a physical basis: these children have abnormal brain function. Overall brain metabolism was 8 percent lower than normal children. ADHD especially involves the areas of the brain that regulate attention and muscle control.[265]

Does excessive television viewing cause ADHD? We know that mental stress triggers the stress response, whether the stress is real or imagined. Television likely affects some children's mental functioning, perhaps causing problems like ADHD. Television viewing, video game playing, and all other aspects of overstimulation doubtless kick up the stress levels – for adults and children alike.

Another concern is the negative content of television shows. Talk shows and soap operas are on when preschool children are left in front of the television. Some mental health experts say that talk shows are hazardous to mental health. Family experts contend that tabloid talk shows distort reality: they present deviant or criminal lifestyle choices as somehow acceptable or even normal. They believe this has a negative effect on children and adults alike.[266]

Stress and the Computer Culture

Nearly eight in ten households own a computer.[267] Seven in ten households have a computer with Internet access. This number jumps to nine in ten among college graduates. Among teenagers, 63% have their own home computer.[268] Numbers are approaching 100% as schools adopt a policy of providing a computer for each student. Those who have computers often bring work home with them – both adults and children.[269] Everybody uses computers for entertainment.[270]

Computers are helpful, but they also add to the stress of modern life. Learning to operate computers can be difficult. Once you learn the programs, they have periodic upgrades that change how they look and behave. Relearning formerly familiar programs wreaks havoc as users are forced to learn the new version's quirks.

Even experienced operators have a lot of frustration: human error can erase work that took days or months to create. Storage devices are becoming a problem because they eventually become obsolete.[271] Some experts ask if the computer industry itself can keep up with rapidly evolving software.[272]

Another struggle is keeping up with computer hardware. If you use a typical computer, the processor chips inside the newer machines keep changing – due to improving technology. Today's chips run faster than those of five years ago – or even less.[273] It helps to have faster chips, but every improvement makes thousands of older computers obsolete – and everyone must learn the nuances of the new ones.[274]

Keyboard operators, like professional typists, can get painful muscle problems like carpal tunnel syndrome. Repetitive movement using the computer keyboard and mouse causes a new kind of muscle ailment: doctors now report a painful muscle condition of the shoulder called mouse shoulder. Repetitive operation of the computer mouse causes it – at work or at home.[275]

Computers, the Internet, and constant smart phone use make getting information easier than ever. Companies want and often need a lot of information to be competitive. They get what they need – but the process can end up burying people in useless information as well. Sorting through information overload is a major problem. More access to information thus creates more work – and more stress.[276]

For example, a recent advertisement described a stockbroker's computer activities. As he glances at stock market data from an online Web site, he reads stock market stories in an online newspaper updated live. The computer is also sending and receiving email at the same moment. He must wade through the email received, deciding to delete junk mail, and reading what looks useful.[277] This kind of non-stop, intense activity adds to the stress of life.

People are becoming more aware of the stress caused by the modern electronic environment. For example, actor Gates McFadden played Dr. Beverly Crusher in "Star Trek: The Next Generation." She offered these comments in an interview:

> We have such a media bombardment of new information, and things happen so quickly in our lives. You can read the newspaper and all the magazines, and you still don't begin to comprehend the scope of any situation. The exposure to so much information is one of the reasons for so much stress in our lives. It's like computer overload – it comes at us so fast and furious that you can't take it all in.[278]

There is even concern that the electronic environment itself may be hazardous to human health. Computers, telephones, and electric power lines put out low level radiation that may cause leukemia and other malignancies.[279] This raises concern about the long-term effects of computers and other digital devices.[280] The cell phone also is suspected by many health experts to be a health hazard because of their intense microwave radiation.[281]

Stress and the Electronic Tide

As electronic technology changes our world, all is not smooth. One problem is how to deal with those who resist using computers.

While computer users relish the help their machines provide, non-users feel irritated or even threatened by the new technology.

While computer use in some fields is totally optional, people will lose their jobs over this issue in coming years. This is creating a new kind of have and have-not situation based on computer literacy.[282] All this pressure and confusion creates stress that ripples through our whole culture.

The electronic tide is transforming our culture from where we were, to where we are, and to where we are going. This constitutes a major change in the American workforce. For example, in 1901 over 50% of all Americans worked in agriculture. Experts predict that less than 5% of the workforce will be working in agriculture in the future.

In 1950, the blue-collar industrial worker made up over 40% of the workforce – and soon less than 15% of the workforce will be blue-collar. Non-manual, computer-based workers now account for 80% of the American workforce.[283] Worrying about your job creates a lot of stress, and there is plenty of worry as the electronic tide sweeps our culture.

One result of these changes is fewer blue-collar workers being forced to work more days and longer hours. Assembly line worker Anna Coleman is typical. She has worked for General Motors for over 25 years. Lately, she worked over nine hours a day, six days a week for 15 months. "We're not the youngest people anymore," Coleman comments. "And with more demands for production, we need more manpower."[284]

Experts in human resources are certain that people are working harder now than in decades. Workers are spending more hours per day and more days per week than ever. In fact, our workforce – blue-collar and white-collar alike – has not worked so hard since World War II. Many work experts are saying that the answer may be a shorter work week – to preserve our sanity.[285]

The crushing demands on workers are taking a tragic toll on their families. Many parents leave children home alone because both parents work long hours. There simply is no one to care for them, and the parents cannot afford a baby-sitter.[286] The pressures on the family and the individual create more stress than ever.

Another result of the stressed-out lifestyle is domestic violence. Doctors commonly see brutalized victims of physical abuse. The attacker may be their spouse, ex-spouse, family member, or other acquaintance. There are so many of these cases that emergency departments are having a difficult time coping with them.[287] The stress of modern life thus contributes to the rise of domestic violence.

Shifting circumstances of modern life often cause workers to move. When jobs dry up in one area, people must move to find work. This disrupts the family as they move from familiar surroundings to a new town or state. Families forced to move often lose the support of family and friends, adding to their stress.[288]

The sweeping stress of the electronic tide is profound. It is changing human experience forever. Today's high-tech lifestyle stresses people beyond their ability to adapt. All this adds to the Adaptation Crisis.

Stress and Changeable Schedules

Another source of stress is today's artificial cycle of day and night. Before electric lighting, people went to bed soon after dark and rose with the sun. The modern environment allows people to create day in the middle of the night. This makes possible night shifts at work and social events at any hour. The 24-hour availability of cable and satellite television further encourages staying up late. These factors converge, causing people to sleep irregular hours.

One result of irregular sleeping is a crisis in occupations that require alertness.[289] Over two thirds of professional truck drivers admit they sometimes feel sleepy at the wheel. As many as eleven per cent of railroad engineers fall asleep on most, if not all, their night shifts. Over fifty per cent of night shift workers in industry admit they doze on the job – at least once a week.

These sleepy people may be uncomfortable but fighting nature's sleep cycle is dangerous.[290] How many traffic accidents, train derailments, and industrial disasters result from hapless workers fighting sleep?[291]

Time-related sleep disorders are now a national epidemic. The National Commission on Sleep Disorders Research recently issued a report that estimates there are 40 million Americans suffering from some type of sleeping disorder. These sleeping problems include insomnia, breathing problems, and falling asleep any time without warning. Sleep disorders also affect teenagers, who report falling asleep during school at least once per week.[292]

Sleep related problems cost Americans nearly $16 million per year in medical care and medications. We doubtless lose tens of billions more – in lost work time, lost productivity, and accident losses. We this see that this is a major problem – and a huge economic drain.[293] Why are sleep disorders so common?

People live arbitrary daylight hours, but our biology does not change so easily. Looking at the human past, people lived a great span of time in the natural environment. Our ancestors lived the day-night cycle. When the sun went down, they naturally went to sleep. At sunrise, the cycle started all over again.

Scientists have studied the effects of daylight on humans. They know that humans have a biological clock that is triggered by daylight.[294] Morning daylight triggers the brain. The brain then activates the pineal, pituitary, and other glands, preparing for a new day.[295] Many scientists now believe that irregular sleeping habits disrupt health and cause disease. [296] All this adds stress to our lives.

Doctors have discovered a daylight-oriented disorder called Seasonal Affect Disorder, or SAD.[297] People with SAD suffer depression during the winter months with fewer hours of daylight per day.[298] Depression in this case is caused by the stress of fewer hours of sunlight.[299] The remedy for SAD is for patients to spend several hours a day in a room lit by lamps that approximate sunlight.[300]

Does conflict with the natural day and night cycle cause health problems? Recently I saw a patient with high blood pressure. He had good control of blood pressure for over two years using a low dose of blood pressure medicine. His blood pressure had stayed normal and was quite stable. When I saw him this time, however, his blood pressure was markedly high.

Previously, he was always very energetic and healthy in appearance. Now he looked noticeably tired and washed out – like he needed to catch up on sleep. I asked him what had changed in his life. He told me he had been switched from day to night shift, and he just hated it. He could not sleep well and constantly felt under pressure.

I increased his medicine to get the blood pressure under control, but the root problem was obvious. This patient was forced to live outside the normal day and night cycle he had lived with all his life. The stress of straining to accommodate the night shift was aggravating high blood pressure. We thus see that shifting our day-night cycle worsens high blood pressure – and that is a major risk factor for heart attack, stroke, and sudden death.

Sleep disturbance causes other problems. Researchers found that short sleeping hours cause accelerated hardening of coronary arteries – the clogged pipes problem we have discussed. This leads to greater likelihood of fatal heart attack. Longer sleeping hours – closer to the recommended 8 hours per night – is associated with lower calcification of the coronary arteries.[301] This is why getting a good night's sleep is vital to health – and may even save your life.

Finally, sleep deprivation has been shown to accelerate the aging process. Poor quality of sleep slows glucose metabolism by up to 40%. Poor sleep also increases levels of the stress chemical cortisol. These changes cause memory impairment – a symptom of advanced aging. This is how people too young to normally have such findings are being crippled by poor sleep. When they improve their sleep, they reverse these problems.[302]

Even ignoring shift changes and poor sleep, job strain itself is of concern. Job strain results when there is friction between workers. It also occurs with stressful work conditions of any kind. The resulting stress has been shown to cause elevated blood pressure.[303]

Job strain has also been shown to directly affect the heart, increasing muscle wall thickness of the left ventricle. This shows that stress at the job not only elevates blood pressure, but also strains the heart as it beats against resistance caused by high blood pressure.[304] Job strain has also been shown to accelerate hardening of the arteries. Taken together, this all amounts to accelerated aging.[305]

The Timing of Nature

Scientists have found clues that many other body functions are cued by natural cycles in nature. There is an entire medical science that studies these natural body cycles. This is chronobiology, or the science of biology as it relates to time.

Research worldwide shows that disrupting the natural waking-sleeping cycle profoundly disturbs mental and physical health.[306] Unfortunately, today's high-tech electronic environment excels in separating people from natural cycles like day and night.

We now see that modern life depends on technology – and technology causes stress. For example, in 1880 a person took a week to travel by horse from Eastern Pennsylvania to Ohio. Now we drive a car the same distance in a few hours, often fighting traffic all the way.

Last century's office worker filed papers by hand, at a steady pace. Today's office worker struggles to keep up with computers, changing hardware and software, and smart phones.

Yesterday's factory worker used simple tools and kept pace with human workers. Today's manufacturing worker suffers endless repetition of machinelike movements – while struggling to keep up with machines.

Research shows that mental stress and physical stress both disrupt Self-Referral and cause deadly health effects. We know that today's electronic and mechanical environment increases both kinds of stress. This is why the human race is in a true Adaptation Crisis. The result is stress, stress, and more stress.

All these pressures in our culture cause more stress than human beings have ever endured in recorded history. Modern life, by its very nature, creates unprecedented stress that impacts every man, woman and child who lives in it.

The Adaptation Crisis is Real

Our biology has utterly been outstripped and overcome by the high-tech demands of modern life. Alvin Toffler described our situation brilliantly in *Future Shock*:

> Future shock is the dizzying disorientation brought on by the premature arrival of the future. When diversity converges with transience and novelty, we rocket the society toward an historical crisis of adaptation. We create an environment so ephemeral, unfamiliar, and complex as to threaten millions with adaptive breakdown. This breakdown is called *Future Shock*.[307]

We have come far in identifying what disrupts Self-Referral. Today's Adaptation Crisis is caused by the stress of modern life. Knowing the problem will help us seek a solution to it.

We now know the source of today's Adaptation Crisis. Modern life, with its unique demands, is creating more stress than human beings can handle. Today's stress is literally destroying lives and killing people. This crisis is killing us by accelerating our pace of life beyond what our biology can tolerate.

We must find a solution to the Adaptation Crisis – or, in the long run, we will not survive as a species. To find the solution to the Adaptation Crisis we must look for ways to improve our ability to cope with stress. What do we know about how our bodies cope with stress? Can we learn ways to improve our ability to cope with stress? And can we find and apply this knowledge to head off the Adaptation Crisis? We had better get to work and find effective answers to these challenges; our very survival depends on it.

Self-Referral

Maximum Health

Chapter 7

Self-Referral and the Adaptation Crisis

Humanity is now in an Adaptation Crisis that destroys Self-Referral and creates disease. How does modern life impact the human body? How does modern life destroy Self-Referral?

Self-Referral and the Adaptation Crisis

When we seek *Self-Referral/Maximum Health*, we look for ways to help the body govern itself. The body governs itself through elegantly designed feedback loops. These feedback loops are the mechanisms of Self-Referral. They maintain health and prevent disease.

Adaptation is the ability to adjust to changing conditions. Many sources of stress today converge on peoples' lives, disrupting Self-Referral. The body cannot cope with the extreme amount of incoming stress. The result is the *Adaptation Crisis*. One question that many ask is: are we sure that modern life is the problem?

We could answer this question if we could somehow go back in history. If we time-traveled to a period when humans lived a primitive lifestyle, we could compare their health status to that of today's people. Would we find health differences between ancient people and today's high technology population?

Time travel is presently impractical, but we can still study the effects of modern culture upon today's primitive humans. One informative research project studied people of the African Zulu tribe. The Zulus lived their entire life in the open, following the hunter-gatherer lifestyle as it was thousands of years ago. In the early 1960s, as civilization encroached into the African wild, some Zulus chose to move into the new cities.

The urbanized Zulus soon showed the effects of the modern environment and lifestyle. Their blood pressure was normal at first, but the stress of urban life soon took its toll. The city-dwelling Zulus soon suffered high blood pressure as a benefit of modern life. Reasons offered for this effect include changes in diet, reduced exercise, and the stress of modern life.[308]

With everything that we know about the stress of modern life, we can conclude that the resulting health hazards are real. We can conclude that Stress Syndrome and the Adaptation Crisis are real. It is no myth that the rush of modern life pushes human biology beyond its ability to cope. Today's lifestyle truly has health hazards attached to it. With all this understood, what can we do about it?

Some Key Questions

Self-Referral creates health, and stress creates disease. Because stress related disease is so important, we must ask some key questions. For example: the stress response occurs in the brain, but the effects of stress show up in all parts of the body. With few exceptions, such as stroke, the stress response – which starts in the brain - usually causes disease elsewhere in the body. How is stress distributed to different parts of the body?

Another question is why stressed people have different diseases. We have described a bewildering list of stress-related diseases - heart attack, asthma, ulcers, and irritable bowel syndrome, to name a few. Why does stress cause asthma in one-person, high blood pressure in another, and heart attack in a third? Why do different people with the same stress have different diseases?

There are differences in stress tolerance between people. Some people tolerate high levels of stress without disease, while others have disease with even a little stress. That is, two people, under the same amount of stress, react differently. One may thrive while the other develops disease. Why is each person's response to stress so unique?

These questions suggest that the stress of life causes a single, whole-body effect. This whole-body effect disrupts Self-Referral, destroys health, and creates disease. We know the brain coordinates the body's normal functions. By examining the relationship between stress, brain, and body we may find answers to these key questions.

The Brain-Stress Connection

The brain plays a critical role in Self-Referral. As a thermostat regulates the furnace to heat a room, the brain regulates the body to promote health. Feedback loops are the mechanisms of Self-Referral.

Feedback loops, working through the nervous system, supply the brain with the moment-to-moment status of the body. The brain compares the body's current status with set-points that maintain health; then the brain sends orders to the body, creating ideal conditions - maintaining health. This is how brain and body interact, creating health through Self-Referral.[309] What do we know about brain disorders caused by stress? Can these disorders disrupt Self-Referral?

Depression is a common mood disorder. Depressed people feel listless, low on energy, and emotionally blue. Patients with depression often have severe sleep disturbance such as waking up in early morning hours and being unable to go back to sleep. Over time these people become more and more sleep deprived and their mental functions – mediated by the brain – become more and more abnormal.

Depression disrupts people's lives and can lead to poor judgment, deteriorating interpersonal relationships, poor job performance, and even suicide.[310] But does stress play a role in causing depression? Research proves the stress of life can cause severe depression[311] through creating extreme fatigue of the brain. The result is abnormal brain function, and the symptoms we call depression.[312]

How real is stress-related depression? What about people in high stress jobs that require them to make life or death decisions? An article in *Emergency Medical News* talked about stress-related depression in New York City Emergency Medical Technicians. These are the EMTs who respond with the ambulance when we call 911 for assistance.

Unbelievable stress is the EMT's daily life. Long shifts, life or death situations, and lack of emotional support cause tremendous stress. Does all this stress affect the EMTs? Three EMTs committed suicide in one year recently. Experts believe this was a direct result of job stress.[313] Depression itself is also a major health threat: research proves that people who suffer from depression have an increased risk of heart attack and death.[314]

Physicians experience a lot of stress in their work. The more stressful the medical work, the more likely depression will be a problem for the doctor. For example, patients with cancer are very ill and require more care. They often have a difficult time recovering from illness and often get worse. This is why doctors who treat cancer patients suffer high levels of stress and may suffer depression.[315]

What happens to people who suffer severe stress and depression? The additional mental and emotional pressure from stressful life events overworks the brain. Nearly everyone experiences this when we have a stressful day at work. After such a day, we feel drained of energy, listless, and more negative in our outlook. Most people throw off the effects of stress through sleep and recreational activities. But if stress keeps coming hard and often enough, many people will become depressed.

Is depression just a fleeting emotion or a physical reality? Scientists found they can measure physical effects of depression. Stress-induced depression disrupts the brain's electrical activity. This is so pronounced that doctors can distinguish depressed from normal patients by brain wave pattern alone.[316] Depressed patients also have abnormally high levels of cortisol – one of the main stress chemicals - in their urine.[317] This unique biochemical change is a clear indicator of stress.[318]

Earlier medications like amitriptyline (Elavil) normalize the brain's chemical imbalance and improve depression.[319] Later drugs like fluoxetine (Prozac), sertraline (Zoloft), and duloxetine (Cymbalta) also treat depression by improving the brain's chemistry.[320] Each drug works a little differently, but they all restore normal brain function by correcting stress-induced chemical imbalances. Like the many cardiovascular drugs, these medications correct the effects of stress.

There are indications that stress – in addition to affecting the brain - also causes disease elsewhere in the body. We know that stress causes depression; we also know that stress causes ulcers. As with different types of cardiovascular disease, there is a stress link that connects treatment of depression and ulcers.

The antidepressant drug amitriptyline (Elavil) reduces excess stomach acid at the same time it treats depression.[321] The H-2 Blockers cimetidine (Tagamet) and ranitidine (Zantac), designed to reduce stomach acid, also affect brain chemistry, and improve depression.[322] This proves a link between stress, abnormal brain chemistry, depression, and excess acid problems like ulcers and acid reflux disease.[323]

Another example relating stress, depression, and other disorders is asthma. The lung's bronchi - lined with muscular tissue - sometimes go into spasm, much like vasospasm in the arteries. This bronchospasm causes the wheezing of asthma and can lead to serious breathing problems or death. Depression and asthma often occur together - another link between depression and another stress related disease. This is another clue that stress lies behind many apparently unrelated disorders.[324]

Yet another link between stress, depression and disease is that of the ACE Inhibitor drugs. These medications help those with heart failure and high blood pressure. We now know these drugs also improve depression.[325]

We clearly see how stress causes depression - and depression in turn is linked with many other stress related diseases. The interruption of Self-Referral thus causes the apparently unrelated disorders of vasospasm, bronchospasm, and bowel spasm. This is how we can trace the true origin of heart disease, hypertension, asthma, most G.I. disease, and depression to the effects of stress.[326] What other brain disorders are linked to stress?

Beyond Depression

Anxiety is another brain disorder caused by stress.[327] Nearly the opposite of depression, anxiety causes extreme nervousness and can be paralyzing. People can be so overcome with anxiety that they cannot think, move, or act. Anxiety, like depression, causes abnormal brain waves. These EEG changes indicate abnormal brain function.[328]

Researchers link anxiety with many symptoms all over the body. These include irritable bowel syndrome - cramps and spasm of the muscular intestines. The mechanism for this bowel spasm is identical to vasospasm and bronchospasm. Anxiety also is linked to excess stomach acid.[329] Effects of anxiety are, in this fashion, very similar to depression.

Like depression, anxiety can ruin people's lives: its many symptoms can be very troublesome. Doctors treat anxiety with medications like lorazepam (Ativan) and similar drugs that also treat depression - like escitalopram (Lexapro) and buspirone (BuSpar).[330] These drugs reverse stress related brain imbalances and, like amitriptyline (Elavil), reverse abnormal brain chemistry.[331]

Depression and anxiety are common disorders. Patients with these problems are difficult to treat because they have seemingly unrelated symptoms. This is why doctors see them as problem patients. There is more to this story, however. The evidence shows that stress causes the so-called mental problems of depression and anxiety. Stress also causes the many so-called physical problems all over the body. This is why patients with either anxiety or depression have many medical complaints. Is it any wonder that doctors and patients alike find the situation confusing?

The brain connects with all the body's organ systems through nerves. When stress causes abnormal brain function, Self-Referral suffers. The brain likely is getting inaccurate information about body status due to chaotic operations. This is why the brain cannot regulate the body to create health through Self-Referral.

Instead, the brain sends out faulty and erroneous commands to the body and creates disease. This is how the central brain-stress connection distributes stress effects throughout the body as disease.

Common emotional stress provokes angina pectoris and silent ischemia.[332],[333] Everyday stress also causes anxiety and depression – which often predicts high blood pressure or even heart attack.[334] While everyone experiences stress, most people do not develop anxiety, depression, or heart attack. Why do some people fall prey to anxiety, depression - or even sudden death?

The Brain, Stress, and Experience

Why do some people become depressed? Why do others suffer anxiety? Does the stress of life cause these illnesses? Evidence suggests that stressful life events provoke these brain disorders. Are there known stress related diseases that illustrate this? The best example is Post-Traumatic Stress Disorder, also known as PTSD.

Post-Traumatic Stress Disorder is a disturbing mental condition first noticed in war veterans.[335] People with PTSD have profound anxiety and depression. PTSD patients report disturbing mental replays of wartime experiences. These vivid, dreamlike replays occur during sleep as nightmares and while awake as daydreams. These replays can be severely upsetting, and often interfere with job duties and family life.[336] There is a strong link between the stressful life events experienced in war and PTSD.[337]

War veterans are not the only people who suffer from PTSD.[338] Many people suffer PTSD following violent, shocking events such as terrible auto accidents, severe injuries, or torture. The common element in all cases of PTSD is a traumatic experience that overwhelms the person's ability to cope.[339] PTSD patients uniformly suffer emotionally disabling stress. Memories of these terrifying events haunt the PTSD patient day and night.

For example, a 19-year-old woman was driving an automobile on slippery pavement. She approached a curve in the road and the brakes failed. Her car slid out of control, overturning several times. The accident severed the woman's left arm just below the shoulder joint. Surgeons reattached the arm and it healed well. The woman's physical recovery was good. However, she developed a severe mental problem: she suffered from Post-Traumatic Stress Disorder.[340]

Soon after the accident, she described waking flashback experiences. She vividly relived the accident, time after time. She feared sleep because of recurrent nightmares that replayed the accident. She was reluctant to take part in physical therapy for fear the arm would fall off. She described brief periods of unreality during which she felt her arm would detach and wave good-bye to her. Through counseling and the passage of time, the woman overcame her PTSD symptoms. She eventually regained her physical and mental health and led a happy life.[341]

Abused children are now being diagnosed as suffering from PTSD. Experts estimate that 40 million Americans may have been abused as children. Today, that translates to about 2 million children every year. These children, like the woman in the auto accident, were never near a war. Nevertheless, the high stress experiences they lived through caused the same PTSD problems as war veterans.[342]

Engrams: The Building Blocks of Memory

What causes Post-Traumatic Stress Disorder? To understand PTSD, we must examine how the brain stores experiences as memory. Scientists are only beginning to understand how memory works. Why do we remember some things and forget others? Why do some memories provoke PTSD and others are harmless?

We do not remember every detail of the world around us. If we did, sensory overload would quickly disable our brains. There are just too many details in experience and the environment to maintain normal thought. The brain automatically retains some memories and forgets others. The brain protects itself - by reflex - from being overwhelmed by experience.[343,344]

The average person stores about 1% of available information as memory. That includes sensory input like odors, taste, sound, visual information, and tactile sensations.[345] Exactly how does the brain remember?

We can understand memory through the action of brain cells, or neurons. Information from the senses triggers neurons, and those neurons send impulses to many other neurons. Scientists call this sequential firing of neurons *reverberating excitation.* Many neurons firing together in this process create a stronger effect than a few neurons firing alone. This intense group firing of neurons is how the brain processes sensory input from the outside world.[346]

The brain is virtually a mass of nerve cells that form pathways in all directions. Any reverberating excitation will cause a group of neurons to fire. These firing neurons form a pattern in three-dimensional space. This is how the brain processes sight, smell, sound, taste, and touch into patterns of firing neurons. Scientists call this pattern an *engram.* The engram is the building block of memory.[347]

When we remember something, the brain works like a computer. A computer electronically stores information for later reference. Each piece of information has a unique pattern. When we request information, the computer searches for the pattern. Once found, the computer retrieves the information.[348] *The engram is the brain's storage pattern.* When we try to remember, the brain searches engram patterns. Once the brain finds the pattern, it remembers. The engram fires - and the memory returns.[349]

Memory often works as a reflex. For example, we may drive half an hour to work but remember little of the trip. We stopped at red lights and navigated traffic but remember nothing of it. Did we do anything wrong? No, this is an example of memory as a reflex. Our brain's memory of many drives to work served as an automatic pilot. This is how memory as a reflex serves us well throughout our lives.

Once the brain stores an experience as an engram, similar sensory input will stimulate that engram - and we experience the memory. For example, odors are strong stimulators of memory. To test this, find a baseball glove. Close your eyes and inhale the odor. If you played baseball as a youngster, memories will flood into your mind about baseball and related experiences. The same is true for the other senses; this is how sensory input stimulates a memory.

An average person will store many millions of engrams in a lifetime.[350] With that many engrams to coordinate, normal memory function is nothing short of amazing. How does the brain coordinate memory? I point out the Self-Referral quality of memory function. We may remember by choice or by reflex, but the mechanism is the same. The brain refers to itself. If it finds a matching engram, we remember; we cannot remember if we cannot find a match.

Stress Syndrome and Engrams

If ordinary life events create engrams, stressful life events must create even stronger engrams. Since memory often works as a reflex, *stressful life events* create *stressful engrams*. Stressful engrams cause exaggerated and delayed stress response. The way Post-Traumatic Stress Disorder works supports this idea. When we refer to a vivid memory, we say that "it made a strong impression on me." This saying is virtually true when we understand engram formation.

Some stressful life events are extremely disturbing. These often-horrible events create equally unpleasant engrams. Can such experiences cause physical damage to the body?

We know life-threatening experiences can destroy heart muscle. How does this happen? The stress response begins in the brain as it reacts to a strongly stressful event. Overcome by extreme stress, the brain creates an extremely powerful stress response. That causes a sudden outpouring of stress chemicals – creating lethal catastrophic damage to the heart. In such a situation, the brain is just as vulnerable as the heart to damage of this kind.

This explains how all interruptions of Self-Referral affect us so strongly. As people live their lives, stressful life events gradually disrupt Self-Referral. Depending on the severity of the experiences, stress may have major or minor effects. Disruption may only affect the brain – but stress also can affect any part of the body. This is how Stress Syndrome disrupts feedback loops; as mechanisms of Self-Referral break down, disease or even death will result.

Stress Syndrome is the most elementary mechanism for disrupting Self-Referral.[351] This is the fundamental mechanism of disease distribution in response to stress overload. In Stress Syndrome the brain acts as primary mediator between stress and the body. When stress overwhelms us, body damage will surely follow. Sometimes the brain takes the damage - but the brain can pass on the stress to any part of the body.

Stress Syndrome thus explains both disease and the aging process. This is how the body loses health and gains disease – or we say we just get older. The body collapses over a lifespan of ninety some years like a blimp with a slow leak. Occasionally, the blimp may catch fire and go down quickly, as in a heart attack or a stroke. If the aging process proceeds unchecked, it often is a slow but inexorable downhill ride.

The Brain: A Closer Look

We now see that the brain acts as the master coordinator of the body. On one hand, this is an internal relationship between brain and body. On the other hand, the brain also stands as the receiver of information – via the senses - from the outside world. That is a very complex arrangement; how does all this work?

Most people think of the brain as a featureless lump of gray tissue. It seems to carry out miraculous tasks in an unknown way. We often express this idea in slang, as in using our gray matter to solve a problem. How does this miraculous organ carry out its work? Much of the brain remains unknown, but science continues to discover more.

The brain appears to be a solid object - but it is far from solid. It is actually a concentrated mass of nerve cells, or neurons. The human brain weighs about three pounds,[352] but it contains about 90 billion neurons.[353] Billions of neurons form trillions of neuronal pathways. These allow communication and control between brain and body. These are a critical part of the millions of feedback loops that make Self-Referral possible.

When we look at the brain closely, it resembles a long tube repeatedly folded over itself. That is exactly what it is. A human being in the womb begins as a collection of cells. Soon the cells organize to form one long tube. During the fourth month of pregnancy, this tube begins to change. The tube folds and loops over itself. It eventually forms the brain and spinal cord - a thick bundle of neuronal pathways.[354]

By the time a baby is born, the brain is fully formed. The spinal cord and various nerves connect the brain with the rest of the body. The spinal cord has large nerves branching from it – much like the branches of a tree. These are the spinal nerves, and they connect the spine with the rest of the body. There also are nerves that connect brain and body directly; these are the cranial nerves.[355] The cranial and spinal nerves are the main conduits of Self-Referral between brain and body.

To live in the world, we must interact with it. An important source of information to the brain are the five senses: sight, sound, smell, taste, and touch. Each of these senses brings information to the brain from the external world - through their own channels of neurons. These channels connect with various parts of the brain that process sensory data. From there, sensory information is collated in the brain's cerebral cortex. The brain, working with the engrams of memory and dynamic information processing – works to construct what we call reality.[356]

When we talk about stressful life events, we refer to the brain interacting with the external environment. When we talk about stress effects in the body, we describe interaction between the brain and body. An important question is: how does the brain interact with the environment – while also interacting with the body as a whole?

The brain-body side of Self-Referral is completely internal and automatic. We cannot consciously regulate heart rate, breathing, and the like. The brain dynamically optimizes these body functions. Nevertheless, these functions are somehow disrupted by stressful life events - that disrupt Self-Referral. How are the automatic functions of the body affected by stressful life events?

The brain constantly sorts through incoming information from the external world. In a single moment our brain processes the fact that it is daytime, we are driving our car, and we have fifteen minutes to get to work. We know it takes us about five minutes to get there from where we are now. All of this is smooth and going according to schedule – and there is no stress.

But what happens if traffic gets thick, and suddenly we can't keep up the pace as expected? We may become stuck in traffic – and it could make us half an hour late for work. That's when we clearly experience stress – from the frustration of needing to get to work on time and being unable to move through traffic as expected.

Sensory data coming into the brain is objective, but the brain's evaluation of the data comes into play here. Understanding the change from driving on time to suddenly becoming late requires what we call thinking. The brain analyzes the data and understands what it means. The brain realizes that changing conditions may make us late for work and identifies this as a problem. The stress response results.

The brain connects with the whole body and governs the body's internal environment. That is why the stress response to being late for work kicks in; the brain understands a problem exists, and this triggers the fight or flight response. That is how external events in the world impact the brain - and the brain responds to what goes on in the external world by preparing for action.

The Brain is the Self-Referral Center

Since the brain acts in such a profoundly powerful way, we must designate the brain itself as the body's *Self-Referral Center*. This is because the brain alone has the ability to keep order among the body's many parts. The brain knows what is going on everywhere in the body – via the myriad feedback loops - and dynamically responds to changing conditions to create health and prevent disease.

However, stressful life events impact all these functions via the brain as the Self-Referral Center. In fact, the pernicious effects of stress on the body prove that this is so. The brain, as the body's Self-Referral Center, experiences stress. If the stress input is powerful or repetitive, it will cause Stress Syndrome. This is what disrupts Self-Referral. Stressful life events impact the Self-Referral Center, and the brain passes the chaos on to the rest of the body - causing aging, disease, or death.

All this is a great theory, but is it consistent with known medical facts? The cerebral cortex is the superficial tissue of the brain most involved with thinking and memory. We know it is intimately related to various parts of the body through studying people with brain disease. Scientists found that the cerebral cortex controls various parts of the body.[357]

The brain as Self-Referral Center processes all sensory input coming into the body – and it sends all orders out to the body. We rely on this critical feedback loop of Self-Referral constantly. Breakdown of this feedback loop seriously interferes with normal life.

We rely on close coordination between the brain as Self-Referral Center and the body for everything we experience and do. When we drink a glass of water or walk down the street, we see the constant flow of feedback loops with the brain as the Self-Referral Center.

The Self-Referral Center also is at work when we engage in complex actions. Once learned, we never think about riding a bicycle or playing the piano – we just do it. Self-Referral is the silent, underlying mechanism that makes all this possible. We know that stress disrupts all this effortless brain function. What goes wrong with the brain's Self-Referral Center when stressful life events overcome it?

The Brain, Stress and Memory

Doctors have documented many cases of Post-Traumatic Stress Disorder, but exactly what causes it? How do stressful life events trigger the stress response long after their occurrence? What is the process that lies behind PTSD?

Stressful life events cause Stress Syndrome. When this process creates *stressful engrams*, it essentially creates *stored stress*. These stressful engrams, if triggered, cause the original events to replay – along with the negative body problems that came with it. This is why Stress Syndrome continues to trigger stress, long after the original events that formed the engram. This exactly explains how PTSD causes ongoing problems long after the original stressful life events. Scientists believe this is what triggers and drives Post-Traumatic Stress Disorder.

As we discussed before, engrams are patterns of memory caused by many neurons firing at once. The stronger the experience, the more neurons fire - and the more powerful the engram that forms. Scientists believe the brain stores memory engrams in two areas: the amygdala and the hippocampus. Both areas lie deep inside the brain, and both interact with the cerebral cortex.[358] Scientists thus suggest that the cerebral cortex is the coordinator of memory.[359] How does the brain carry out this coordination?

The cerebral cortex processes experience. For example: one experience provokes strong emotional reaction, like fear of a dangerous animal. The brain stores that memory in the amygdala. Another experience is spatial - say, learning the layout of your house. Our brain stores that memory in the hippocampus.[360]

Research with monkeys proves these facts. When scientists remove the amygdala from monkeys, they no longer react with fear when confronted by previously known predators. Monkeys without their hippocampus cannot remember how to get around in their previously well-known cage. Scientists believe our brains work the same way.[361]

Experiments with rats show that stress affects memory. Rats injected with adrenaline, a key stress chemical, are much more likely to remember and avoid a shock wire in a maze than normal rats. Scientists believe that adrenaline heightens the impact of experience.[362] We know that stress causes high adrenaline blood levels in humans. Could stress caused by strongly unpleasant experiences work the same way with humans as it does in rats?

PTSD: A Closer Look

In his fascinating book *The Brain*, Dr. Richard Restak describes how stress affected a young English electrical engineer named Terry Boucher. Boucher enjoyed parachute jumping as a hobby. When Boucher made his first jump, his parachute opened as planned and all was going well. Then he got conflicting instructions from people on the ground. He panicked, opened his reserve parachute, and the wind blew him off course into an airport building. Fortunately, he only suffered a few scratches and a bruised ego. After he was back on the ground,

> Boucher was at first calm. Then he described his experience to bystanders. He quickly became visibly upset. Boucher talked animatedly as his pulse raced at 170 beats per minute. He relived the stressful experience, even though he was safe on the ground.[363]

This is how stressful life experiences literally make a strong impression on us. Whether by losing an arm in a car accident, being traumatized by childhood abuse, or experiencing the horrible events of warfare – the result is the same. Adrenaline-enhanced engrams leave their mark. We are left with lasting effects mediated by the brain, interfering with Self-Referral on some level.

That is why many veterans report delayed stress response, even years after wartime events. Fred Gusman is a clinical social worker. He works in a Veterans Administration treatment center for Post-Traumatic Stress Disorder in Menlo Park, California. One former soldier told Gusman that he could not tolerate holding his wife's hand while shopping. "If something goes wrong," he explained, "I need to feel free to react." Though the war was over many years previously, this veteran was still reacting to stress engrams caused by the war.[364] How is it that the events of experience – a close shave in a parachute or wartime experiences – end up causing such problems for people? How exactly does this occur?

We know the cerebral cortex is the coordinator of memory. We also know that PTSD affects the brain as the Self-Referral Center. We have thoroughly examined the connection between stressful life events and disease; let's specifically look at the PTSD process in more detail.

The Brain as a Computer

A clear way to understand how intense mental stress causes PTSD is to compare how the brain works with the operations of a computer. The physical computer itself is the hardware. That includes the CPU, circuit boards, memory chips, video monitor, keyboard, mouse, and storage devices.[365]

To be useful, the computer depends on programs - coded sets of instructions that tell the hardware what to do. Programs put words and pictures on the screen and allow data entry from the keyboard. Programs calculate, store, and retrieve information. We call programs as a whole software.[366] Software runs inside the computer's hardware and is regarded as separate from the hardware.

Scientists often use the computer as a model to understand the human brain. They describe the brain's physical structure as the hardware. Thoughts, memories, emotions, and similar mental processes are the software. The brain is seen as an organic machine within which the software functions.[367]

Let's use computer operations to better understand the brain. We may run a computer program to find a list of people named Baker. The computer follows our program and searches a large data base. Finding people named Baker, the computer ignores other names – and produces a list of people named Baker – which we can examine and use as needed.

Human thinking works the same way. For example, we make a shopping list for the grocery store. Then we drive to the store, get a shopping cart, and move up and down the aisles. Ignoring items that we don't need, we put what we want in the cart. We confirm choices by referring to our list. In this sense, brain operations are very much like computer operations.

Since we know that stressful life events cause disease, we might wonder about the mental aspects of this phenomenon. Nearly everyone has some stressful life events, and they are mentally disturbing at a deep level. We might ask: how can thoughts - or software - damage the hardware? How can something as fleeting and temporary as a thought damage flesh and blood?

The Brain Crashes

Let's reexamine the computer. How can software - mere electrical impulses dancing inside circuits - damage hardware made of metal and silicon? The answer is: all computers depend on a delicate system of electronic checks and balances. Conflicting instructions destroy this delicate balance. This causes an electronic lockup, called a system crash.

When a computer crashes, the monitor screen freezes, goes black, or fills up with random figures. A crashed computer will not respond to keyboard control. The only solution is to turn the computer off and start over. This can ruin hours or even days of work.[368]

When a computer program crashes, it can damage the hardware. For example, a storage device is writing data and the program locks up. The storage device loses control, writing meaningless garbage to itself. This can ruin the storage device by making it unreadable.[369]

Researchers now believe Post-Traumatic Stress Disorder works the same way. Intensely stressful life events like war experiences, robbery at gunpoint, or violent injuries overwhelm the brain. The victim's thoughts spin out of control, overcome by events. Like the out-of-control storage device, the brain strongly imprints harmful memories during those adrenalin-enhanced events. This is how thought - the brain's software - damages the hardware: the brain itself.[370]

This is an interesting idea, but does it relate to known facts? Let's examine stroke, a well-known example of brain damage. Can we connect stressful life events and stroke?

Stress, Stroke, and Aging

A stroke occurs when the brain is cut off from oxygen long enough to cause tissue death. The time required is about four minutes. When a stroke occurs, the damage reflects what part of the brain is affected. One stroke victim cannot read a book. Another cannot move an arm, a leg, or both. Others cannot speak clearly. Still others lose control of their urine or bowel functions.

The stroke is a truly catastrophic event that often kills the patient or leaves them disabled to some extent[371].

What causes a stroke? A stroke results from a blood clot, gradual hardening of the arteries, high blood pressure, or vasospasm.[372] Stroke typically affects the brain – the body's Self-Referral Center. Is there a connection between Stress Syndrome – repetitive firing of stored stress engrams – and stroke?

Stressful life events, especially those involving strong emotions, contribute heavily to stroke. The cerebral cortex is the processor of memory. When strong stressful life events occur, the brain stores adrenaline-enhanced memories as engrams. Over time, such engrams become more numerous and overlap. At some point, one more stressful life event occurs – whether real or replayed via adrenaline-enhanced engram – and the brain as the Self-Referral Center spins out of control. Like the storage device in a computer crash, the brain creates physiologic chaos. This is the basis of stroke, and this is how mental events can cause physical damage to the body.

Short of a stroke, can this mechanism still cause ongoing brain damage? We have discussed the idea of mini-infarcts. These are small areas of tissue that may be killed off by fleeting vasospasm anywhere in the body. As the brain operates as the Self-Referral Center, it distributes the effects of stress to anywhere in the body – including the brain itself.

Such progressive microscopic brain damage is likely to be the basis of the aging process. Little by little, the stress of life strains the brain. Microscopic bits of tissue become damaged by mini-infarcts. This can happen at the brain level and anywhere else in the body. *This is what we call the aging process.*

PTSD Proves Stress Causes Brain Changes

Adrenaline enhanced memories are the cause of Post-Traumatic Stress Disorder, creating *stored stress* as *severely stressful engrams*. These stressful engrams are so strong that they replay themselves at any time, causing the disturbing symptoms of PTSD. This again demonstrates the link between mental events and subsequent brain dysfunction. This is how memories of strong stressful life events cause PTSD, even years after traumatic experiences.

To illustrate, many PTSD victims suffer sleeplessness, headache, and a disturbing restlessness. Veterans Administration psychologist Erwin Parson recalls treating a six-year-old boy with PTSD. The boy had watched his father fatally stab his mother. Parson remembers the boy as hopelessly restless:

> He kept jumping up and down, rattling drawers. I would bribe him with cookies to sit still for ten minutes. One day, after a year and a half of therapy, the youngster told Parson: "When I sit, I get too sad."

Parson suddenly understood. The constant movement was the boy's way of managing delayed stress. He was having the same symptoms as combat veterans. No one in 1975 had a name for Post-Traumatic Stress Disorder, but this boy had it.[373]

Few stressful life events are worse than a child watching his father brutally murder his mother. The boy suffered severe stress response during the incident. Witnessing the murder caused an adrenaline-driven system crash of the brain, resulting in abnormally strong, upsetting memories. Subsequent replay of these stressful engrams caused the boy's later behavior problems. This phenomenon has commonly been found in children exposed to violent event trauma.[374]

Can stressful life events cause brain damage as I have suggested? Dr. Lawrence C. Kolb has advanced such a theory. Dr. Kolb works with PTSD patients at the Veterans Administration Hospital in Albany, New York. In 1986 he suggested that stress causes changes in the cerebral cortex. These changes in turn cause PTSD.

> Adrenaline enhanced memories result from strong stressful life experiences, like those in wartime. Dr. Kolb says that these changes cause impaired coordination of the cerebral cortex with other parts of the brain.[375]

So far, we have focused on the brain's cerebral cortex. Stress affects the entire brain as the Self-Referral Center. It also can damage any other part of the brain or – through the brain – any part of the body. Every interference with Self-Referral, no matter how small, will have a domino effect. Damage collects over time, like sand in an hourglass, until disease becomes obvious.

This explains disease – but it also explains the aging process. Aging is a direct result of mini-infarcts caused by the stress of life. We may never develop an obvious disease or illness; we may never even need a doctor or a hospital. Nevertheless - most people notice, as the years go by, we are older than we used to be. *Aging is a result of progressive disruption of Self-Referral.*

Is there proof of these ideas? Studies found increased levels of stress chemicals in the urine of combat veterans. The higher these chemical levels were, the worse the PTSD problems.[376] Scientists also found a clear association between PTSD and dementia: combat veterans with PTSD were studied over time. These soldiers were *200% more likely to suffer dementia in older age*. These are strong indications that *stressful life events impact the brain, causing PTSD – and these long-term effects connect to early dementia.*[377]

Seeking a Stress Remedy

With a clearer understanding of the negative effects of stress, what can we do about the stress of modern life? Some people advocate abandoning modern life altogether. This is undesirable because we rely on technology for our high standard of living. Does anyone really want to give up antibiotics, phone communications, the Internet, or automobiles?

In this brave new world, where more is different and less remains the same, we do not need a retreat from reality. The crises our world faces requires as many healthy people as possible. *Humans desperately need a practical way to improve their ability to cope with stress.*

How can we restore Self-Referral? What are we looking for when we try to cope with stress? Today's medical approach primarily uses drugs to control feedback loops. This often improves symptoms but fails to solve the underlying problem.

We must somehow immunize people against the accelerated stress of modern life.

Many today point out the side effects of prescription drugs. The medicines save lives, but they all have side effects. If medication corrects a feedback loop, isn't that the end of the problem?

All drugs correct a specific bit of disharmony, but the body is designed to work as a unit. When we correct one problem, other problems result. Say we use a Beta Blocker to control fast heart rate – but Beta Blockers can cause weakness that interferes with exercise. They also can cause asthma, depression, and impotence.[378] Nearly every prescription drug has negative side effects we must avoid - even though the drug saves our life.

No Self-Referral feedback loop operates by itself; rather, it is part of the vast and complex physiology. That is, you can't change one feedback loop without accidentally interfering with many other feedback loops. This is why drug intervention in the body's complex system is so difficult. *This is a clear indication of the genius of researchers in the pharmaceutical indus*try; *getting any medication to do one thing to remedy a health problem while leaving the rest of the physiology alone is an amazing feat.*

Restoring Self-Referral

When we seek *Self-Referral/Maximum Health*, we look for ways to restore the body's harmony. Restoring Self-Referral is the opposite of tinkering with feedback loops. If we fail to create whole body harmony, disharmony results – in spite of our best efforts.

Today's prescription drugs correct symptoms but do little to restore whole body harmony. This sounds paradoxical, but do not be surprised. When we seek Self-Referral, we must often blend logic with art, and science with expanded perceptions. Lao-Tzu comments:

> Governing a large country is like frying a small fish. You spoil it with too much poking. Center your country in the Tao and evil will have no power. Not that it isn't there, but you'll be able to step out of its way. Give evil nothing to oppose and it will disappear by itself.[379]

When we view the body from the perspective of a single cell, the body is a large country indeed. Doctors cause more problems than they solve if they are too quick to prescribe strong drugs. Patients destroy their own health when they insist on drugs for minor but irritating symptoms. It is better to take as few prescription drugs as possible to avoid side effects.

We are missing something, however, if we only focus on avoiding unneeded medications. How can we center our bodies in Self-Referral so disease will have no power? Remembering the Tao of the warrior, let's review what we have learned about stress.

The stress response is a natural feedback loop that responds to stressful life events. It is logical that the opposite is true. *The body must have some mechanism to counteract stress. We must find an anti-stress feedback loop to counteract the stress of modern life.*

Finding an anti-stress feedback loop could solve the Adaptation Crisis. Locating the body's anti-stress switch should be helpful, but we must be careful. We know there are a myriad of feedback loops. Reckless tinkering with the anti-stress switch may cause more problems than it cures. People need a safe and effective way to promote Self-Referral. Can we find a way to promote total body harmony? Is it somehow possible to restore Self-Referral?

Chapter 8

Seeking a Stress Remedy

We know Stress Syndrome destroys Self-Referral and disrupts the body's feedback loops, creating disease instead of health. We must find a safe and effective remedy for the stress of life.

Self-Referral and Rest

Self-Referral is dynamic and responds instantly to changing conditions. It senses and changes our myriad body settings from moment to moment. Self-Referral is completely natural, requires no conscious effort, and operates day and night. We are seldom aware of Self-Referral at all - unless it stops working.

When stress disrupts Self-Referral, it causes disharmony. The range of problems caused by stress is formidable. The chaotic effects of stress can cause an unexpected illness, provoke a heart attack, or simply add to the aging process. Disrupted Self-Referral causes high blood pressure, dangerous heart rhythms, and many other disorders. The words disease, death and aging simply describe various specific interruptions of Self-Referral.

The stress of life often interrupts Self-Referral, but people are healthy most of their lives. The body must have a natural anti-stress feedback loop. If it did not, the constant stress of life would quickly overpower the body. How does the body recover from daily stress?

We know the demands of life cause stress. One way to avoid demands - and stress - is to separate yourself from activity. For example, anyone who stays up late inevitably feels the call of sleep. We spend six to eight hours sleeping and wake up refreshed. This is one way the body maintains balance between the opposites of sleep and wakefulness, between being alone and being with others. Lao-Tzu tells us in the *Tao te Ching*:

> Ordinary men hate solitude. But the Master makes use of it, embracing his aloneness, realizing he is one with the whole universe.[380]

This sounds more like the life of a monk than the life that modern people live. Is this aloneness something reserved only for saints in distant monasteries? Stress experts agree that modern people need inner peace and relief from stress. Everyone sleeps for a time during each 24-hour period. Is sleep enough to repair the damage caused by today's daily stress?

The Sleep Feedback Loop

The average adult spends about seven hours of every day sleeping. Some people require more sleep than others. Females generally require one more hour of sleep per day than males. This is why we spend nearly one-third of our lives sleeping.[381]

Sleep is unavoidable. When sleep is necessary, we sleep whether we want to or not. Why? We can only stay awake for so long, and the need for sleep overpowers us. When we fall asleep, we are unaware of our surroundings. What do we gain by these periods of forced dormancy?

Sleep, like Self-Referral, is a natural process and requires no conscious effort. The body automatically sets aside time for rest and repair through sleep. During sleep the body slows down many energy-consuming activities. This allows repair of the effects of stress.[382] Sleep restores a tired mind and body to a rested state - but how does this happen?

Sleep produces a whole-body state of rest.[383] During sleep, the autonomic nervous system relaxes: blood pressure drops, heart rate slows, and most muscles relax. Muscles in the stomach and intestines become more active, especially if food is present. The body's total energy use is called metabolism - and metabolism drops by 10 per cent during sleep.[384] This indicates that sleep causes the body's energy-consuming activities to drop substantially.

Sleeping also allows rest for the nervous system, notably the brain.[385] Since the brain constantly coordinates the body's functions, fatigue profoundly affects its efficiency. Sleep allows the brain to throw off the effects of fatigue. How does this occur?

We can compare the brain to early mechanical computers. These machines used vacuum tubes. These are the glass, filament-filled tubes used in radios before transistors, solid state electronics, and printed chips were invented.

Scientists found they could only use the computer's vacuum tubes for a short time. The tubes became unreliable because they developed electrical imbalances. Through trial and error, the scientists found a way to correct these imbalances: they turned the computers off at regular intervals. The tube imbalances disappeared - and the computers worked again. In a similar way, the brain turns itself off to recover from the stress of life.[386]

Sleep deprivation clearly shows the brain's need for sleep. Animals die within days if forced to stay awake - even when we give them adequate food, water, and shelter. Humans kept awake for long periods do not die, but they suffer unpleasant effects. Everyone knows the fatigue and sluggish thought that follows a long day's work. When we miss sleep for longer periods, the effects are more severe.

People forced to stay awake past 24 hours soon lose the ability to think clearly. Kept awake past 60 hours, people suffer fatigue, irritability, and poor concentration. Hallucinations involving the senses of sight and touch are common. Extreme lack of sleep can cause psychotic episodes: these are a complete break with reality. People suddenly go berserk, screaming and sobbing about unseen dangers.[387]

Doing without sleep causes stress as indicated by body chemistry changes. People suffering from sleep deprivation have increased blood levels of cortisol and epinephrine.[388] These stress chemicals interfere with brain function. This loss of brain efficiency disrupts Self-Referral. This is why sleep deprivation has a profoundly negative effect on the brain, nervous system, and the entire body.[389]

Self-Referral requires a rested brain and body. That is why the urge to sleep is so hard to fight. When we need sleep, we sleep to survive and wake up feeling rested. In Cybernetic terms, this is the Sleep Feedback Loop. The brain shuts down for sleep when it needs to recover from stress. Once rested, we wake up and life resumes.

Sleep Is Not Enough

Change in life causes stress, and every change we face forces our bodies to adapt to it. Change can be physical, like riding a bicycle - or it can be mental, like a timed arithmetic test. The more change we encounter, the harder our bodies work to adapt.[390] Why is this so?

Studies of deer, dogs, mice, and human beings prove that living things operate best within an adaptive range. There is a limit to how much change our bodies can accommodate. Beyond the adaptive range, our bodies begin to degenerate.[391] Aging, disease or death is the result.[392]

There are many indications that the stress of modern life pushes people *beyond their adaptive range*. Sleep reverses stress by forcing us to sleep part of every 24-hour day, but modern people often feel tired anyway. The reason is clear: our high-tech culture has outstripped the body's ability to cope with the onslaught of too-busy schedules and technology. Evidence is mounting that sleep alone does not provide enough rest for the stress of modern life.

The modern lifestyle seems deliberately designed to produce stress. Change is the common thread that connects the many sources of modern stress. People often change jobs due to hard economic times or for better pay or benefits. This causes them to move out of town, out of state, or even out of the country. When families move, they lose their home, family, friends, and familiar surroundings. They are thrust into unfamiliar territory filled with strangers. This kind of change is common today, and it pushes people beyond their adaptive range.[393]

Fragmentation of the family, caused in part by mobility pressures, has become critical. Divorce rates are well over 50% in many areas, producing many single parents. These struggling individuals must work and somehow provide parental care. The upbringing many children receive today concerns many experts on family issues as family pressures push people beyond their adaptive range.[394]

Technology itself makes often impossible demands. Radio, television, and video players create stress. Add to this smart phones, computers, and game devices and we have a constant barrage of sound, picture, and stimulation. The sights and sounds may be pleasant, but they force the body to adapt to busy surroundings. This constantly changing plugged-in electronic environment pushes people beyond their adaptive range.[395]

Inhumanly fast and efficient machines that were supposed to be our servants are now our masters. Driving cars demands split-second decisions. Office workers cope with computers, voice mail, Internet work, and texting. Factory workers cope with automation and keeping up with machines. Jangling phones interrupt us everywhere: movie theaters ban cell phone use on the premises - just so their patrons can enjoy the show without interruptions. All these changes, many of them irritating, push people beyond their adaptive range.[396]

These modern sources of stress converge to place unprecedented demands on the human body. Research shows that mental stress and physical stress are equally deadly.[397] We are adding to our own stress by our lifestyle choices. The cell phone or late-night movie may be fun - but they cause plenty of stress. This is how our own conveniences cause disease or even sudden death.[398]

The Search for Stress Relief

The work of Selye and others proves the deadly effects of stress. Stress causes disease, but what can we do about it? We must face reality - it is too late to turn back the clock. Technology may stress us, but we depend upon it daily. Few would put the genie back in the bottle and opt for a technology-free culture to avoid stress.

A better solution is to improve people's ability to cope with stress. *Can we improve the human body's ability to cope with change - and avoid the problems that stress causes? Answering this question effectively is critical to surviving the times in which we live.*

The search is now on to find better ways to cope with stress. Many offer stress reduction techniques designed to help people cope with modern life. We will examine the most used stress reduction techniques and evaluate their effectiveness. We will categorize these techniques as follows:

Behavior Modification

Biofeedback

Progressive Muscle Relaxation

Hypnosis

Isolation Tank

Meditation

Some of these techniques provide daily periods of rest that supplement sleep. Others work to change the way people think about stress. Still other techniques seek to change specific habits associated with stress and disease.

The differences between these techniques seem bewildering, but they are all different roads trying to reach the same destination. All have the same goal: they seek to reverse the stress-generating effects of modern life. We will now discuss each of these stress reduction techniques in more detail; surely one or more of these techniques will prove useful.

Behavioral Modification

Behavioral Modification is an educational process. People learn about stress and what behavior increases stress. Behavioral Modification instructors teach people to change their behavior to reduce stress. Once informed of dangerous habits, they assume, people will change their behavior for the better.[399] This sounds logical. If we can change stress producing behavior, it should reduce people's stress. Less stress should mean better health.

To illustrate, Type A people set vague, poorly defined goals. Making the situation worse, they impose unrealistic deadlines on themselves. Studies show that more heart attack victims have Type A behavior than the risk factors of smoking or being overweight.[400]

Behavioral Modification teaches Type A people that they promote their own heart attack with their behavior. It teaches better planning techniques such as setting clear goals and ways to better pace their work.[401] This is one way people can remove stress from their lives - and live longer.[402]

Behavioral Modification sounds useful, but does it work? Researchers studied 862 heart attack victims and found Type A behavior in almost 99% of the patients. The researchers trained 592 of these patients with Behavioral Modification. About 45% of the trained group reduced their Type A behavior because of the training.[403]

The researchers studied the same patients three years later. About 7% of the Behavioral Modification trained patients had suffered a second heart attack compared to 13.2% of the untrained patients. The trained patients thus cut the risk of a second heart attack nearly in half. These findings prove that Behavioral Modification works well with some patients.[404]

Scientists use Behavioral Modification to treat high blood pressure, although with less success.[405] Critics caution that Behavioral Modification is no substitute for medication.[406] Some studies confuse issues by combining Behavioral Modification with other stress reduction techniques. Such studies make it unclear which technique produced the results.[407]

Biofeedback

Biofeedback uses a mechanical device to help the brain work with the body.[408] For example, some people suffer headaches from tight forehead muscles. Scientists can treat these headaches with Biofeedback. They place a sensor on the patient's forehead and connect it to equipment that senses tight muscles. The equipment beeps when the muscles relax. No sound occurs when the muscles are tight.[409]

The patient sits quietly with the equipment in place, listening for the beep. The beep sounds when the forehead muscles relax. When the beep stops, the patient tries to make the beep sound again. Biofeedback theory assumes that patients learn to relax with repeated practice. This relaxes the tight forehead muscles. Scientists also believe that Biofeedback reverses the general effects of stress.[410]

Clinicians use Biofeedback to treat headache,[411] ringing of the ears,[412] insomnia,[413] the stress of cancer,[414] sexual problems,[415] asthma,[416] hypertension,[417] motion sickness,[418] athletic muscle training,[419] and spinal injury rehabilitation.[420] Biofeedback helps some problems[421] but is of questionable value in others.[422]

Progressive Muscle Relaxation

Progressive Muscle Relaxation (or PMR) uses conscious relaxation of muscles to provide whole body relaxation. The patient sits in a comfortable position and alternately tightens and relaxes various muscle groups of the body. A common pattern is to begin at the top of the head and work down the neck. Then attention shifts to the arms, trunk, legs, and ends with the feet.[423]

Progressive Muscle Relaxation works to produce a state of whole-body relaxation. Proponents believe that relaxing the muscles will benefit the whole body. Like Biofeedback, Progressive Muscle Relaxation theory assumes the patient will learn to relax. Progressive Muscle Relaxation thus reverses the general effects of stress.[424] Therapists use Progressive Muscle Relaxation to treat the general stress of life,[425] the stress of diabetes,[426] nausea from cancer chemotherapy,[427] migraine headache,[428] insomnia,[429] and hypertension.[430]

Hypnosis

Hypnosis requires a therapist to place the patient in a hypnotic trance. Working with the therapist, proponents believe the patient processes stressful life events while in the trance. As the patient comes out of the trance, the therapist gives a posthypnotic suggestion to relax. Therapists believe these suggestions reverse the effects of stress.[431]

For example, a patient might have Post-Traumatic Stress Disorder. The hypnotist puts the patient into a trance state. During the trance state, the therapist directs the patient to remember traumatic experiences. The patient better assimilates the experiences during Hypnosis. Before bringing the patient out of the trance, the therapist gives the patient a suggestion to relax.[432] Therapists use Hypnosis to treat many health problems. These include irritable bowel syndrome,[433] Post-Traumatic Stress Disorder,[434] stress related memory loss,[435] the stress of cancer pain,[436] asthma,[437] and the general stress of life.[438]

Isolation Tank

Isolation Tank technique uses withdrawal from the outside world to reduce stress. The equipment needed is formidable. Isolation Tank setups include a large tub enclosed by a metal cabinet. Therapists fill the tub with warm, salty water. Patients enter the cabinet and close the door. The cabinet provides an isolated environment because it is sound and light proof. Patients float face up in the water, experiencing silence.[439]

The Isolation Tank works to reverse the effects of stress with a comfortable, relaxing environment.[440] Like Progressive Muscle Relaxation, the Isolation Tank promotes whole body relaxation. Sessions may last from a few minutes to an hour or more. Therapists sometimes combine tank sessions with psychotherapy or other counseling.[441] Isolation Tank technique produces a state of generalized relaxation.[442] Advocates make wide reaching claims[443] of therapeutic benefit,[444] but the technique has received little scientific study.[445]

Meditation

Meditation describes a cluster of stress reduction techniques. While apparently very different, all types of Meditation are mental procedures that work toward whole body relaxation. Transcendental Meditation, or TM, is the most widely known type of Meditation.[446] Other forms of Meditation are Buddhist Meditation,[447] the

Relaxation Response,[448] Mindfulness,[449] and various schools of Yoga.[450]

Meditation techniques employ a specific mental procedure. This often involves the mental repetition of a sound, word, or phrase. Sitting in a comfortable position, the patient performs the mental technique. Meditation produces whole body relaxation. Advocates claim that Meditation reverses the effects of stress.[451]

Patients use Meditation techniques to treat hypertension,[452] the stress of work,[453] psychiatric illness,[454] drug abuse,[455] prevention of alcoholism,[456] insomnia,[457] asthma,[458] angina pectoris,[459] and the general stress of life.[460]

Which Stress Reduction Techniques Work?

Confusion reigns about how to treat stress. Everyone wants to be an expert about how to treat stress. The so-called "experts" often disagree and contradict one another. That is why even well-educated people are confused how to relieve stress and look for answers.

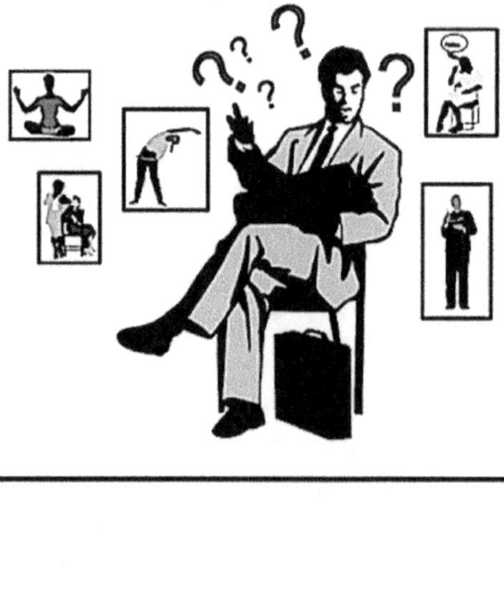

Stress Therapy: Confusion Reigns

Doctors and patients agree that stress is a major health problem. Awareness of stress is at an all-time high, but confusion abounds about how to treat it. What stress reduction techniques work? Which techniques are ineffective? Why does confusion reign in this key area of modern health?[461]

One reason for confusion is there are so many stress reduction techniques. Behavioral Modification, Biofeedback, Progressive Muscle Relaxation, Hypnosis, Isolation Tank, and Meditation are *broad types of techniques*. Each of these has hundreds of individual variations. Physicians and patients often cannot understand what is available. The confusion about which technique is better should not surprise us.[462]

Another reason for confusion is that physicians do not learn enough about stress in medical training. Doctors place medical practice squarely on the foundation of science. Confusion about stress reduction techniques causes many to dismiss them all as unreliable.

This is why medical educators teach little about what many consider a marginally scientific subject. Doctors in training thus learn that stress reduction techniques are useless. Their teachers often advise them simply to refer stressed patients to a psychiatrist or a lay therapist.

These training experiences foster negative doctor attitudes toward stressed patients. Doctors learn to view stressed patients as a nuisance. Adding to these negative attitudes, stressed patients are difficult to treat. They suffer many poorly defined symptoms and demand immediate care.

All this is emotionally draining to the doctor – and when busy physicians cannot find a treatable disease, they often give up in frustration. Doctors often dismiss these patients as hypochondriacs; the doctor prescribes a tranquilizer and moves on to the next patient.[463]

Finally, lack of information is not the only source of confusion about stress reduction techniques. Some people advance nonscientific - and sometimes nonsensical - objections to the techniques themselves. Critics base these objections on ideology (I doubt that can help anyone!), ego (I invented this technique, so it must be the best one!), greed (My clinic teaches this technique, and I will become rich!), and religion (This technique conflicts with religious beliefs.)

Stress Related Drug Abuse

Since doctors offer little relief, many seek stress relief through drugs and alcohol. To illustrate, the late Carrie Fisher was a well-known actor, author, and screenwriter. Most people know her as Princess Leia of the *Star Wars* movies. She also wrote two best-selling novels, *Postcards from the Edge* and *Surrender the Pink.* Her first novel became a successful movie.

Fisher shared her experiences with drugs and alcohol in a *Time* magazine profile. She long abused the prescription drug Percodan for stress-related emotional problems. "I wanted to blunt what was painful," she stated. She also ritually abused LSD, seeking "transcendent illumination."[464]

Fisher's expectations of stress relief and spiritual illumination ended in profound disappointment. "My idea was pain reduction and mind expansion," she admitted, "but I ended up with mind reduction and pain expansion." Learning that alcohol and drug abuse were poor antidotes to stress was a hard lesson: she had to have her stomach pumped to save her life. She later sought treatment and quit drugs.[465]

In my experience, Carrie Fisher's story is far from unique. Stress symptoms are absolutely rampant in most medical practices. This is why patients demand prescription drugs to relieve stress. People often go to the doctor's office to demand prescription medications - *by brand name*. This is not a result of advertising; the patients talk to their friends and often come in asking for what helped people they know – who have similar problems.

Most doctors resist this pressure, but some give in to patient demands. Many doctors cave in to rid themselves of endless visits and countless telephone calls from stressed patients. This is why drug abuse is not confined to mind-expanding experimenters or back-alley dealers. Some of the worst drug abuse occurs through misuse of the doctor's prescription pad.

Our Pill-Popping Society

Another cause of stress-related drug abuse is our pill-popping society. Television and radio advertisements dramatize complaints from heartburn to headache to back pain - all of which, incidentally, are long term effects of stress. Grimacing actors, whose feigned suffering often deserves an Oscar, always achieve perfect health in seconds - thanks to the advertised product. This is why people expect and demand a quick and easy chemical fix for any stress symptom, real or imagined.

Most people periodically need mild over-the-counter medications for minor problems - perhaps a cold or an upset stomach. Media advertisements, however, present an unbalanced view. This very effective propaganda teaches that drugs are a necessity in life. Today's drug culture is a direct result of this barrage of commercials. Most people assume that they must treat every symptom with medications, even if drugless remedies are available.

Patients who demand addictive drugs make me uncomfortable. These people come for their first appointment with no complaint other than a request for diet pills, tranquilizers, or narcotics. After reviewing their case, I politely explain that I do not prescribe such medications freely. Even then, I only prescribe them for a short time. Most of these patients leave and never come back.

Does this mean that doctors should withhold medicines from patients in need? No - patients with terminal cancer, spinal disc, or other terribly painful diseases should be medicated - aggressively, if necessary. People with severe psychiatric problems should get needed medicine to better cope with life. These patients should be under the care of a Psychiatrist or Pain Specialist who can better judge the need for addictive medications. Doctors should otherwise use addictive drugs as seldom as possible, and they should stop them entirely whenever feasible.

Unfortunately, the confusion of how to treat stress effectively leaves no other option than prescription medications. Don't bother examining your lifestyle, this approach implies. Don't live life at a saner pace. Take this pill instead.

During my college days in the 1970s, drug abusers sardonically called this “better living through chemistry.” Treatment of stress by excess medication strikes me as eerily like Aldous Huxley's *Brave New World.* In Huxley’s dystopic future, people are routinely overmedicated to keep them following orders. The rule of that nightmarish fictional society is to see that everyone stays in line, at any cost: “When the individual feels, the community reels.”[466] Are we seeing that today?

The obvious answer to this situation is a stress reduction technique that requires no drugs. This makes confusion about stress reduction techniques of more than academic interest. Millions of patients in all types of medical practice would benefit from such a technique.

Which Stress Reduction Techniques Work?

Ignoring the confusion, consider this: medical science has unraveled answers to many complex health problems. Great minds discovered insulin for diabetes, penicillin for infection, and the Beta Blockers for heart disease. Surely, we can focus the same level of intellectual commitment on stress reduction techniques.

Why is the question “which stress reduction techniques work?” so hard to answer? There are several reasons for this scientific quandary. One reason is that scientists disagree about the definition of stress reduction. Some claim that stress reduction only requires a subjective sense of peace and quiet.[467] Other researchers define success by specific brain wave changes.[468] Still others define success by muscle relaxation[469] or decreased oxygen consumption.[470]

Another reason for confusion in this area is the subjective nature of these techniques. How do we know whether a patient is meditating or sleeping? How can we compare floating in an isolation tank with an educational class on goal setting? With all this confusion, how can we know which stress reduction techniques work?

Finally, many studies combine two or more stress reduction techniques to produce a given result. These studies assume that if one technique is good, several will be better. This approach clouds which techniques produce results, and which are bogus. One such study combined Progressive Muscle Relaxation, Meditation, and Behavioral Modification to treat heart disease.[471] Another study combined Hypnosis, Biofeedback, and Progressive Muscle Relaxation to treat low back pain.[472] This is how many well-meaning studies obscure the issue as to which technique works best.[473]

Self-Referral

Maximum Health

The Glueck and Stroebel Study of Stress Reduction Techniques

REMEMBER: This is one of the first scientific studies to compare stress reduction techniques directly. This head-to-head study compares Biofeedback, Transcendental Meditation, Progressive Muscle Relaxation, and No Technique.

Biofeedback: Patients trained with Biofeedback machines that made an audible tone when the patient was in a relaxed state. The technique was to make the tone sound as often as possible. Patients practiced this for twenty minutes, twice a day.

Transcendental Meditation: Patients learned the TM technique. The technique consisted of mentally repeating a sound, or mantra, for 20 minutes without concentration or effort. Patients practiced this for twenty minutes, twice a day.

Progressive Muscle Relaxation: Patients learned to relax their muscles to produce a whole-body state of relaxation. The technique was to relax various muscles throughout the body. Patients practiced this for twenty minutes, twice a day.

Controls: These were patients with no stress reduction technique. The researchers matched these patients with those in the other groups for factors like age and sex. They were used for comparison purposes only.

Let's Go Head-to-Head

Finding a solution to these problems has been elusive. How can we compare these techniques? The best method would be a simultaneous, head-to-head comparison of several techniques. Dr. Bernard C. Glueck and Dr. Charles F. Stroebel carried out such a study. Without naming it as such, these authors alluded to Self-Referral. They described health as depending on the body's "sophisticated feedback mechanisms" and suggested that stress reduction techniques might reverse autonomic hyper-arousal and improve total health.[474]

These scientists were not content with theoretical poetry; they studied objective physiologic changes. Through examination of previous research, they found measurable indicators of stress. They used these stress indicators to directly compare several techniques at once. They studied psychiatric patients at the Institute for Living in Hartford, Connecticut[475] to evaluate Biofeedback, Transcendental Meditation, Progressive Muscle Relaxation, and No Technique.

The average patient stay was 5.5 months, so everyone had plenty of time to work with the techniques. Instructors carefully taught each patient to perform their technique correctly. Everyone had equal time for personal instruction and ample time to practice their technique. All patients attended group meetings to discuss their practice. The patients were evaluated before, during, and after instruction, with a final evaluation upon hospital discharge.[476] How did the groups compare?

The TM patients showed greater psychiatric improvement than those in the Biofeedback, Progressive Muscle Relaxation, and Control groups. This true head-to-head comparison proved TM to be superior to Biofeedback, Progressive Muscle Relaxation, and No Technique. The findings created quite a stir - why was this so?[477]

When something new works, people notice - it attracts attention. Conventional wisdom assumed that all three stress reduction techniques would work equally. They did not. Why did the TM group improve more than the Biofeedback and Progressive Muscle Relaxation groups?

What Is Different About TM?

Glueck and Stroebel wondered if TM could repair stress damaged feedback loops. They speculated that patients could reverse the long-term effects of stress.[478] The question was: how can we measure physical effects from subjective techniques? The investigators knew several well-known measures of stress and relaxation. They applied these measurements to people performing the various techniques. What were these measurements? How did they carry them out, and what did they mean?

One measure of relaxation is *Galvanic Skin Resistance, or GSR*. Scientists run a tiny electrical charge between two wires placed across the skin. The resistance the current meets in passing across the skin is the GSR. Perspiration on the skin is an indicator of stress. Water conducts electricity, so when sweat is present it decreases the GSR - indicating stress. The higher the GSR, the less perspiration is present – indicating relaxation.[479]

A second measure of relaxation is brain wave activity recorded by electroencephalogram or EEG.[480] Brain waves change during relaxation, and previous research found such changes when people practiced TM.[481] The researchers thus recorded EEG changes produced by all three techniques in the study.[482]

This study was a true head-to-head comparison of the physical effects of these techniques. Conventional wisdom predicted that all three techniques would produce the same effects. Was this the case? No - all the techniques produced subjective feelings of relaxation, but they did not produce the same physiological changes. What were the differences between these techniques?

TM produced a consistent increase in GSR, or skin resistance to electricity. This showed that TM produced deep relaxation. Patients learning TM produced this effect immediately, and consistently produced the same effect every TM session afterward. The Biofeedback and Progressive Muscle Relaxation patients were unable to produce consistent GSR changes at all.[483]

TM produced unique EEG changes. TM produced many Alpha brain waves in the more active half of the brain. Within minutes of starting TM, the other half of the brain showed the same Alpha pattern. As TM continued, Theta and Beta waves also appeared throughout the brain. Biofeedback and Progressive Muscle Relaxation produced little increase in Alpha waves, and that was only in the more active half of the brain. Neither Biofeedback nor Progressive Muscle Relaxation produced the other EEG changes seen in patients practicing TM.[484]

The TM patients had greater psychiatric improvement on hospital discharge than the Biofeedback and Progressive Muscle Relaxation patients. TM produced strong measurable body changes that proved deep rest. The Biofeedback and Progressive Muscle Relaxation techniques only produced a subjective sense of rest with few measurable body changes. We conclude that TM, by consistently producing deep rest verified by science, accounts for psychiatric improvement in the TM patients.

Practical Matters

The study's design made other comparisons possible. Glueck and Stroebel reported problems with the Biofeedback and Progressive Muscle Relaxation patients. Both patient groups initially had great enthusiasm for the techniques, but they later lost interest. The problems that arose were due to practical matters.[485]

Progressive Muscle Relaxation patients were enthusiastic for about three weeks following instruction. Then they lost interest and complained of poor subjective experiences. Many patients protested that the technique bored them. All had stopped the practice by the fourth week.[486]

Biofeedback patients learned minimal Alpha wave control, but only after 15 training sessions. They were unable to produce even those meager results without Biofeedback equipment. Many complained that uncertain results only added to their tension and anxiety. This was unfortunate, as Biofeedback's purpose was to reduce those symptoms.[487]

The TM patients, by contrast, consistently produced physiologic changes showing deep rest. Those results required no expensive and cumbersome equipment. TM patients gave uniformly positive reports of relief from stress. Finally, the TM patients showed more improvement upon hospital discharge.[488]

When comparing stress reduction techniques, practical matters become obvious. For example, Behavioral Modification is effective but does not produce distinctive physiological changes. The strength of an educational process lies in the knowledge gained. Once taught about stress producing behavior, most people will try to change and avoid the offending behavior. But when the educational process is over, it is over; it does not compare with a daily practice such as TM.

Biofeedback has major drawbacks as a stress reduction technique. It does not produce specific physiological changes like TM. What little effect it does produce relies on elaborate equipment. Few have access to such equipment - especially for so little benefit.

Hypnosis is also impractical as a routine stress reduction technique. While useful in seriously ill psychiatric patients, it requires hours of sessions with highly trained and expensive therapists. Most people cannot afford the time and money needed to have daily Hypnosis from a therapist.

The Isolation Tank also has major drawbacks as a stress reduction technique. This technique requires expensive equipment that occupies a great deal of space. It takes constant work to maintain water cleanliness and temperature. Isolation Tank also requires a lot of time - something that few busy people have. Finally, there has been little research done to find what - if any - measurable body effects Isolation Tank technique produces.

By contrast, Meditation - specifically Transcendental Meditation - is highly practical as a stress reduction technique. Patients quickly learn TM and it produces consistent stress reducing effects. TM demands no equipment, requires only twenty minutes twice a day, and needs no therapists past a brief initial course of instruction.

Meditation and Self-Referral

When we seek *Self-Referral/Maximum Health*, we look for ways to restore the body's ability to govern itself. Health is the natural result of the body's feedback loops - seamless mechanisms of Self-

Referral. Like a palace guard, these promoters of Self-Referral are always on patrol to maintain health. When disease intrudes, it is always because something disrupts Self-Referral.

We know about the negative health effects of modern life. The modern environment causes more stress than ever before. This is why stress related illness plagues people now more than ever. The resulting Adaptation Crisis is wreaking havoc on individuals, families, and - ultimately - on our whole civilization.

When we examine the many problems that humanity faces, answers often elude us. *We have found a vital answer with TM. This successful stress reduction technique may be the most important discovery of our time.* Bearing this in mind, let us reexamine Lao-Tzu's advice:

> Ordinary men hate solitude. But the Master makes use of it, embracing his aloneness, realizing he is one with the whole universe.[489]

Aloneness is not exclusive to lonely saints in distant monasteries. TM offers an opportunity for anyone to experience aloneness and heal the effects of stress. Taking twenty minutes twice a day does not seem too much to ask to improve our health - or even to save our lives.

When we consider the damage that modern life causes, sleep is no longer enough to combat the devastating ravages of stress. TM offers a unique option to blend today's lifestyle with the ancient art of Meditation. The average person can easily learn TM, and two twenty-minute sessions per day easily fit into the busiest person's routine.

TM provides inner peace - and relief from stress. Scientific studies prove that it is more effective than other stress reduction techniques. They also prove that TM is more practical than other stress reduction techniques. Most importantly, people are more likely to practice TM - and they are more likely to get more reliable results.

TM and Self-Referral

It is interesting that TM first produces its effects in the brain. TM, a simple mental technique, produces consistent brain wave changes in the EEG. Other physiological signs of deep rest follow.

Biofeedback and Progressive Muscle Relaxation, while being superficially similar to TM, do not produce the same EEG changes. They also do not produce TM's deep level of rest.

We know the stress response begins in the brain – the body's Self-Referral Center. Stressful life events cause the brain to trigger the stress response, producing chronic autonomic overstimulation. This is Stress Syndrome – a state of hyper-arousal that disrupts the feedback loops of Self-Referral. The result is disease, aging, or death.

TM is a simple mental technique that produces a state of deep rest via the brain. As a result, the brain - as the body's Self-Referral Center – *triggers the body's anti-stress feedback loop. TM is just as natural to the human body as the stress response.* Practicing TM simply balances out the exaggerated stress response caused by modern life. *TM thus is likely to be what we are looking for to trigger the anti-stress feedback loop – and restore Self-Referral.*

Chapter 9

Solving the Adaptation Crisis

Self-Referral balances the body's feedback loops and creates health. Through dynamic Self-Referral, the body adapts to the changing demands of life. We must restore Self-Referral to solve the Adaptation Crisis.

Self-Referral and Adaptation

Through Self-Referral, the body governs itself. By maintaining an ideal body environment in an ever-changing world, Self-Referral creates health. Feedback loops are the mechanisms of Self-Referral - and they balance the many pairs of opposites: hot-cold, fast-slow, sleep-awake and a myriad of others.

Most people are healthy more often than sick; we reason from this that Self-Referral works more often than not. Why, then, are so many today sick from stress? The level of stress is far worse today than a hundred years ago; it is much worse than even fifty years ago. This is why today's humanity suffers from the Adaptation Crisis.

Self-Referral usually copes with change, but the demands of modern life are far worse than in the past - and often overwhelm Self-Referral. These demands spring from technology, increased mobility of people, strain from stressed lifestyle, and information overload. This unprecedented level of stress disrupts the body's feedback loops, causing disease or even sudden death.

The effects of the Adaptation Crisis go far beyond individual people. Many who cannot cope with the stress of modern life turn to tobacco, alcohol, or drugs. These major public health problems increase the risk of disease and death – and increase the cost of healthcare. In addition, stressed people are unhappy, angry, and sometimes violent. Adding drugs, tobacco and alcohol to this already volatile situation makes family and job problems inevitable.

The rising tide of crime and violence is a direct result of the Adaptation Crisis. Families are breaking apart. Children are not being taught the basic values and skills needed to succeed in today's world. The result is a growing underclass of people who are unfit for employment and who lack basic interpersonal skills. The Adaptation Crisis thus contributes to poor health, increasing Healthcare Expenditures, drug abuse, family failure, crime, violence, and even political chaos.

Human beings today have a clear choice: either retreat from the stress of modern life or find better ways to cope with it. Modern people rely on technology to maintain a high standard of living. Few would choose a more primitive lifestyle. Seeking a better way to cope with stress is a far more practical choice.

This is why *Self-Referral/Maximum Health* has importance far beyond a philosophical discussion. This is not just another subject for coffee house bull sessions; we are talking here about major medical and societal concerns. In fact, restoring Self-Referral is critical to the survival of the human race. Lao-Tzu tells us:

> The Tao is the center of the universe. Thus, when a new leader is chosen, don't offer to help him with your expertise. Offer instead to teach him about the Tao.[490]

The Tao is perfect balance of all opposites, resulting in perfect health, and perfect peace. How do we teach someone about the Tao? People must learn to better plan and organize their lives to reduce stress. Behavioral Modification, Mindfulness, and other educational processes help, but education only goes so far. People need an effective and dependable method that improves their bodies' resistance to stress. *We desperately need a dependable, practical, and scientifically valid way to restore Self-Referral.*

Seeking a Stress Solution

Doctors usually treat stress symptoms and disease with prescription drugs. Beyond medications, a popular health promotion tactic is to teach people healthy habits. Media news and advertising teach us to avoid disease-producing habits like too much salt, excess weight, and lack of exercise. Through healthy lifestyle choices, people can avoid future disease.

Teaching people about risk factors, however, is not enough. Even if we live a healthy lifestyle and avoid Type A behavior, the stress of life continues. Many events are simply outside our control. Answering telephones, driving cars, or working under a deadline are largely unavoidable. Education alone will not improve the hyper-arousal caused by modern living. What can we do to better cope with today's stressful lifestyle?

Learning an effective stress reduction technique is the reasonable solution. This obvious answer, however, has roadblocks. Most stress reduction techniques are impractical. They require expensive equipment, highly trained technicians, or both. And research shows most of the techniques do not provide the deep rest needed. The choice is clear. Scientific research shows that Transcendental Meditation - TM for short - is the most practical and effective stress reduction technique now available.[491]

Today the facts are clear, but confusion remains about stress reduction techniques. Knowledge of the pernicious effects of stress is widespread, but the solution seems mired in confusion – even though research proves that TM is the best solution to the Adaptation Crisis. Why does this quandary persist? The reason is that solutions to health problems are products of current medical knowledge.

When doctors better understood heart disease, improved therapies resulted. First came nitroglycerin, then Beta Blockers, and then the Calcium Channel Blockers and ACE Inhibitors – and all the life-saving drugs that continue to emerge. The same is true regarding other diseases and therapies. Doctors first learned about bacteria before they could develop antibiotics. The results were sulfa, then penicillin – and now we have many antibiotics. Medical therapy thus is a product of advancing medical knowledge.

Doctors have known about stress since the 1930s, but most did not recognize stress as a health menace until the 1970s.[492] TM has been available since 1958[493] but was not widely known until the late 1960s. Serious TM research began in the 1970s.[494] Over forty years of research has proven the value of TM as the most effective stress reduction technique. Only now, in the twenty-first century, can we appreciate TM's true value.

Mind, Body, and Medicine

What is the history of medicine's relationship with Meditation? Associating Modern Medicine and ancient Meditation seems odd. Doctors base Modern Medicine on the scientific model. They will not accept new ideas without scientific proof. Meditation, by contrast, springs from ancient traditions that are, to the Western mind, nonobjective or even mystical.

Complex cultural and language barriers create more problems. How can a Western physician and an Eastern Swami communicate? Just bridging English and Hindi is quite a task. Add a third language like Sanskrit plus ancient traditions, and most doctors will quickly retreat, scratching their heads in frustration.

Another persistent problem is Meditation's credibility. Conservative Western doctors often connect Meditation with bogus techniques taught by unscrupulous and unqualified "experts." *Scientific studies quickly show that ineffective Meditation techniques just do not work.*

These obstacles together create a large barrier to understanding. This is why staid Western doctors have a difficult time grappling with ideas from the East. This confusion prevents many people from taking Meditation seriously. As a result, doctors and patients alike doubt that Meditation has any value.

This situation is very unfortunate because we may overlook a priceless stress reduction technique – one that is desperately needed to combat the Adaptation Crisis. Can we find common ground between Modern Medicine's approach to the body and ancient meditation's approach to the mind?

Western medical thought always connected mind and body. Modern science owes much to the philosopher-scientists of ancient Greece. Plato wrote that people should cultivate both mind and body for ideal health.[495] Aristotle taught that the mental activities of thought and emotion are products of biological processes.[496]

Eastern medical tradition also teaches the unity of mind and body. Ancient Indian medicine teaches that mind and body are parts of one whole. This unity is the basis of health. Divisions between mind and body create chaos that brings disease. Strong emotions disrupt health and cause disease and suffering. The ancients of India developed the science of Meditation to restore the unity of mind and body.[497]

Ancient Chinese medicine teaches that mind and body work together for ideal health. Ancient Chinese doctors also referred to negative emotions, stress, and disease. They called strong emotions the enemies of health and the cause of disease. They believed that excitement, sadness, desires, and pain reduced the body's ability to cope with change. They used Meditation and related practices to improve the health of mind and body.[498]

We see that *Self-Referral/Maximum Health* used to be part of mainstream medical thought. How did this central idea of medical philosophy become lost? Medical knowledge is vast. An entire life is not enough time to learn the whole field of medicine. The ancient Greek physician Hippocrates offers one explanation: "The life so short, the craft so long to learn."[499] This is how important ideas become lost in the crush of medical knowledge.

Mind and Body: Separate or Whole?

Modern Medicine's very structure teaches that mind and body are separate. Most doctors treat what we define as body diseases. These include specialists of Family Practice, Internal Medicine, Surgery, Pediatrics, Orthopedics, and others. By contrast, only the specialties of Neurology, Neurosurgery, and Psychiatry work with the mind – and then often indirectly. What explains this surprising situation?

Modern Medicine's view of mind and body is a product of recent history. Since the industrial revolution, most people have likened the brain's complex work to that of a machine. We express this idea through figures of speech. When tired, we say my mind is rusty or my mind isn't sharp. If someone becomes extremely stressed, we may say his mind has broken down.[500]

A machine lacks any ability of self-regulation beyond the rudimentary controls built into it. We cannot work *with a machine*; we can only work *on a machine*. Today, most medical therapies are products of this assumption. Doctors assume the brain is a machine, so they work on it. Doctors thus alter brain chemistry with drugs or change brain structure by surgery.

In addition, doctors are practical; they seek remedies for definable disease. In the past, a sore throat was more real than the stress of a new job. Medical research has only recently shown the link between *subjective stress* and *objective disease*. We cannot blame physicians for failing to treat a condition they consider unimportant.

The Disease Approach to medicine puts undue focus on disease. Doctors and patients are in such a hurry to diagnose, prescribe, or operate that we neglect the unity of mind and body. *This is why doctors seldom consider using the mind to promote health in the body.*

Rediscovering Wholeness

Is there a better way? We know that stress produces strong brain-body effects. These include negative emotions and deadly diseases like high blood pressure, stroke, and heart attack.

Stress reduction techniques work with the mind to reduce the pernicious effects of stress. The new connections we see forged by scientific research are exciting. The search for the unity of mind and body can begin anew. Instead of maintaining the fiction that mind and body are separate, we can work with both. By rediscovering mind-body wholeness, medicine is returning to its historical roots; medicine is coming home.

TM research has reintroduced an ancient aspiration as a practical reality. *We can work with the mind to improve our body's health.* In this way we can work with the brain instead of only working on it. This easily learned technique is not only useful but revolutionary. *Humans can, by working directly with their brain, better adapt to the stress of modern life.*

The Glueck and Stroebel study proves that TM is easy to learn and produces deep rest. One study, however, does not decide an issue. We need to closely examine the TM technique. Is TM only useful for psychiatric patients, or can it help other people? TM produces brain wave changes, but does it have broader effects on health? Are these effects helpful or harmful? Finally, many other Meditation techniques exist. How do they compare with TM?

Past Meditation Research

Doctors and scientists have examined Meditation since the 1800s.[501] During the colonial period, many Western people encountered Far Eastern cultures for the first time.[502] Many European and American travelers were first exposed to Meditation in India, China, or Japan.[503] Many Western doctors saw the possible value of Meditation and tried to learn more about it. What did early researchers learn about Meditation?

Questions asked by early researchers are the same that we ask today. People who meditate sit quietly with their eyes closed. Does Meditation accomplish anything unique, or is it just an extra nap? Assuming it works, can a mental technique produce physical changes that we can measure with scientific devices?

Dr. Therese Brosse was a French cardiologist of the 1930s. She heard about Meditation through stories brought back from India. The doctor was curious about claims made by Indian Yogis. These are Indian individuals who practice Meditation and related disciplines. The Yogis claimed they could control their heart and breathing in unusual ways. Dr. Brosse wondered if Meditation could improve patients with heart disease.

To evaluate the claims, she traveled to India to study the Yogis. Dr. Brosse then carried out one of the first scientific studies of

Meditation in 1935. Her equipment was primitive by today's standards, but she recorded heart activity. She found that a subject could stop his heart for a time during Meditation. This was of doubtful medical use, but it suggested that Meditation could produce measurable body effects.[504]

This stimulated interest in the possibility that Meditation could improve health, and other research followed. Dr. M. A. Wenger studied Indian subjects in 1955. Meditation produced physical effects of slow and shallow breathing and decreased skin resistance to electrical current.[505] Wenger was so impressed with his results that he wrote a book exploring the relationship of psychology and physiology.[506] Dr. J. G. Henrotte studied Indian subjects in 1957. These studies found that Meditation caused decreased breathing and decreased stomach activity – again, evidence that Meditation produced physical effects.

Later research focused on brain wave changes, which better reflect mental activity. Scientists studied Meditation using the electroencephalogram, or EEG. The French researchers Dr. N. N. Das and Dr. H. Gastaut conducted early EEG studies of Indian subjects in 1957. They reported an increase of alpha brain waves during Meditation. Later researchers proved that alpha waves indicate deep rest.[507] Dr. B. K. Anand reported similar findings on Indian subjects in 1961.[508]

Dr. Therese Brosse published further findings in 1963. She found that Meditation caused decreased breathing, but also affected heart rate and brain waves. She had hopes that Meditation would improve health in people with heart disease.[509] She was not able to realize that application, but her findings did prove that Meditation - a mental technique - somehow caused deep physical rest.[510]

Researchers also studied Meditation in other countries.[511] Japanese researchers A. Kasamatsu and T. Hitai studied Zen Meditation in 1966. They also found that Meditation produced increased alpha wave activity in the brain.[512] Follow-up work in 1968 showed that experienced meditators achieved more alpha activity and deeper rest. The experienced meditators also produced physical changes including decreased oxygen use, shallower breathing, and slow heart rate.[513]

Problems in Meditation Research

These early studies showed that Meditation produces measurable body changes - but research on a new subject often raises more questions than it answers. Several problems were obvious.

One problem was how to compare many different Meditation techniques. Although all the studies examined Meditation, subjects used many different Meditation techniques. To illustrate, one technique was to force all thoughts from the mind. Another technique was to think about body parts to make them "come alive." Still another technique allowed the mind to wander among various positive ideas. All techniques involved thinking, but they otherwise had little in common.

A second problem was sensationalism. Early studies often focused on bizarre claims of body control. For example, one researcher buried a subject alive to prove that Meditation reduces the body's use of oxygen. Fortunately, a large crowd found him alive but unconscious 72 hours later.[514] This sensational style of research did little to advance the credibility of Meditation.

Finally, early studies often combined mental and physical techniques. Researchers studied subjects while they were meditating, but also while they performed breathing and stretching exercises. It was unclear whether Meditation or physical exertion produced the results in question.[515]

Some experts predicted that Meditation would be extremely useful,[516] while others were scornful.[517] This controversy is why doctors often view Meditation as little more than a medical curiosity. Recent interest in stress management brought Meditation back to center stage. By the late 1960s, many studies proved the negative health effects of stress. There was an obvious need for a practical stress reduction technique. The confused state of Meditation research was equally clear. It was time to reexamine Meditation in modern terms.

Early TM Research

By the late 1960s, many studies proved the negative health effects of stress. There was an obvious need for a practical stress reduction technique. The confused state of Meditation research was equally clear. It was time to reexamine Meditation in modern terms.

In 1968 Robert Keith Wallace was completing Ph.D. work at the University of California, Los Angeles. After reviewing previous stress reduction technique research, he decided to study Meditation. He used modern methods to carry out the most complete Meditation research at that time.[518]

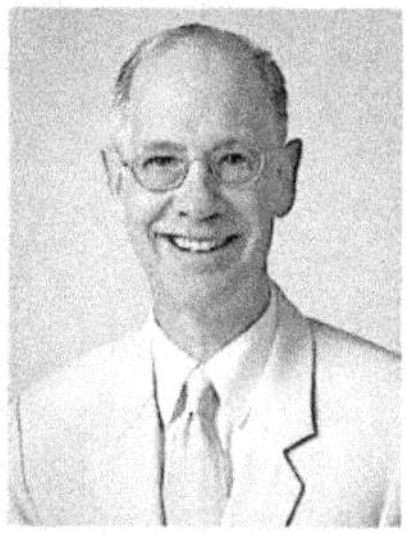

Pioneer TM Researcher
Dr. R. Keith Wallace

Wallace studied Transcendental Meditation because it was well known and available. TM was easy to learn and practice. Practitioners said that TM had immediate effects. There also were many TM meditators living in the Los Angeles area. Wallace studied a group of 15 college students that were in good mental and physical health. All had practiced TM from six to thirty-six months before the study.[519]

Wallace used state-of-the-art equipment and methods. He tested each subject while resting with eyes open and closed, before and after TM. He also tested the subjects during a 30-minute session of TM. Clear measurements thus compared the effects of TM versus simply sitting and resting. Wallace's also study tested TM's effects on the body. Previous studies set only vague ideas of what they were studying. Wallace was more specific in his research design.

What did Wallace find? The study proved that TM produces unique body changes. Oxygen consumption dropped, heart rate slowed, GSR increased, and the EEG showed an increase in Alpha wave activity. These changes define a unique state of deep rest. Wallace thus found that TM produces physical effects that were measurable and distinctly different from simply resting with eyes closed. These findings were to ignite a firestorm of scientific research that followed that thoroughly investigated Transcendental Meditation's short-term and long-term effects.

This study was titled "The Physiological Effects of Transcendental Meditation" and appeared in the prestigious journal *Science* in 1970.[520] The paper caused quite a stir in the scientific community. Wallace had studied Meditation in modern terms, and it produced body changes never before documented. Wallace's work inspired the large body of scientific TM research that followed.[521]

Self-Referral

Maximum Health

The First Wallace Study

REMEMBER: This is the first scientific study that showed the body effects of Meditation - specifically Transcendental Meditation, or TM. This proved that a mental technique - TM Meditation - produced physical changes typical of deep rest. These changes were the opposite of those caused by stress.

Oxygen Consumption: All work of the human body consumes oxygen. We breathe in oxygen via the lungs. Oxygen consumption measures the total activity of the body. Deep rest decreases oxygen consumption; activity increases oxygen consumption. TM produced a marked decrease in oxygen consumption in the meditators.

Heart Rate: The heart beats faster to pump more blood through the arteries and increase blood pressure. This propels oxygen to all parts of the body. Deep rest slows the heart; activity speeds up the heart. TM produced a marked decrease in the heart rate of the meditators.

Galvanic Skin Resistance (GSR): Skin resistance to electricity measures how much perspiration is present. Perspiration is a measure of how stressed the body is. Deep rest decreases GSR; activity increases GSR. TM produced a marked decrease in the GSR of the meditators.

EEG Changes: Previous studies showed that meditation increases alpha brain waves. Activity decreases alpha waves; deep rest increases alpha waves. TM produced a marked increase in alpha waves that indicated deep rest.

Wallace's findings caused researchers to ask many questions. First, were Wallace's findings reproducible? Were his results a one-time fluke, or would other scientists produce the same results when they repeated the experiment?

Another question was: how did TM produce the effects shown in the study? Scientists previously assumed no one could consciously affect breathing, heart rate, GSR, or brain waves. All these activities are automatic functions of the body. Wallace's work changed everything because TM somehow accessed and changed these autonomic nervous system functions.

Finally, was TM the only technique that could produce such results? This question stemmed from curiosity, but other questions emerged. Some scientists questioned the secrecy of TM instruction. Many scientists also wanted to automate Meditation. They wanted to create a Meditation machine, like that of Biofeedback. They believed machine-based Meditation would be easier to understand and administer to patients.

TM: A Closer Look

To answer these questions, we must take a closer look at TM. What is TM? How do we learn TM? How do we practice TM? What more do we know about TM's effects on the human body?

TM is a mental technique that produces a deep state of rest. Maharishi Mahesh Yogi brought TM from India to the West in 1959. TM is the most widely known Meditation technique in the world. As of 2017, over six million people practiced TM worldwide.[522] Over one million of the TM meditators are in the United States.[523] TM meditators include people from every age, sex, profession, educational background, and religion.[524]

People learn TM from TM Instructors. These TM instructors are trained through the tradition of Maharishi Mahesh Yogi to ensure that they teach TM correctly. People cannot learn TM from a book or other source. Why? Personal instruction ensures that the novice masters the TM technique. In addition, TM is mentally dynamic. Common experiences occur at various stages of the practice. Thus, it is best to have frequent interaction with a trained TM instructor during early practice for best results.[525]

During instruction, the TM instructor teaches the meditator a *mantra*, or sound. The mantra has no cognitive meaning. Mantra is a word in the Sanskrit language. The word mantra translates as *a sound, the effect of which is known.* The mental repetition of the mantra triggers the deep rest that TM produces.[526]

Meditators practice the TM technique while sitting upright in a comfortable position. They close their eyes to avoid distraction and mentally repeat the mantra for 20 minutes as learned privately from a trained TM instructor. TM does not involve concentration or contemplation. It is an effortless mental technique and requires no forcing or straining.

This is how people practice TM twice daily - twenty minutes, morning and evening. The key requirements are the correct mantra and the correct procedure, learned from an authorized TM instructor. The technique is dynamic, natural, and effortless.[527]

To understand TM's effects on the human body, we must review the scientific research that followed Wallace's initial work. Does TM reliably produce the body changes reported by Wallace? What are other short-term and long-term effects of TM? How does TM compare to other Meditation techniques?

Later TM Research

Many scientists became interested in studying TM's effects after Wallace's work. The first point of interest was: would repeat studies duplicate Wallace's results, or would they show different effects? Wallace continued extensive TM research while other scientists also studied TM.

Wallace followed his initial work by extending his studies through 1970.[528] He published this work in 1971[529] and 1972.[530] These studies reproduced the previous results involving heart rate, oxygen consumption, skin resistance (GSR), and Alpha brain wave changes.

Wallace found that TM caused changes in the body's chemistry.[531] The human body constantly uses oxygen for digestion, muscle activity, and heart function. Blood lactate and carbon dioxide are two key waste products. The wear and tear of stress increases these chemicals; Wallace showed that TM lowers the levels of these stress indicators. This proved that TM produces a true stress-reduction response in the body.[532]

Scientists around the world became interested in studying TM. Researchers replicated Wallace's findings at the University of Alberta in Edmonton, Canada[533] in 1973. Other scientists reproduced Wallace's findings at California State College at Sonoma, California[534] in 1974. Still other scientists also repeated Wallace's findings at Maharishi European Research University in Switzerland in 1975.[535]

These studies attracted interest from researchers in clinical medicine. The findings all prove that TM provides deep rest and reverses the effects of stress. The findings of Wallace and others are inarguably true and well-grounded in the scientific method with solid research design.

One more link will prove TM's value to medicine: can we use TM to treat specific health problems? What do we know about TM's effects on specific stress related diseases?

TM and Hypertension

We have discussed the relationship between stress and cardiovascular disease. It is clear that stress causes increased blood pressure, heart regulation problems, stroke, and vasospasm anywhere in the body. These stress effects cause major disease and are frequently direct causes of sudden death.

This is the basis of the ubiquitous vasospasm caused by Stress Syndrome – and this is the cause of the aging process, disease, and sudden death. This is exactly the sequence of events caused by today's Adaptation Crisis. It seems logical to specifically use TM to counteract stress related disease. What do we know about TM's effect on cardiovascular disease?

In 1972, Dr. Herbert Benson and Dr. R. Keith Wallace studied TM's effect on high blood pressure patients in Boston. They measured patients' blood pressure over sixty days following TM instruction. The TM patients had markedly lower blood pressure after learning TM. This improvement was independent of medications and judged to be positive effects of TM.[536]

Dr. David B. Simon and others studied TM's effect on high blood pressure in Chicago in 1975. After checking the patients' high blood pressure over six weeks, they taught patients the TM technique. Following 60 days of TM, blood pressure improved – again due to positive effects of TM.[537]

Dr. Barry Blackwell and others studied TM's effect on high blood pressure in 1975 in Cincinnati. They studied high blood pressure patients, checking their blood pressure for a month. Then they taught the patients TM. The results were the same: TM improved the patient's blood pressure.[538]

Since the 1970s, researchers across the world verified TM's clear success at lowering blood pressure. Dr. J. W. Anderson carried out a meta-analysis of these studies in 2008. He used advanced statistical analysis to measure the results of studies carried out worldwide and found that TM consistently reduces blood pressure.[539] Finally, in 2013 the American Heart Association reported in its journal *Hypertension*:

> The TM technique is the only meditation practice shown to lower blood pressure.[540]

TM's effectiveness in treating hypertension was further confirmed when the editors of *The Manual of Hypertension of the European Society of Hypertension* included a chapter about TM's effectiveness in treating high blood pressure. This book is the definitive textbook on hypertension relied on by European specialists. One of the book's chapters outlines stress as the cause of hypertension and explains how TM reverses stress and normalizes high blood pressure.[541]

TM and Angina Pectoris

We know that stress causes high blood pressure and vasospasm. Vasospasm is the common cause of angina pectoris, stroke, and sudden death. TM was proven by solid scientific studies to reduce high blood pressure; many wondered: would TM improve angina pectoris?

Dr. John W. Zamarra studied TM's effect on angina pectoris patients in 1975. Dr. Zamarra taught one group TM and a second control group read about TM but did not learn it. Zamarra tested all the patients by EKG and exercise testing before and after TM instruction. Eight months passed. Zamarra then compared the two groups.[542] Did TM make a difference?

Dr. Zamarra found the TM patients clearly improved - both physically and mentally. The TM patients had more exercise tolerance; that is, they could ride an exercise bicycle much longer without chest pain. The non-TM patients had no improvement in exercise tolerance. Doctors reported the TM patients had less anxiety, needed fewer tranquilizers, and slept better. Finally, they had better relations with other people. The non-TM group had no mental improvements.[543]

TM and All Cardiovascular Disease

The relationship between stress and high cholesterol is well known. High cholesterol is known to be a huge risk factor in blood vessel plaque formation or atherosclerosis. TM has been proven to reduce cholesterol over time as meditators continue TM.[544] TM also has been proven to reduce thickening of the carotid artery in the neck. Such carotid plaquing is known to be a major risk factor and a common cause of stroke.[545]

What do all these positive effects of TM accomplish when examined all together? A study published in 2012 proves that TM provided a 48% reduction in heart attack, stroke, and sudden death for TM meditators versus an equally matched non-meditating population.[546] This proves that TM not only solves Stress Syndrome and the Adaptation Crisis, but TM also greatly improves the very diseases that are caused by these scourges of modern life. In short, *TM is extremely effective in treating cardiovascular system disease.*

All this research has caused quite a stir in the medical community. Many research projects are either underway now or planned for the near future. The National Institutes of Health has awarded over $25 million in grant support for research on the benefits of the TM technique in treatment and prevention of cardiovascular disease.[547]

TM's effect on exercise tolerance in angina patients is extremely important - but only if we understand vasospasm. When Dr. Zamarra studied his patients in 1975, doctors knew little about coronary artery spasm. The clogged pipes theory still held sway. Only a few researchers suspected vasospasm. We now know that hyper-arousal of the autonomic nervous system causes vasospasm of the coronary arteries.

A recent study underlined TM's positive effects on the cardiovascular system. The researchers taught TM to cardiac rehabilitation patients. Some of these patients used TM alone and some had TM plus the usual physical exercise rehabilitation. The rehabilitation progress of both these groups was compared to controls. What did they find?

Using advanced Positronic Emission Tomography (PET) imaging, researchers found that both groups of TM patients had significant improvement of blood flow to the heart. This confirms that TM has a beneficial effect when used with physical rehabilitation. The fact that TM also improved circulation as verified by PET imaging proves the value of TM in cardiac rehabilitation.[548]

TM – Far Ahead of Its Time

We often hear abstract ideas long before we appreciate their practical value. Scientists suspected that vasospasm caused sudden death long before anyone could prove it. Working to combat vasospasm, scientists developed Beta Blocker drugs – and found they improved high blood pressure and angina pectoris. Similarly, scientists long suspected that stress caused heart disease. Most doctors are only now taking this idea seriously. And only now can we see that TM brings a clear answer to these problems.

Maharishi Mahesh Yogi, Dr. R. Keith Wallace, and a handful of scientists suggested in the 1970s that TM would improve heart disease. This suggestion made little sense until doctors understood vasospasm. Medicine's paradigm had to shift and expand to include vasospasm to recognize TM's value. *It has taken medical research over forty years to understand TM's usefulness. In that sense, TM was far ahead of its time.*

There are profound implications in the TM research. TM improves high blood pressure, angina pectoris, vasospasm, stroke, high cholesterol, and hardening of the arteries. TM apparently reverses the sustained hyper-arousal that lies behind these conditions. TM truly saves lives. And most importantly – TM counteracts Stress Syndrome and the Adaptation Crisis that threatens humanity's very survival.

> *That is why the mental improvement in Dr. Zamarra's TM patients is just as important as their physical improvement.*

TM reduces explosive emotions like anger, anxiety, and worry. These strong emotions cause vasospasm - and it is critical to curtail those emotions before they create heart attack, stroke, or sudden death. That is why Dr. Zamarra's report of improved anxiety, sleep, and better interpersonal relations are just as important as improved exercise tolerance.

TM and the Quality of Life

Dr. Zamarra's TM patients improved their quality of life because they decreased their level of stress. Why did their quality of life improve? All living things operate best within an adaptation range. Humanity now is in an Adaptation Crisis: the overwhelming stress of modern life constantly exceeds our adaptation range, wreaking havoc on human health. TM counteracts the stress of modern life by providing two periods of uniquely deep rest per day. These TM sessions reverse the effects of stress and counteract the pernicious effects of modern life. As time goes on, TM also improves the body's ability to cope with future stress.

Modern life produces a high standard of living, but a low quality of life. Why is this true? Modern life originated in the Western industrial nations of Europe and North America. This culture now is spreading through the Middle East, Africa, Central and South America, and Asia. People living the modern lifestyle often have more abundance of food and material goods, but that is not all that modern life brings.

Modern people live in an environment that is too busy for their own good. They sleep irregular hours - and often do not get enough sleep. Tired people have dull minds. Research shows the brain suffers most from inadequate rest. Poor rest causes the stress response, increasing stress chemicals in the blood stream.

Stress causes depression, anxiety, and other mental illnesses. Modern people are nervous and irritable because of chemical brain imbalances caused by stress.[549] These mental illnesses are so common that we fail to notice them anymore. We just accept these abnormal mental states as normal. *This is why I call the stress of modern life subclinical mental illness.*

TM reverses the effects of stress, including its underlying strain of blood chemistry. If we tame the stress response, abnormal brain chemistry will improve as well. This is why TM will be of great benefit to those with mental illness.[550] What do we know about TM and mental illness?

TM and Sleep Disorders

How rested we are strongly affects our quality of life. Sleep is the body's chief repair mechanism. Sleep is vital to health; if the body cannot repair itself, stress does more damage at a faster rate. Sleep disorders are irritating, but they also add to the stress of life – and create disease.

Insomnia is a disturbing sleep disorder where people can't easily fall asleep. Some insomnia patients can't fall asleep for hours; others do not sleep for days on end.[551] They often require strong medication to fall asleep. Sleep drugs are known to interfere with normal brain function, making a bad situation worse.[552] These drugs are addictive and can add to the problem; that is why a drugless cure for insomnia is very desirable.

Canadian psychologist Donald E. Miskiman studied TM and insomnia in 1972 at the University of Alberta. The insomnia patients recorded the time needed to fall asleep for one month. Then the researchers taught the patients TM. The patients continued recording for three months. Miskiman's patients needed far less time to fall asleep after learning TM.[553] A follow-up study in 1975 showed the TM patients continued to have insomnia relief.[554]

Many people have annoying but less serious problems falling asleep. These people sleep poorly but do not consult a doctor.[555] Sleep disorders are more than just an annoyance. Many people who have poor sleep are more likely to develop more serious psychiatric disorders. These include major depression, anxiety, and personality disorders. Experts believe that treating sleep disorders early literally prevents future mental illness.[556]

This brings more immediacy to the use of TM. If TM helps insomnia patients, it will surely help people with less severe sleep disorders. Improved sleep with TM accounts for improved quality of life – and prevention of major mental illness is a high priority. What do we know about stress and other kinds of mental disease?

Stress causes anxiety in many people. Research shows that anxious people are more likely to have poor mental health.[557] People with anxiety often need medications like Ativan (Lorazepam) or Xanax (Aprazolam) just to cope with day-to-day life. Stressed people may become addicted to these drugs.[558] The side effects of anti-anxiety drugs often worsen the quality of life.

Psychologist Jean Ross studied TM and anxiety in 1972 at the University of Edinburgh, Scotland. She tested patients for anxiety. Then she taught the patients the TM technique. They retested the patients for anxiety three and four months later. The tests showed clear improvement in anxiety and related mental health. This was more obvious for those who practiced TM regularly than those who were not regular.[559]

TM and Drug Abuse

One measure of mental health is whether people abuse alcohol, marijuana, and other drugs. People often use drugs to cope with stress. Flirtation with drugs often results in lifetime addiction and misery. Drugs ruin lives, generate enormous medical expenses, and undermine the legal system that holds our culture together.

Dr. Herbert Benson and Dr. R. Keith Wallace studied TM's effect on drug abuse in 1970. Working in Boston, they surveyed 1,862 subjects on drug abuse and attitudes toward drugs before learning TM. They repeated the survey thirty-three months later. Drug abuse among the TM meditators dropped markedly - including marijuana, LSD, and narcotics. Subjects also developed more anti-drug attitudes – likely because they had learned first-hand that TM was a better answer to stress than drugs.[560]

Dr. Mohammed Shafii studied TM and marijuana use in 1974 at the University of Michigan Medical School, Ann Arbor. They surveyed 126 TM subjects on marijuana use before and after instruction in TM. Then they compared TM subjects to 90 non-TM subjects. A significant decrease in marijuana use occurred in the TM group; they found little change in the non-TM group.[561]

Many experts believe that stress contributes strongly to alcoholism; many alcoholics use alcohol specifically for stress relief. Using the same methods to study TM's effect on alcohol use that he used to study marijuana, Dr. Shafii noted a major change among TM subjects. The TM group showed a sharp decrease in alcohol use; no changes occurred in the control group. He concluded that TM prevents alcoholism because it effectively counteracts the stress of life.[562]

A 2018 study evaluated TM's effect upon heavy alcohol abusers. A group of alcohol abuse patients were taught TM and compared to a control group who were treated only with counseling and related measures. Patients in both groups were evaluated after discharge at 30 and 90 days. The TM patients had eliminated heavy drinking, had far less urge to return to drinking, and markedly decreased stress. All this is consistent with the idea that people drink to relieve stress, and TM removes the stress that drives the drinking.[563]

Alcohol and drug abuse are commonly recognized as a way that people cope with the stress of life. People naturally want relief from the unrelenting stress of modern life, and alcohol and drugs can be an easy way to get relief. TM's ability to offer stress relief to replace the need for alcohol and drugs is medically important. *But TM also offers relief from the endless misery caused by alcohol and drug abuse – along with the legal and social chaos that it creates.*

TM and the Nervous System

Perhaps the biggest question we might ask in terms of TM's value lies in its effects on the brain and nervous system. We have reviewed a huge number of positive TM effects on reversing the negative effects of stress, but how exactly does TM accomplish this? We can answer this question by looking more closely at TM's effects on the brain and nervous system.

We know the stress response occurs in the brain itself. When stimulated by stressful life events, the brain reacts with the fight or flight response. It is the unrelenting stimulation of modern life that causes Stress Syndrome - the basis of all disease and the aging process.

The result of all this is today's Adaptation Crisis. Human beings can no longer keep up with the stress of life. TM counteracts all this; TM produces an anti-stress response, and studies show unique brain wave changes during TM. What do these changes mean?

Dr. Jean-Paul Banquet studied TM's brain wave effects in 1972 at Massachusetts General Hospital and Harvard Medical School in Boston. He studied ten subjects while they practiced TM. The researchers compared the TM subjects' EEG to non-TM patients. TM produced unique brain wave patterns. TM subjects showed brain wave patterns typical of deep rest - but brain waves showing alertness also were present.[564]

These findings were unusual. Resting subjects typically have a much different EEG pattern than alert subjects. The EEG patterns were contradictory. How could someone be resting while they were alert? Dr. Banquet followed his initial work with a more detailed study in 1973. Their findings were the same: *TM produced a unique brain wave pattern called restful alertness.*[565]

Dr. Banquet carried out a third study in 1974. Working with Dr. Maurice Sailhan in France, they studied 15 subjects with EEG. The scientists recorded brain wave changes during TM. They also recorded their EEG while the subjects were alert, sleeping, and resting. The results again showed that TM produced restful alertness. This unique state was different from sleep, resting, and alertness.[566]

Dr. Mark Westcott studied TM's effects on the brain in 1973 in Durham, England. He studied subjects who practiced TM and compared their measurements with people who relaxed with eyes closed. Non-TM subjects in a third group concentrated on mentally composing a letter. They compared the EEG records, looking for the effects of TM on brain function.[567]

TM subjects showed increased brain wave coordination between the two hemispheres of the brain. The right and left sides of the brain during TM showed strong EEG similarity. They did not find these changes in the resting or concentration groups. Banquet believes that *the EEG shows increased internal coordination of the brain.*[568]

Dr. Paul H. Levine studied TM and brain coherence in 1974 and 1975 at Maharishi European Research University in Switzerland. They studied subjects while they practiced the TM technique - looking for signs of brain coherence in the EEG Records.[569] *Their study showed strong evidence of whole brain coherence during TM.* Brain waves in the right hemisphere became like those of the left. Brain waves in the top of the brain became like those in the bottom of the brain. Brain waves in the front of the brain became like those at the back.[570]

These studies showed that TM produces unique brain wave changes. One major finding is TM's unique EEG effect. This is why a scientist can easily distinguish TM from the waking state, resting with eyes closed, and sleep. Why is this so?

These very different subjective experiences produce objective brain waves on the EEG record. If a subject is out of sight but connected with the EEG, a scientist can tell what the person is doing. The EEG accurately distinguishes between TM, resting, sleeping, or simply sitting awake.

A second major finding is that TM improves the brain's internal coordination. Stress causes chaotic brain function; TM causes the brain to organize itself and become more coherent. TM seems to cause the brain to get back in touch with itself. *TM thus provides deep whole-body rest but also improves the brain's Self-Referral – its coherence - as well.*

The Coherence Effect

Dr. R. Keith Wallace came together with Dr. Christopher Clark and Jay B. Marcus to write a brilliant book called *The Coherence Effect*. This book makes the convincing statement that coherence of the brain - as evidenced by coherent brainwaves – is one of the single most important indicators of health. He writes:

> Brain wave coherence, for example, is the new frontier in brain science. When studying brain waves, the term "coherence" means that the cells in different parts of the brain are firing at the same time in the same way . . . This is important because one part of the brain is responsible for memory, one for moral reasoning, and several parts for creativity and other functions. Because success requires many different areas of the brain to work together, the different areas need to be communicating with each other. And they communicate by a synchronous, or coherent, firing. Brain coherence improves mental functioning and is associated with reduced anxiety, depression, PTSD, high blood pressure, high cholesterol, and other disorders. Conversely, the absence of brain wave coherence is associated with autism, schizophrenia, and Alzheimer's disease. These findings are why researchers today are looking so closely at brain wave coherence.[571]

Transcendental Meditation is the only proven effective stress reduction technique. While its physiologic effects show indications of profound deep rest, the brain wave changes show even more profound effects. TM causes the brain to literally get in touch with itself, get synchronized, and work better. The result is better Self-Referral in the brain itself – and as the brain coordinates all Self-Referral, this is of critical importance. When the brain operates with greater coherence, a new level of health has been reached. That is what we call Maximum Health.

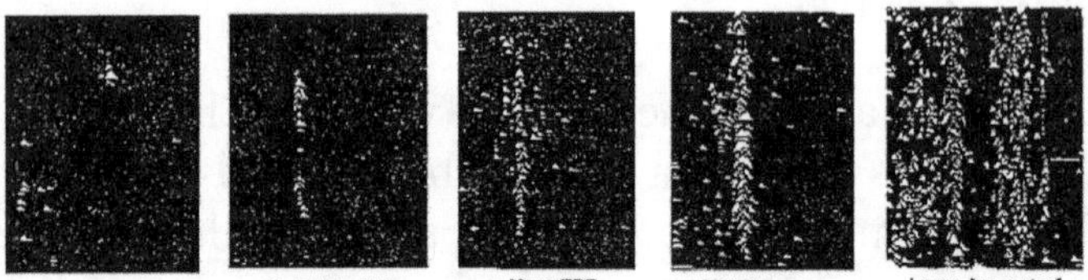

Low EEG Coherence Non-Meditator Sleep | Noticable EEG Coherence With 2 Weeks TM | More EEG Coherence at 4 Months TM | EEG Coherence Increased With 5 Years TM | Large Amount of EEG Coherence With 15 Years TM

Proof of TM's Improvement of Brain Function

Research proves that brainwave coherence is a direct result of practicing Transcendental Meditation. The above series of graphs shows that the practice of TM immediately creates measurable brainwave coherence at two weeks of practicing TM versus the low brainwave coherence of sleep. Progression of brainwave coherence is even more pronounced at 4 months of TM. The progression continues as shown at 5 years of TM. The 15-year TM meditator has remarkably coherent brainwave function. All this indicates that brain function is becoming more orderly with practice of TM. That orderliness is indicative of SELF-REFERRAL steadily improving over time. This is the basis of incredibly positive health benefits of practicing Transcendental Meditation. No other meditation technique - Mindfulness or otherwise - has been proven to cause these kind of improvements.

TM and Post-Traumatic Stress Disorder

Recent research has revealed that TM is extremely effective treating Post-Traumatic Stress Disorder. Given our recent extensive discussion about PTSD, this should be no surprise. We understand that extreme stressful life events like war experiences or violent life-threatening injuries cause Stress Syndrome - storing these memories as stressful engrams. These stressful engrams can retrigger at any time, causing vivid reexperiencing of the original events.

Whether the PTSD patient is a war veteran, has lived through life-threatening situations, or has suffered abuse - the effect is the same. The PTSD patient is haunted by recurring mental replays of stressful life events in dreams or while awake. They often suffer from anxiety, depression, and insomnia. All of this causes constant disruption of their lives. We know that PTSD is a stress-storage problem; what do we know about treating PTSD with TM?

A common method used to treat PTSD is exposure therapy. The PTSD patient is taught by counselors to consciously confront what is bothering them, the assumption being that as time goes on the patient will learn to better cope with the troubling memories.

A 2018 study compared a group of veterans with PTSD who were taught TM with veterans treated via standard exposure therapy. The results showed that 61% of veterans who learned TM had clinically significant improvement versus 42% treated with exposure therapy, and 32% with health education alone.[572] PTSD expert Dr. Vernon Barnes of Augusta University wrote in an editorial in the same issue of *Lancet*:

> The current study . . . advances the field, reporting benefit of the Transcendental Meditation Program in reducing PTSD in veterans . . . Consistent with military culture, the TM technique is self-administered, self-empowering, completely transportable, and inconspicuous.[573]

This study offered several examples of PTSD relief from TM. Following several tours of duty in Iraq and Afghanistan, a 33-year-old male Marine veteran suffered from depression and PTSD.

> I had a problem going to sleep and staying asleep on a regular basis. My mind was clouded with regrets and uncertainties. On some occasions I would think that I was better off dead, so I don't have to deal with it.

He learned Transcendental Meditation and very soon found that he was able to sleep through the night.

> Now, my mind is not as clouded as it was before. TM has helped me feel less stress and be more energized. With regular practice I've been able to manage myself and live a life that I enjoy.[574]

Another TM patient was a 32-year-old female Navy veteran diagnosed with military sexual trauma, which became PTSD following her discharge.

> I would drink alcohol in excess to numb the pain of loneliness I felt from isolation. I was afraid to venture out of my house or drive or do anything that included interaction with people.

Within a few days of meditating, she reported feeling calmer, and then, in the following weeks, she said,

> I began to trust and heal. I began to drive again, And I enrolled in community college. The TM Program has given me my life back.

TM is quite effective for PTSD, but there are more benefits. TM also reduces the need for psychotropic or mind-altering medications while under treatment for PTSD. Because TM reduces the stress that drives PTSD, patients under treatment often need fewer drugs, and even then, at lower doses.[575]

TM and Non-Veteran Post-Traumatic Stress Disorder

Finding severe, life-disrupting PTSD in military veterans is readily understandable. But what about PTSD caused by other severe stressful life events? Is TM useful in treating people with those problems?

People living in the African country of Uganda are frequently subjected to all manner of physical and psychological trauma because of frequent violent warfare there. Researchers studied PTSD in Congolese refugees who had survived the difficult situations in those areas. Some refugees were taught TM, and some were followed as controls. Those people who learned TM had a markedly rapid decrease in PTSD symptoms over time when compared to the non-meditating control group.[576]

People living in Japan suffered a severe earthquake-tsunami disaster in 2011. Two cities, Sendai and Ishinomaki, were strongly affected by the upheaval. Homes and workplaces were destroyed, and many people injured and killed. TM was taught to people who had survived the disaster. A control group was not taught TM. The TM groups in the two cities showed major reduction in stress levels after learning TM. The control groups had no changes and continued to have stress effects due to the disaster.[577]

People imprisoned in the penal system suffer severe stress. Crowded conditions, lack of privacy, forced regimented living, and a dangerous environment converge to create a lot of inmate stress. It should be no surprise that PTSD is a frequent result of the prison experience.

Researchers taught a large group of Oregon state correctional inmates TM. The prisoners were then followed over time to gauge the effects of TM. Those prisoners who practiced TM saw clear improvement in PTSD symptoms. There were strong and specific improvements in anxiety, depression, disassociation, and sleep disturbances. The control group had no such changes. These findings were true for both male[578] and female[579] prisoners.

TM and the Stress of Medical Practice

Everyone knows there are extraordinarily high levels of stress in rendering medical care. Doctors, nurses, and caregivers all work with sick and injured people. The job is physically and emotionally demanding. The work shifts are long, and the pressure never lets up. Can TM be of assistance to medical personnel?

Researchers taught doctors TM and tested them before instruction for signs of physician burnout, including depression and insomnia. The doctors practiced TM and were retested at 30-day and 90-day intervals. Comparing the TM doctors to controls, there was significant improvement in physician burnout, depression, and insomnia. This suggests that physicians everywhere would greatly benefit from learning the TM Technique.[580]

Like doctors, nurses work long hours with endless stress. Changing shift times and duties add to the pressures of the job. Would TM be of benefit to nursing personnel? A group of nurses were taught TM and followed over time. After four months practice of TM, the nurses showed marked improvement in burnout, secondary traumatic stress, and showed evidence of increased resilience – the ability to effectively meet new challenges. There also was reduced compassion fatigue, indicating improved ability to have caring feelings for patients.[581]

Another challenge for medical care personnel is the stress encountered by caregivers. These are support people who care for patients in hospitals, nursing homes, and home care. Some patients are unable to care for themselves, and caregivers have the often-demanding job of supplying care that debilitated patients need. Family caregivers are often under even more stress. They are responsible for care of needful family members at home. They are often not formally trained and work very hard to meet the needs of their ailing family members. The result is a lot of stress and hopelessness.

In this context, family caregivers were taught TM and allowed to practice it for two months. The results were dramatic. When compared to original measurements, there was significant improvement in their mood. They had clear improvement in anxiety, depression, confusion/bewilderment, anger and hostility, and fatigue. This resulted in the caregivers having a much better quality of life coping with their demanding duties.[582]

One of the most important ways to improve the healthcare system is to help those people who are stressed find effective stress relief. Everyone from doctors to nurses to caregivers report big improvements in their quality of life after learning TM. It is thus clear that the Transcendental Meditation Technique will be of great benefit to all personnel in the medical care delivery system.

TM and Stress in the Educational System

Everyone in the American educational system is aware of major difficulties in schools across the country. Poor academic performance, increasing failure rates, dropping out before graduation, and inability to gain entrance to higher education institutions are on the rise. All of this is directly or indirectly connected to the stress of modern life. Can TM help this concerning situation?

Children in grade school are at the beginning of their academic career. They are also learning critical interpersonal skills they will depend on for future success. A growing part of the educational literature call this social-emotional learning or SEM. Education professionals know that SEM forms the basis of student social behavior, academic performance, and emotional health.

A recent study taught TM to a large group of grade school students. They practiced TM twice a day for four months. The researchers measured their SEM levels and compared them to a control group who had never learned TM. The results were quite striking.

The TM students showed significantly higher SEMl learning skills. The TM students had better social skills, better ability to manage their feelings, and were better able to navigate social environments. They showed better ability to learn and solve problems. They were better able to control their own impulsive behavior and showed more care about themselves and others.[583]

A critical time in the lives of children growing up is junior and senior high school. Anxiety in response to the demands of school is very common. Many students become anxious from the demanding social and academic environment. Does TM help students with those problems? Researchers studied a group of 195 ninth graders in a California school district. They practiced TM regularly during school and on the weekends. Comparing them to a non-meditating control group from another school in the same district was very informative.

Over the six-month study period, there was a clear decrease in anxiety in the TM students. Their resilience was also measured; that is, the student's ability to encounter new stressful situations and adapt without anxiety. It is known that greater resilience indicates greater emotional capability to cope with stress.[584]

Do these improvements in TM students translate into improved academic performance? Students who do not perform well in school often have low grades and a tendency to fail. While grades are not everything, they are an important indicator of student success. Does learning TM help students improve their academic performance?

Students who are at-risk include those known to be living with many disadvantages. Such students may come from broken families, may be afflicted with poverty, prone to crime, or have exposure to drug abuse. Researchers taught TM to a group of at-risk students and then measured their subsequent academic performance three months later. The at-risk students had significant improvements in academic performance. Specifically, their improvements were in both mathematics achievement and language skills.[585]

Improving academic performance is wonderful, but at-risk students also have a strong association with failing to complete school and graduating. Following the same students through completion of high school, *the TM students had an 89% decrease in drop-out rate*. Finally, at-risk students are known to stop school early and not go on to higher education. *The same group of students had a 59.3% acceptance rate to college or other postsecondary schools compared to the non-TM rate of 33.3%.*[586]

Another part of the crisis in the educational system is teacher and school administrator burnout. Because of increasing stress from student social pressures, many teachers and administrators report burnout. This is identical to the problems encountered by veterans, doctors, nurses, and caregivers. The common denominator is high-stress work, day after day. Can TM help teachers and administrators?

Researchers taught TM to school administrators and teachers. After a four-month period, they compared stress-related emotional factors with the numbers from the beginning of the study. The findings were well-defined. *There was significant improvement in the educational professionals' ability to cope with stress*. The improvements included less depression, less teacher burnout, and improved perception of stress and how to handle it.[587]

Does TM help students at the college level? The Brain Integration Scale consists of measuring brain response while completing a performance test. Higher BIS scores indicate more comprehensive and effective brain operation during testing. Students who were taught TM increased their BIS score by 59% - indicating they were better able to take tests and have good scores. The TM students were also significantly less likely to be sleepy, which often interferes with studying and test taking.[588]

Just as strong brain integration supports students in college-level academics, experts are now saying it also correlates strongly with creativity and success in many professions. This includes top managers, world-class athletes, professional musicians, successful police, and creativity in general. *Based on the above findings, a strong argument can be made that TM is a major tool to unlock the best in human potential.*

The Basis for All This Success

Identifying the wide-ranging success of TM in combatting so many negative effects of stress is quite eye-opening. *We see here that many aspects of the negative impact of stress upon our culture, minds and bodies is completely treatable – and likely curable.* Further, it is obvious that people with normal brain function have better lives, better health, and more success in general than people who suffer brain deficit due to the negative effects of stress. These are strong conclusions, but can we find evidence that this is true?

We previously reviewed the facts concerning TM and brain physiology. Research studies have shown that EEG brain wave patterns show distinct changes as people practice TM. Specifically, the brain shows signs of getting in touch with itself. The brain waves on the right synchronize with those on the left. Synchronization also occurs between brain waves on the top and bottom of the brain, and front to back.

Another finding in many studies was that TM causes a unique physiologic state called restful alertness. That means that, during TM, the body goes into a profoundly deep state of physical rest while the conscious mind stays lively. That contrasts sharply with the states of being awake, sitting with eyes closed, or sleeping. This state of restful alertness is believed responsible for the many positive effects of TM.

Exciting new research takes these findings to a new level. Using an advanced imaging system called fMRI, researchers studied meditators as they practiced TM. They were studying brain circulation while people practiced TM. What did they find?

Brain circulation changed markedly during TM as seen by fMRI imaging. The fMRI images show in great detail what goes on with the circulation of the brain from moment to moment. During TM, the circulation to the pons, cerebellum, and brainstem at the back of the brain slowed down. At the same time circulation to the front of the brain increased. What does that mean?

The frontal area of the brain is the location for inner awareness, which indicates the restful alertness reported in previous studies has a real basis in fact. That is, the mental state areas of the brain are receiving more blood flow. At the same time, the areas of the brain associated with action - regulating blood pressure, heart rate, and other vital functions - are receiving comparatively less blood flow. *This confirms sharp mental alertness occurring simultaneously with deep rest. This is exactly the state of restful alertness reported during the practice of TM.*[589]

We Must Inoculate Against Stress

With what we know of the Adaptation Crisis, it is obvious that the stress of modern life is the root of our health problems. Stress also drives many of the social, legal, and even political problems that we face. I suggest – as Maharishi did - that we need to inoculate against the stress of modern life.

The way immunization works is we inject a substance that causes the body to produce antibodies against what we are immunizing against. This is a well-known medical principle. Using that approach, we have seen eradication of many diseases that used to exact a terrible cost in suffering. Diseases largely banished by this treatment include polio, diptheria, smallpox, and many others. This is so common that we just take it for granted.

I submit that we are at precisely the same place with stress. Is there evidence that this is true?

Serum cortisol is one of the stress chemicals, and one of the best indicators of chronic stress. It is a well-known fact that stress chemicals peak in the early morning hours. Researchers taught college students TM and checked their morning serum cortisol levels. With only four weeks of TM practice, their morning serum cortisol levels were significantly reduced compared to that of a control group, who were not taught TM. That means *TM not only worked to reduce stress immediately, but in only four weeks was reducing the effects of chronic stress.*[590]

Subsequent testing of the TM students versus controls also was impressive. Researchers measured the stress response in both the TM and control groups by exposing them to unexpected loud noise. The TM students had significantly less stress response to the loud noise compared with controls. *Again, this was only four weeks after learning TM.*

I submit that we have found the inoculation to protect against the stress of modern life. Teaching people TM will accomplish that quickly and effectively. *Learning TM is the critical way to immunize human beings from the negative effects of stress.*

An enormous literature now exists that verifies that TM improves the notorious hyper-arousal state of the autonomic nervous system. We now see that TM does this within four weeks of starting TM. With regular practice, TM rests and revives the autonomic nervous system - reversing the effects of stress.[591]

TM Solves the Adaptation Crisis

Adaptation is the body's ability to cope with the stress of life. Today's modern lifestyle stresses the human body beyond tolerance. The result is a myriad of chronic health problems caused by Stress Syndrome. This disruption of Self-Referral by stress causes all disease and the aging process. That single mechanism is the cause of so much misery and mischief that we can no longer ignore it.

The body depends on Self-Referral to cope with stress. Self-Referral works to maintain an ideal body environment in a constantly changing world. If stress disrupts any of the body's many feedback loops, disease results. Disease is the disharmony that results when Self-Referral can no longer maintain harmony.

Let us restate this in terms of Cybernetics. Returning to the example of thermostat and furnace, the brain is the thermostat, and the body is the furnace. Modern life simply sets the thermostat at an abnormally high setting. Stress Syndrome is like setting a thermostat at 110 degrees when the room only needs to be 70 degrees. The body is working too hard, and too hot - no wonder it breaks down and frequently wears out early.

This is the basis of the Adaptation Crisis – and this crisis is the enemy of human health; it also is the central challenge to the survival of the human race in our present historical moment.

The logical answer to the Adaptation Crisis is a stress reduction technique that reverses the pernicious effects of stress. Extensive scientific research proves that Transcendental Meditation (TM) is that technique. That TM reverses the hyper-arousal state is interesting. It is exceptional that stress related diseases respond so well to TM. Realizing that TM reverses the effects of stress is staggering. Is TM the answer to the Adaptation Crisis?

Dr. Harold H. Bloomfield, Michael Peter Cain, and Dennis T. Jaffe wrote the landmark best seller *TM: Discovering Inner Energy and Overcoming Stress*. This book made an eloquent case for TM as the logical answer to the Adaptation Crisis. Dr. Hans Selye - the father of the stress concept - wrote the book's forward[592] to plead the same case:

> TM's physiologic effects on metabolism, breathing, skin resistance, blood lactate, brain waves, and the cardiovascular system - are exactly the opposite to those identified by medicine as being characteristic of stress. Similarly, the therapeutic effect of TM on bodily derangements is most evident on those conditions known as "diseases of stress" or "diseases of adaptation" (especially mental, cardiovascular, gastrointestinal, and hypersensitivity ailments) which are caused by inappropriate adaptive responses to the stressors of everyday life.

TM's effects on stress related diseases are of great importance. TM is the key to the human body's anti-stress response, a critically needed therapeutic tool to supplement today's medical therapies.

TM offers the needed answer to the stress of modern life.

Self-Referral/Maximum Health seeks ways to help the body restore its harmony and promote health. When we look for ways to improve the body's ability to govern itself, TM is impressive. The TM technique is easy to learn and requires no therapist or special equipment. TM produces a state of deep rest that is distinct from being awake, sleeping, dreaming, or simply resting. TM reverses the pernicious effects of stress.

Common diseases related to stress improve with regular practice of TM. TM has no negative side effects and produces consistently positive results. Which stress reduction technique is most effective? *Volumes of scientific research answer this question: the TM technique is proven to be most effective.* This is why I clearly state: *TM solves the Adaptation Crisis.*

Today's scientific knowledge acknowledges TM as the single effective cure for Stress Syndrome, stress in the individual, and – ultimately – the Adaptation Crisis. Listing the prestigious scientific journals who have published articles of scientific research verifying and supporting TM is quite a formidable task. Those journals include[593]:

> Science, Lancet, Scientific American, American Journal of Physiology, International Journal of Neuroscience, Experimental Neurology, Electroencephalography and Clinical Neurophysiology, Psychosomatic Medicine, Canadian Medical Association Journal, American Psychologist, British Journal of Educational Psychology, Journal of Counseling Psychology, The Journal of Mind and Behavior, Academy of Management Journal, Journal of Conflict Resolution, Perceptual and Motor Skills, Criminal Justice and Behavior, Journal of Crime and Justice, Proceedings of the Endocrine Society, Journal of Clinical Psychiatry, and Social Indicators Research.[594]

To specifically access this vast library of scientific research, articles have been reproduced and bound in seven volumes as *Scientific Research on the Transcendental Meditation Program.* Anyone having an interest in TM and the research associated with it would find these large books both extremely educational and a gold mine of useful information.[595]

There can be no better validation than that of today's medical authorities. These are the institutions of medical knowledge and medical care that doctors and patients alike look to for the most accurate and up-to-date advice for medical care.

Positive recommendation from the Mayo Clinic:

> Transcendental meditation is a simple, natural technique... This form of meditation allows your body to settle into a state of profound rest and relaxation and your mind to achieve a state of inner peace, without needing to use concentration or effort."[596]

Positive recommendation from the Cleveland Clinic:

> Transcendental Meditation doesn't focus on breathing or chanting, like other forms of meditation. Instead, it encourages a restful state of mind beyond thinking... A 2009 study found Transcendental Meditation helped alleviate stress in college students, while another found it helped reduce blood pressure, anxiety, depression, and anger."[597]

The popular press has also picked up on the value of TM. From *Forbes Magazine*: "Perhaps its greatest benefit is that it's relatively quick to learn and easy to master. No waiting weeks or months of practice before you see results: TM cuts right to the chase, taking only days — or for some, minutes — before one feels reprieve from their painful and overwhelming thoughts."[598]

Self-Referral

Maximum Health

Chapter 10

Meditation and Health

The stress of modern life causes today's Adaptation Crisis. To better understand how Transcendental Meditation solves the Adaptation Crisis, we must know more about Transcendental Meditation.

Self-Referral and Modern Life

When we search for *Self-Referral/Maximum Health* we look for ways to help the body govern itself. The body governs itself through elegantly designed feedback loops. These mechanisms of Self-Referral promote health and prevent disease. Modern life challenges the body's ability to govern itself more than ever before, provoking today's Adaptation Crisis.

Humanity is now in an Adaptation Crisis caused by the pressures of modern life. The stress of modern life outstrips the body's ability to cope with it. This is why so many suffer from stress related diseases like high blood pressure, heart attack, stroke, ulcers, and mental illness. Stress also contributes to drug abuse, crime, violence, and disintegration of the family. This is how stress is killing people and destroying our culture.

Why can't Self-Referral keep up with the demands of modern life? Remember: Self-Referral is the balance of opposites. A very important pair of opposites is activity-rest. Self-Referral depends on a rested brain and body. This is why we must balance activity and rest to stay healthy.

How does modern life interfere with our ability to rest? Modern life is packed with change. Change challenges us from when the morning alarm goes off, wading through morning television and Internet news, looking through Facebook, and travelling to work. We meet more change at work through the day's job demands. Change challenges us after work when we try to wind down, get some rest, and fulfill family duties. By the time we go to bed, we often have problems sleeping thanks to the challenges of the day we just lived - and worrying about the challenges of tomorrow.

Change repeatedly triggers the brain's stress response, causing Stress Syndrome. This repeated firing of the stress response damages the brain. The brain, as the Self-Referral Center, passes damage elsewhere – anywhere in the body. This is how the constant barrage of sight, sound and experience disrupts health. Because of the challenges of modern life, today's people have more change per unit time than any population in known history – all provoking stress.

People learn about stress through television, newspapers, magazines, and online information. They want to improve their quality of life by reducing stress. There are many stress reduction techniques, but most are impractical. We know from scientific studies that Transcendental Meditation is today's most effective stress-reduction technique. TM has much to recommend it. It is easy to learn and needs no special equipment. TM requires only twenty minutes, twice a day.

Restoring Self-Referral

When we consider the stress of modern life, flexibility to change is critical. Self-Referral depends on constant communication between brain and body. We depend on Self-Referral every moment we live to maintain health. This is why health depends on flexibility of the nervous system. Lao-Tzu tells us:

> Men are born soft and supple; dead, they are stiff and hard. Plants are born tender and pliant; dead, they are brittle and dry. Thus whoever is stiff and inflexible is a disciple of death. Whoever is soft

> and yielding is a disciple of life. The hard and stiff will be broken. The soft and supple will prevail.[599]

To apply these ideas to our daily life, just think of the last time you missed a lot of sleep. It was difficult to wake up and hard to get out of bed. Even the shower was little help. You forced yourself to stay awake via will power and caffeine. You could only get the day out of the way and catch up on sleep later. You were not aware of it, but people thought you were irritable that day. Why? Lack of sleep made you inflexible.

Today's tension-packed society makes a night's sleep obsolete. Sleep no longer provides enough rest for today's stressful lifestyle. The pressures of modern life wear us down, even when we get plenty of sleep. The result is millions of people trying to carry on in a state of exhaustion.

Modern life stresses people more than ever. The pressure of this lifestyle also fatigues people. Today's stressed population suffers constant frustration as they struggle to keep up with life's demands. Stress cripples people, and they do not even know it. This is why so many people today assume that life is a struggle. Their own inflexibility prevents success and happiness.

Modern life disrupts Self-Referral between brain and body. Stress overloads the nervous system's ability to cope. This is how stress makes us inflexible. Lao-Tzu tells us the soft and supple will live, and the brittle and stiff will be broken. When we consider the deadly effects of stress, we see the accuracy of Lao-Tzu's words.

There is an ancient story about a mighty oak tree and a humble blade of grass:

> The oak tree was so large that it nearly blocked the sun from a tiny blade of grass growing at the edge of its shadow. The powerful oak, proud of its broad trunk and enormous branches, spoke to the insignificant blade of grass:

"Look at me, puny grass," the oak boasted. "My roots are deep, and I have grown strong. Nothing can hurt me, and I am lord of all I survey."

"You are right, Mighty Sir," the grass replied, feeling more insignificant than ever. "Your size and strength are without equal."

The oak tree smugly enjoyed his moment of power. The grass humbly went about the business of being a blade of grass. The days passed.

Suddenly, a great storm moved through the forest. A great wind with thunder and lightning turned the peaceful setting into a howling assault on the usual order of things. The oak tree felt the wind but strained to hold its ground. The grass did not resist the wind; rather, it moved without resistance as the windy blasts buffeted the hapless plant.

Without warning, the wind tore the oak tree out of the ground by its roots. The howling tempest tore the doomed tree in half. Then the branches gave way. One by one, the pieces of the tree splintered and blew out of sight. The storm raged all day and all night; then morning came.

The blade of grass that grew in the oak tree's shadow was still alive. Rather than being destroyed, the grass survived and thrived.[600]

Why did the wind destroy the oak while the grass survived? *The oak proved inflexible, while the blade of grass was flexible.* The grass was able to go with the wind's flow. The storm proved that flexibility counts far more than rigid strength. Through this story, we can better understand Lao-Tzu's warning:

> The hard and stiff will be broken.
> The soft and supple will prevail.[601]

I have heard so many people say, "that heart attack came from nowhere!" or "who could have seen that stroke coming?" These major health problems do not come suddenly; they come from the cumulative effects of stress. Little by little, one day at a time, the human body loses flexibility - and that loss over time brings the health disaster.

Stopping catastrophic events thus comes into focus as a necessity in medical care, and *stress reduction is the central issue*. This is exactly why restoring the body's flexibility is critical to maintaining health and preventing disease. Our bodies constantly create health through the flexibility of Self-Referral. Self-Referral allows moment-to-moment communication between brain and body. Self-Referral allows the body to quickly respond to life's demands. *This is why health depends on the flexibility provided by Self-Referral.*

TM Restores Flexibility

Research proves that TM restores flexibility because it restores Self-Referral. TM provides two periods of deep rest per day. This deep rest is unique and measurably different from sleep, resting with eyes closed, or other meditation techniques. TM's unique state of deep rest reverses the negative effects of stress. TM solves the Adaptation Crisis by restoring flexibility to people who have lost it.

To understand how TM works, we must examine TM in its own context. Where did TM originate? Who discovered TM? How did Western scientists come to study TM's effects?

Maharishi Mahesh Yogi, or Maharishi for short, was a Hindu monk from Northern India. It is through Maharishi's efforts that TM became available to the West. Leaving India in 1958, he traveled to Hawaii. In 1959 he moved to San Francisco. Maharishi then traveled all over the world, teaching TM wherever he went. Western scientists learned of TM through Maharishi's teaching.[602]

Maharishi brought TM to the West, but he was quick to say that he did not discover it. He learned TM from his Master, His Divinity

Swami Brahmananda Saraswati Maharaj, Shankaracharya of Jyotir Math. Maharishi referred to his Master by the shorter name of Guru Dev.

His Holiness
Maharishi Mahesh Yogi

After studying extensively with his Master, Guru Dev, Maharishi left India in 1958 to teach his Master's knowledge - touring the world five times from the years 1958 to 1965.

Maharishi's tireless lecturing, teaching, and organizing skills brought India's Vedic knowledge to the West. It is due to his infinite patience and tireless effort that TM and all related knowledge is available to everyone in the world today.

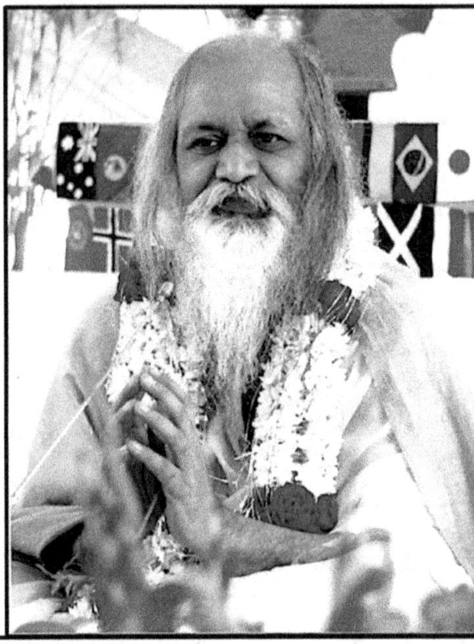

Guru Dev was the latest in an unbroken succession of Masters that monastic records trace to antiquity. These Masters taught students their knowledge for thousands of years, generation after generation. Maharishi studied with Guru Dev for thirteen years and then brought TM to the West.[603] This is why TM is not new; it is only new to the Western world, especially to Modern Medicine.

TM allows the mind to experience the whole range of itself. This is what the term Transcendental Meditation implies. Meditation means thinking or thought. Transcendental means beyond. Transcendental Meditation thus is a thinking technique that allows the mind to go beyond the usual range of thought.[604] What does this mean?

TM springs from an oral tradition that is at least six thousand years old. This is why Maharishi used many illustrative stories and figures of speech. He commonly explained how TM works through allegories.[605] We find many of these colorful stories in his books and lectures.[606] Let us examine some of Maharishi's stories that illustrate how TM works.

The Pond and the Swimmer

To illustrate how TM is different from ordinary thought, Maharishi suggested that we imagine the mind as a pond. Ordinary everyday thinking, he taught, is like swimming at the pond's surface.

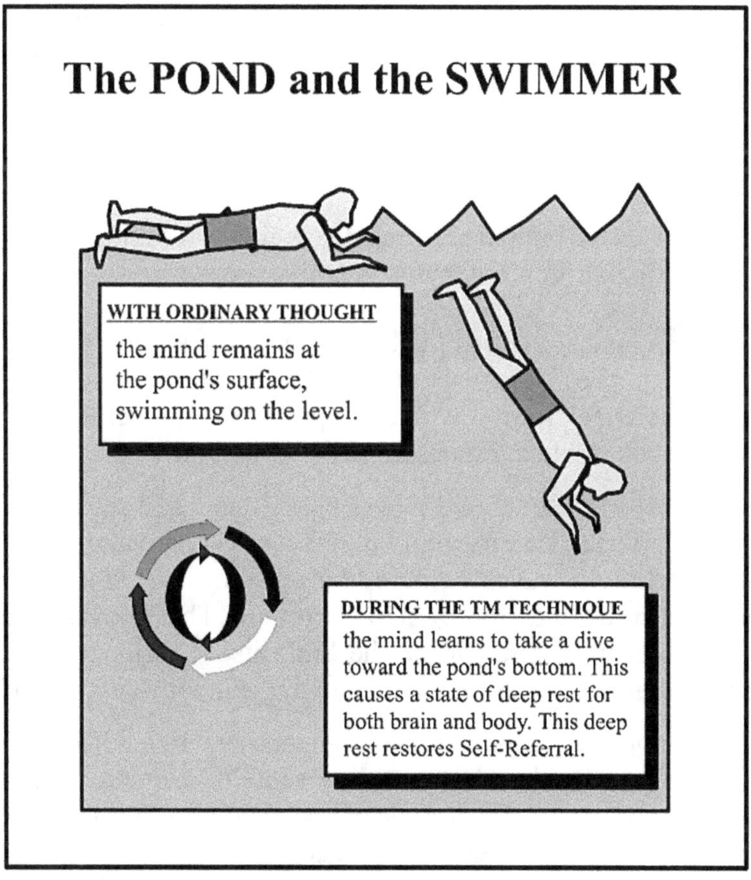
The POND and the SWIMMER
WITH ORDINARY THOUGHT
the mind remains at
the pond's surface,
swimming on the level.
DURING THE TM TECHNIQUE
the mind learns to take a dive
toward the pond's bottom. This
causes a state of deep rest for
both brain and body. This deep
rest restores Self-Referral.

Swimming at that level is the common experience of moving through the water, but we only stay at the water's surface. In this way we learn a little about the pond's waves and perhaps a small amount about the water a foot or two below the surface.

Maharishi said this is fine, but the experience is limited. If one learns to do a surface dive, he taught, then the whole experience of swimming changes. Instead of staying at the pond's surface, we change direction and dive into the pond's depths. Maharishi pointed out that when we learn TM, it is like learning to dive deeper toward the pond's bottom. Once we know how to dive, we can explore and enjoy more of the pond. This ancient allegory thus explains how TM allows our minds to experience deeper levels of thought.[607]

This is an excellent allegory, but can we apply it to today's knowledge about thinking and the brain? Doctors are only beginning to comprehend the human brain. Some scientists believe the brain is so complex that no one can understand it. Others say we can only know a small part of the brain's workings. For example, Professor David Hubel writes in the Scientific American book *The Brain*:

> Can the brain understand the brain? Is it some kind of giant computer, or something more?[608]

Research suggests that the brain can interact with itself directly. How can this be? Humans, through TM, trigger a high level of brain wave coherence. Brain wave studies prove that TM helps the brain to get more coordinated with itself. How do we know this?

Studies by Banquet and others prove that TM synchronizes the brain with itself. That is, front brain waves become like those in the back. Left brain waves become like those on the right. Top brain waves become like those in the bottom. This proves that TM promotes Self-Referral inside the brain itself. Stripping away the technical jargon, TM allows the brain to get in touch with itself.

The subjective experience of someone practicing TM is that of calming down inside. There is a deep sense of relaxation. Breathing and heart rate settle down in deep rest. The phrase "taking a dive" accurately describes this experience. We know from scientific research that the brain becomes more coherent and coordinated with itself. The description of a swimmer exploring more of the pond after taking a surface dive thus is also uncannily accurate.

Critics say the allegory of the pond and swimmer is not scientific. Of course, it is not scientific; *it is a subjective explanation - of a subjective experience!* It is only through the scientific study of TM that we appreciate the allegory's truth. The research done with TM is exciting. Why did it take so long to do the research that validates TM?

It is common to propose new ideas - but it may take a long time for them to be proven. Albert Einstein had important subjective ideas as far back as 1916 - early in his life.[609] Many ridiculed him for suggesting new explanations for how the universe works.

Scientists did not accept Einstein's published ideas until objective research proved what his subjective theories predicted.[610] That process continues today, with headlines still being generated by yet another scientific study proving Einstein's theories to be true through ongoing research.[611]

Maharishi, like Albert Einstein, perceived many universal truths early in life. He connected these principles with Modern Medicine in a practical way. The TM technique, while ancient in origin, is ultimately contemporary. It has taken modern science over 350 scientific studies to verify what Maharishi explained with simple stories and allegories during the 1950s and 1960s.[612]

The Bubble Diagram

Teachers of TM often use Maharishi's Bubble Diagram to explain how TM works. The pond represents the mind. Imagine a bubble rising from the bottom of the pond to the surface. The bubble represents a thought. The pond's surface represents the level of conscious thought. We usually become aware of the thought bubble only as it breaks at the pond's surface.[613] Why is this so?

Maharishi held that the average person's mind is only aware of the pond's surface and a shallow portion below it. Modern psychologists agree, saying that people typically use only a small part of the brain's potential. The thought bubble emerges at a very deep level, so we do not notice it until it rises to the surface.

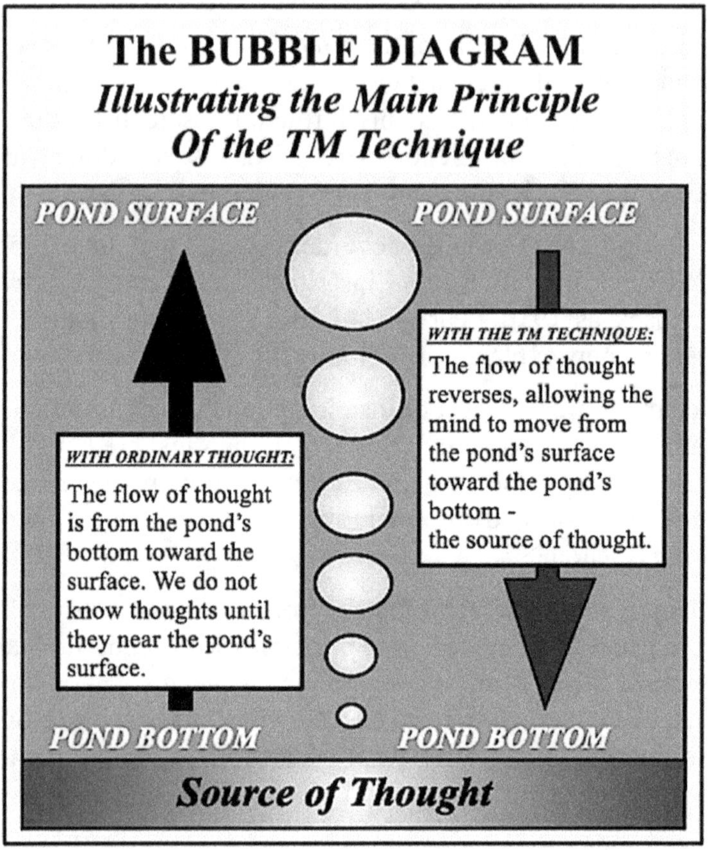

TM allows the meditator to reverse this process. This technique allows us to become aware of deeper levels of thought. We eventually go beyond, or transcend, thought itself. The mind then directly experiences the source of thought.

Maharishi allegorically placed the source of thought at the pond's bottom. When we practice TM, he said the mind has a natural tendency to move toward the source of thought. Why is this so? Maharishi said the closer the mind gets to the source of thought, the more pleasant the experience.

This explanation of TM is very ancient. While couched in modern terms, it is likely to be well over six thousand years old. Many will say that six-thousand-year-old ideas are of little use to today's medicine, chemistry, or engineering. The Bubble Diagram is a good teaching aid, but is it accurate?

The Bubble Diagram illustrates the overall physiologic effects of TM. The pond's surface corresponds to waking metabolism. As the mind moves toward the pond's bottom, body metabolism drops. This provides deep rest.

This ancient story also describes other physiologic changes. Maharishi calls the pond's surface gross, or easily perceived. He calls the deeper levels subtle, or less easily perceived. Heartbeat and breathing in the waking state are easily detectable. They thus are more gross than the subtle slow heartbeat and shallow breathing produced by TM's deep rest. TM produces deep rest, a pleasant experience. The person meditating would experience the deep rest as attractive.

Modern research thus confirms the ancient Bubble Diagram explanation. Maharishi refers to this as the main principle underlying TM. *This is the principle of transcending.* TM's oral tradition is thousands of years old – and we now see the ancient sages were uncannily accurate in their knowledge of human physiology.[614]

TM and Self-Referral

The Bubble Diagram explains how TM works, but it does not convey some aspects of TM. It shows mind and body moving from normal thought and metabolism to quieter thought and lower metabolism, and back. This gives a false impression that TM simply moves the body's metabolism up or down like an elevator. TM is a dynamic process and more complex than the Bubble Diagram suggests.[615]

Thinking does not require planning or effort on our part; it just happens. In the waking state, our minds spontaneously move from one thought to another. We may think of a camera we want to buy. Then we think about grocery shopping. After a while, we think about the air hammer we hear across the street.

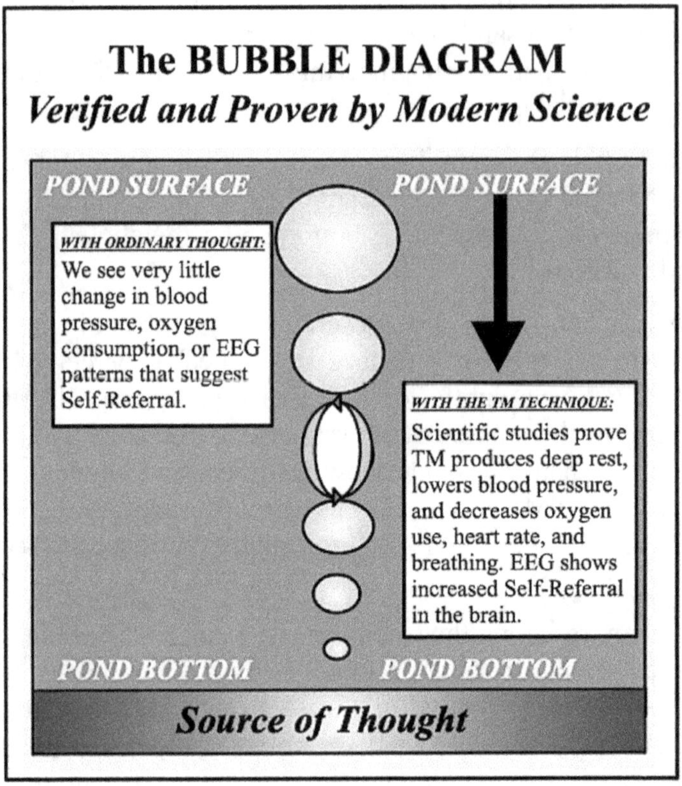

This is like the swimmer in the pond. While swimming at the surface level, one thought is like a wave - first we meet one, then another, then another.[616] Most people's thinking is like this; we can call this horizontal thinking.

Like the swimmer, if we learn to dive - new possibilities open to us. We are no longer limited to meeting thought waves sequentially, one at a time. What is the result? TM provides deep rest for brain and body, but there is much more to it. We begin to explore deeper levels of the pond: we begin to know more and more of our own awareness. In this sense, *TM introduces a vertical component to a normally horizontal situation; it is a truly novel mode of mind-body operation.*

Seen through Cybernetics, *we can define TM as a feedback loop between our conscious mind and the source of thought*. We thus can diagram TM as a circle. Half the circle represents the mind and body settling down to a state of deep rest; the other half circle represents the return to activity at the pond's surface. This circular process of alternating deep rest and activity restores Self-Referral. Maharishi said that the mind simply does what it needs to get deep rest. *This process is a natural tendency of the human mind.*[617]

TM and Stress Storage

We know the brain stores experiences as memory. Most memories are harmless, creating normal engrams. Strong stressful life events cause *stressful engrams*, triggering Stress Syndrome – and this causes problems like Post-Traumatic Stress Disorder. Extremely disturbing events literally become engraved in the brain. These adrenaline-etched memories cause disquieting repeated mental playbacks. These memory playbacks cause repeating stress response, long after the event is past – disrupting Self-Referral. Is there some description of this process in TM's ancient knowledge?

Maharishi described such a stress storage mechanism. Referring to the allegory of the pond, he said stressful life events create impressions at the finest level of the mind. In the Bubble Diagram, this is at the pond's bottom.[618] When a person is strained and fatigued, Maharishi said, stressful experiences add to these impressions. These impressions interfere with normal operation of the nervous system.[619] Regular practice of TM, he said, restores Self-Referral and promotes health.[620]

The ancient knowledge that stands behind TM deserves careful examination. Investigating these ideas in the light of modern science reveals valuable insights. Can we learn more about stress storage from this ancient oral tradition?

Patanjali was a Maharishi of ancient India. The dates of his life are uncertain. Estimated dates of his written works are from 400 B.C. to 400 A.D. Other than his written works, we know little of Patanjali the man. Like our era's Maharishi, he worked to define and teach meditation during his life.[621]

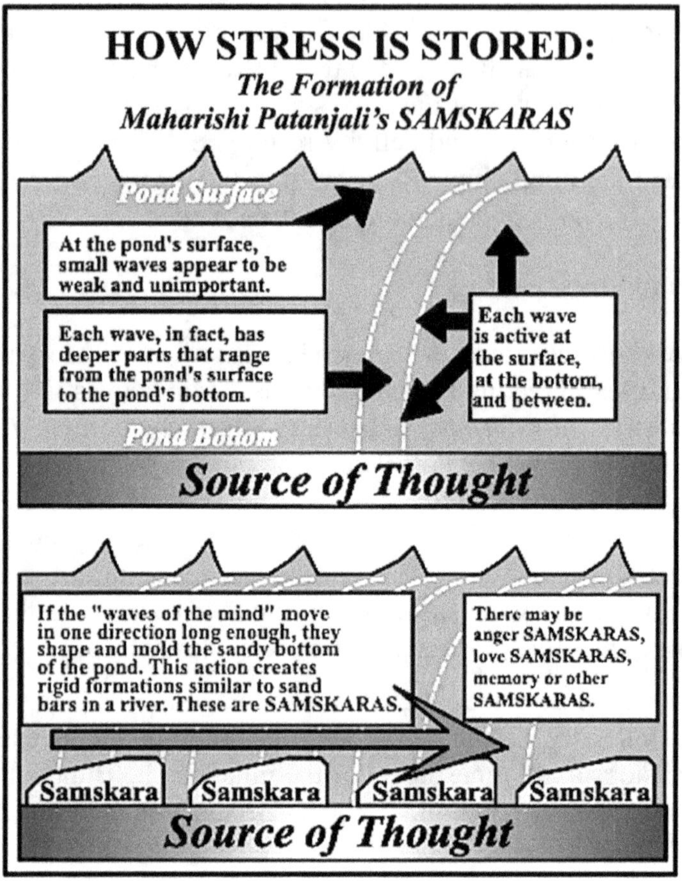

Like the Maharishi of our times, Patanjali used the example of a pond. The pond represents the brain; thoughts are waves passing through the pond. A wave at the surface may appear weak - but the wave extends into deeper levels of the pond. He said that small waves at the surface are actually deep and powerful.[622]

Patanjali's pond has a sandy bottom. Waves passing through the pond create banks of sand on the pond's bottom. These sandy banks at the bottom are more permanent than waves passing over them. Repeated passing of similar waves creates the pond's sand bars. Patanjali said *the sand bars represent the tendencies of the mind*.[623]

Patanjali called these sand bar patterns *Samskaras*. Sustained thought waves in one direction, he said, may add to existing Samskaras – or create new Samskaras. He also noted that Samskaras can influence future thought waves - just by their presence.

How can Samskaras affect future thoughts? Remember: all surface waves, no matter how small, extend to the pond's bottom. A large sand bar in a river affects the river's flow – guiding all passing waves in its direction. That is how Samskaras affect thought waves. Even if a thought wave begins in a different direction, the Samskaras at the bottom will redirect the wave in their predominant direction.[624]

Patanjali taught that Samskaras form the basis of personality.[625] To illustrate, we all know people with a bad temper. Why do these people get mad so easily? Patanjali said that these people have many anger Samskaras. Sometime in the past, this person repeatedly experienced anger. Repeated temporary thought waves of anger shaped the sandy bottom into permanent patterns of anger. As time went on, patterns favorable to anger become permanent and made the person prone to anger.[626] The same is true of other aspects of personality and thinking.

Good Waves, Bad Waves

This would sound like another quaint allegory if we did not know about Post-Traumatic Stress Disorder. We know terrible stress like that produced experiencing war affects the brain. The stress of modern life is seldom as intense as wartime experiences, but over time, it also creates negative effects. This is how the accelerated change of modern life badly stresses most people. Today's stressful lifestyle is far more intense than that of the rural, agricultural life lived by people in Patanjali's time. If Samskaras were significant in Patanjali's time, they must be even more significant today.

People today spend hundreds of hours per year watching television, movies, and rented videos. I wonder about the stress created by this viewing. Today's television and movies contain acts of violence, sexuality, and coarse language unheard of thirty years ago. Horror, science fiction, and action-adventure films feature shootings, stabbings, and even decapitations as standard fare shown in grisly detail.

We know these events are fictional, but they must have some effect on our nervous system. Special effects simulate such horrors, but our minds reflexively accept them as real. What kind of Samskaras are we burning into our brains with this material? How much disease does this stress add to our bodies?

This toxic material poses a problem for consenting adults – but modern technology brings this material to anyone, no matter how old they are, or whether they are ready for it. Most homes today have a television set with cable, satellite, or streaming services and a video player. This exposes many innocent children to disturbing events that seem real – and in former times would have been far from their experience. Easy access via the Internet and streaming cell phones magnifies this problem exponentially.

Even ignoring stressors like excesses in entertainment, the pace of modern life is relentless. Modern life creates stress that is beyond our control. The phone rings. We must meet an impossible deadline. The children need to get to school on time. All this daily stress contributes to Samskara patterns.

I was recently given a valuable insight from a friend regarding the pace and demands of modern life. He works in sales and service in the Recreational Vehicle manufacturing industry. He told me that people are getting more and more demanding. When people ordered parts ten years ago, they understood it would take some time to make and deliver the parts. Today, he tells me, people just go ballistic if there is delay of any kind. As a result, it is push, push - and no quarter given – making it much harder on everyone.

People I know in the field of medical care tell me the same story. Patients are getting more and more demanding. Any delay in service or less than perfect performance provokes a severe anger reaction. This is often way out of proportion to the actual situation.

On the other end of the system, looking from healthcare management down to medical care providers, leadership is getting more and more oriented to numbers driven and highly scripted goals. All of this puts undue pressure on everyone providing medical care to the public – and destroys patient-doctor relationships.

Nearly everyone can tell stories about the clear ratcheting up of pressure on people throughout modern culture. Part of this is doubtless technology driven. That is, people work with computers to study how to do things better. Then leadership does what the study suggests, trying to improve operations. This often changes how people do their jobs. Before you know it, the easy way to do an effective job gets changed all around. One job is moved into three jobs that involve making everyone miserable in the process.

This is how the stress of life shapes - and often distorts - the nervous system. For example, stressful life events cause some Samskara patterns. Negative emotions like anger, anxiety or worry form other patterns. Bad habits like Type A behavior add to Samskara patterns. And – through it all – the relentless stress of modern life impacts us all.

TM Dissolves Stored Stress

This is why Maharishi said that the stress of modern life creates deep exhaustion. Fatigue builds up over time, wearing down the nervous system.[627] TM provides deep rest supplemental to sleep. Regular TM also removes accumulated stress.[628] However, TM is not a quick fix, Maharishi maintained. *It is the repeated practice of TM that gradually releases stored stress.*

Why is this true? Stress builds Samskaras gradually over time. The gentle removal of Samskaras by TM also takes time. When mind and body settle down during TM, the body gets deep rest – and repairs Samskara damage caused by stress.[629] During this process the brain optimizes its own operation, restoring its own Self-Referral. With repeated practice, Maharishi said that TM will gradually wear away all patterns of stored stress, restoring complete Self-Referral.[630]

As one practices TM twice a day over time, one slowly wears away the Samskaras caused by stress. We can imagine a pond bottom that is smooth and without sand bars. This corresponds to a perfectly functioning brain and nervous system. Self-Referral would then be free of all obstruction. This is the ultimate restoral of Self-Referral.

TM Removes Stored Stress
and Restores SELF-REFERRAL

Regular practice of the TM Technique provides deep rest – and as the body rests, TM allows the body to wear away the SAMSKARAS, leaving a stress-free nervous system and better health.

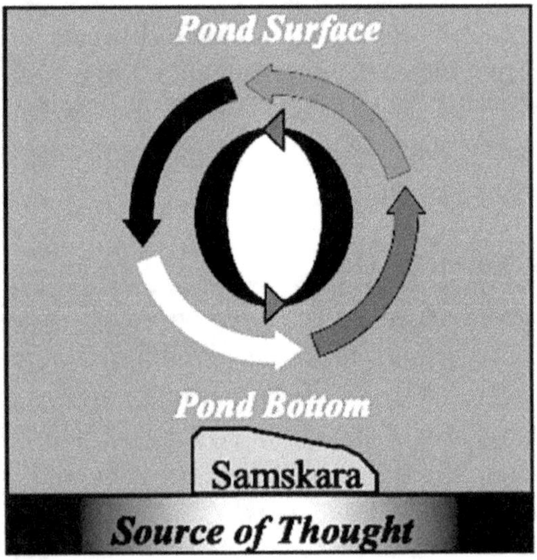

631

Maharishi called this the state of Enlightenment. This sounds like an unattainable goal to many, but Maharishi insisted that Enlightenment is the normal state of human life. He said *the daily experience that most humans today accept as normal is, in reality, far below normal.*

After reviewing state of the art stress research, these ideas are clear and timely. Please remember, however, that these ideas are from a book published in 1968. Type A and Type B personalities were only ideas. The clogged pipes theory was still the commonly accepted theory of angina pectoris. Vasospasm, Beta Blockers, ACE Inhibitors, and all the other stress-treating medications were far in the future. *We see again that TM was far ahead of its time.*

TM Versus Other Meditation Techniques – Again

Several competing Meditation techniques exist today – notably the *Relaxation Response* and *Mindfulness*. Scientific research proves that TM works, but what about these Meditation techniques? Do they also relieve stress?

Following Wallace's work, doctors and patients only heard part of the news. Meditation was good, they heard, but they thought TM was one among many Meditation techniques. One type of Meditation was as good as another, they reasoned. Besides, it might be cheaper and easier to learn it from a book. Dr. Herbert Benson was one of the first to suggest this.[632]

In 1968, Dr. Benson was associated with The Harvard Medical School and Beth Israel Hospital in Boston. He studied TM's effect on high blood pressure.[633] He co-authored several articles with TM pioneer Dr. Robert Keith Wallace. These studies proved TM's stress reduction effects[634] including improved body chemistry,[635] improved high blood pressure,[636] and reduction in drug abuse.[637]

Dr. Benson later published a book called *The Relaxation Response* in 1976. He made a good case for a link between stress and cardiovascular disease - specifically heart attack, high blood pressure, and stroke. He reasoned from animal studies that the body must have a natural anti-stress mechanism for relaxation. He called this the *Relaxation Response*.[638]

Dr. Benson believed that TM was not unique in producing the Relaxation Response. He argued that several stress reduction techniques also produce the Relaxation Response. These included Zen meditation, Hypnosis, and Progressive Muscle Relaxation.[639] Benson offered his own technique called The Relaxation Response, stating that it did not matter which stress reduction technique anyone used – all of them worked, based on the Relaxation Response mechanism.[640]

Benson claimed the Relaxation Response reduced blood pressure, heart rate, oxygen consumption, and blood lactate levels.[641] Preliminary studies showed that it also improved high blood pressure.[642] These effects were like those produced by TM, but the similarity ended there. Later research testing these techniques - reviewed in previous chapters of this book - proved the other techniques were vastly inferior to TM.

We know the stress response begins in the brain. A stress reduction technique thus should affect the brain in measurable ways. TM produces whole body rest, but it also produces unique EEG brain wave changes distinct from resting, sleeping, and dreaming.[643] TM also produces brain wave changes that restore the brain's Self-Referral.[644] Benson's Relaxation Response does not produce these unique brain wave changes.[645]

Moreover, researchers have not adequately studied the long-term effects of the Relaxation Response. Hundreds of international studies prove that TM improves hypertension, angina pectoris, asthma, mental illness, and the quality of life. The same studies prove that TM has no unpleasant or dangerous side effects. The Relaxation Response has not had one-tenth the study that TM has. Benson's claim that the Relaxation Response is equivalent to TM thus is highly questionable.[646]

Benson did bring up one important point. He believed that the specific sound, or mantra, used during meditation was not important. Benson wrote that a person could choose any mantra, such as a simple word like "One." Was he correct?[647]

Does the Mantra Matter?

Misinformation about Meditation techniques misleads many people. There is little superficial difference between TM and Benson's Relaxation Response. Both require one to sit still, close the eyes, and perform a simple mental technique. This confusion has led to hundreds of copycat meditation techniques.

Yet despite these similarities, scientific studies show that TM produces unique body changes that the Relaxation Response does not. The key difference is that TM reverses the autonomic hyper-arousal that causes so many stress-related disorders - and the Relaxation Response does not.[648]

What is special about TM that produces such unique effects? Glueck and Stroebel concluded that it was the unique effect of TM's sound, or *mantra*. Meditators mentally repeat the mantra during TM. They speculated that the mantra stimulates the limbic system of the brain in a unique way. *They believed the mantra is the key that unlocks the complete anti-stress response in the human body.*[649]

Suggesting that TM's mantra is a key to unlock the body's anti-stress response at first sounds fanciful. Is this just another Eastern allegory? I think not. To illustrate, enzymes are chemicals found throughout the body. Enzymes are critical to many chemical reactions that maintain health. One such enzyme allows oxygen to bind to hemoglobin in our red blood cells. This enzyme works to get the oxygen we need to live.[650]

There are many such enzymes in the body. If there are many enzymes at work, why do they always work correctly? Do the chemical reactions ever become confused? That is, why does *only* one enzyme work in one situation and *only* a second enzyme works in another?

Biochemists know that *each enzyme has a unique structure*. This structure exactly matches the molecular structure of the other chemicals involved in the reaction. *It is the unique lock and key operation of enzymes that prevent enzyme errors throughout the body.*[651]

We know that thought is closely related to brain chemistry. Thought occurs through the chemical activity of brain neurons. Brain chemistry also influences the quality of thought. For example, brain chemistry imbalances cause both depression and anxiety. Stress causes these disorders, and medications correct these specific chemical imbalances.

This is how TM's mantra - a thought - provokes a physical response in the brain. This response optimizes brain wave activity and provides deep rest. *The special mantras used in TM thus are thought equivalents of a biochemical enzyme.* We know that only certain enzymes - specific as a lock and key - will trigger a given biochemical reaction, and no other. Likewise, *only the correct mantra will trigger TM's deep rest.* What is unique about the TM mantras?

The mantras and their proper use are an oral tradition that originates in India. Masters passed this knowledge to their students for at least six thousand years. TM instructors report they are sounds without intellectual meaning, and they assign different mantras to different people. TM instructors and meditators keep the mantras secret to preserve their effectiveness.[652]

Some people experiment with a mantra from a book or elsewhere. This is exactly what Dr. Benson advocates in *The Relaxation Response*. Benson suggests mentally repeating the word "One." Many TM critics point out that even if the Relaxation Response is less effective, surely practicing it is harmless.

Nothing could be farther from the truth. *Using the wrong mantra causes many problems - some minor and others major*. People have picked nonsense syllables, pleasant sounds, or words with pleasant meanings. They mentally repeat these sounds in the style of TM. Reported effects have included headaches, poor attention span, and anxiety.[653]

One example is the mantra OM. Many people have chosen this mantra, mentally repeating it while resting with their eyes closed. People often report negative results from this practice. One 28-year-old individual offered the following experience:

> I was into an Om meditation [Using "Om" as the mantra] . . While I was doing it, I would be in a beautiful mood, but if I left my room or had to deal with everyday things I was definitely incapacitated. After six months, I felt an incredible conflict. I got to the point where I couldn't do anything - I was so split.[654]

These effects are logical in the light of modern Meditation research. We know that TM produces profound body changes, especially in the brain. We also know that TM improves health and the quality of life. *The correct mantra produces positive body changes. A wrong mantra likely causes negative body changes*. This is why using a wrong mantra is extremely unwise and possibly injurious. The person troubled by the OM meditation started TM with the correct mantra and instruction. The change was immediate:

> After I started TM every day just got brighter. I was finally getting what I was looking for but was always missing. Now I'm working again and just got promoted. My energy level has increased at least 200%.655

Unfortunately, many in medical circles still accept Benson's opinion that the mantra does not matter. This is why so many mistakenly assume that any Meditation technique is equivalent to TM. When non-TM Meditation does not produce the expected benefits, many take it as proof that TM does not work.

For example, researchers studied Meditation's effect on high blood pressure at Wright-Patterson Air Force Base in 1980. Working with 55 patients, they taught half the patients a non-TM meditation technique. The Meditation group used the mantra "Baba Nam Kevalam." This translates as "Love is all there is."[656] The control patients attended lectures on health topics.

The results were clear: non-TM Meditation produced little change in the patients' high blood pressure. Unfortunately, many who read the article also assumed that TM did not work.[657] This was not true, but the confusion created by Benson and others made many readers assume this was the case.

TM Vs. Other Meditation Techniques

Mindfulness is a system of thinking and lifestyle practice that uses the conscious mind to transform health – both mental and physical – for the better. Mindfulness is a practice of realigning thinking to be more aware of ourselves, our surroundings, and other people.

Mindfulness is an intentional way of thinking and doing that works to help us see life and our place in it. By seeing ourselves more clearly and understanding better that we are part of the greater universe, Mindfulness works to help us better understand others and thus become less judgmental and harsh – on ourselves and others. All these ideas are very positive and have much in common with teachings of the major religions of the world. Mindfulness thus would doubtless improve anyone's life who learned to apply and live these principles.

Central to the practice of Mindfulness is mindfulness-based stress reduction (MBSR) and mindfulness-based cognitive therapy (MBCT).[658] Both techniques and practices rely on use of the conscious mind and therefore have nothing in common with Transcendental Meditation. No technique of Mindfulness produces TM's deep rest or restoration of the brain's Self-Referral. *By contrast, many brain studies clearly show that TM brings synchronization of brain waves side to side, top to bottom, and front to back. No other technique has been shown to do this.*

Finally, meta-analysis is a powerful tool that statisticians use to study complex issues in research. Researchers now use Meta-analysis to study questions like which high blood pressure medication works best. Using meta-analysis, researchers can add the results from many individual experimental studies together. With advanced mathematics, they can treat all the data as though it were part of one big experiment. Then they can come to authoritative conclusions.

There have been many research studies published since the 1960s studying relaxation techniques. TM researchers Dr. Michael C. Dillbeck and Dr. David W. Orme-Johnson conducted a meta-analysis of all the TM research versus that done with other relaxation techniques. *They found that TM produced twice the deep rest that other techniques provided.*[659] Recent meta-analysis research has even further refined the contrast between TM, Mindfulness, and other meditation techniques.

Meta-analysis research clearly shows that TM reduces anxiety more effectively than Mindfulness,[660] both in people who suffered excess anxiety before learning TM and in those who started TM without excess anxiety.[661] A meta-analysis done at the Chemnitz University of Technology in Germany found that *TM has far more effect than Mindfulness and other meditation techniques in reducing negative emotions like anger, confusion, depression, guilt, fatigue, tension, distrust, suspiciousness, and frustration.*[662] All this confirms that TM is by far the most effective stress reduction technique available today.

The Burden of Proof

Regarding claims to be equivalent to TM in stress reduction effectiveness, the burden of proof clearly is with the challenger. Doctors and patients should no longer accept claims that unproven meditation techniques are just as effective as TM. Dr. Benson's Relaxation Response, advocates of Mindfulness, and others have challenged TM on the field of science. Very well, this is as it should be. If these critics want to claim equivalence of the Relaxation Response or Mindfulness with TM, they will need an ambitious research program to match the research done on TM. *And they need to prove their claims.*

TM now has many imitators. Supermarket checkout counters often sell books that teach Meditation. Bookstore shelves often feature self-proclaimed Meditation "masters." Celebrities pump out Meditation books and audio CDs on a regular basis.

These well-meaning people are contributing to the stress problem; when they teach bogus techniques to stressed individuals, the pseudo-Meditation will not help them. As we have seen through the research described earlier, such bogus techniques will likely have negative effects, making a bad problem worse.

> *Why would anyone risk their mental and physical health with unproven Meditation techniques?*

Meditation is no longer an unscientific subject. In previous times, one opinion was as good as another. This is no longer the case. More than fifty years of research proves that Meditation has powerful effects on the brain and body. Using a poorly studied technique is like taking medicine from an unlabeled jar, hoping it will help you. The bogus pills not only fail to work as advertised – they also may harm you.

TM: A Worldwide Success

The Adaptation Crisis is real. Stress is a life-threatening problem in today's world. Many thinking people want to meditate for relief from stress. Those who say "just use any Meditation technique" are giving bad advice. Science proves the ancient tradition that stands behind TM is true and effective. Why accept an ineffective or even dangerous substitute?

As of 2017, over five million people worldwide practice TM.[663] One million of them are in the United States. TM practitioners include people from every age, sex, profession, educational background, and religion. And the number of TM meditators keeps growing.[664]

Why has TM fared so well, especially among the modern, scientific people of the West? One reason is the scientific basis of Transcendental Meditation. Science shows that TM does what it claims. Maharishi was always eager to submit TM to scientific scrutiny[665] - and TM proved itself.

Another reason for success is the secular and nonpolitical nature of TM. Maharishi refused to tie Transcendental Meditation to any system of politics[666] or religion.[667] Maharishi avoided political and religious controversy whenever possible.

Modern Medicine has produced ingenious medications, but doctors often ignore underlying stress. Doctors can turn down the stress thermostat with drugs, but this only masks the real problem.

We can regain true health only by restoring Self-Referral. Doctors prescribing drugs cannot impose this kind of health externally. Patients must restore it from within themselves.

Maharishi often voiced compassion for human suffering. "Dr. Salk invented a vaccine for polio and in months everyone was inoculated," he remarked. "Polio was missing from American life." Maharishi was convinced that TM and related knowledge can ultimately save humanity from the dire problems it now faces. "When something is found to work," he asked, "why delay?"[668]

Chapter 11

Self-Referral and Movement

Movement is one measure of life itself, and we depend upon movement for an active life. Stress disrupts Self-Referral and movement. How can we restore the Self-Referral of movement?

The Self-Referral of Movement

When we seek *Self-Referral/Maximum Health* we look for ways to improve the body's ability to govern itself. Self-Referral maintains an ideal body environment in a constantly changing world. The brain – as the body's Self-Referral Center - coordinates Self-Referral between brain, body, and environment.

The brain as the Self-Referral Center operates by coordinating with the body through nerves. These form feedback loops between brain and body. These elegantly designed mechanisms allow the brain to govern the body, much as a thermostat governs a furnace. Brain and body work together through Self-Referral to maintain health and prevent disease.

Self-Referral balances pairs of opposites like hot-cold and fast-slow. *One important pair of opposites is that of tight-loose.* All the body's muscles can be either *tight* or *loose*. When a muscle becomes tight, we say it contracts; when it becomes loose, we say it relaxes.

Muscles contract or relax to maintain body posture, as in standing or sitting. Muscles also contract and relax whenever we move, as in walking or running. That is why all muscle action depends on communication between brain and muscle.

Whether we stand, sit, walk, or run - constant Self-Referral between brain and muscle is responsible. Muscles and muscle groups are coordinated by the brain to allow these complex actions to run smoothly. This is how the brain as the Self-Referral Center coordinates every muscle in the body.

Modern life generates stress that disrupts Self-Referral, creating an epidemic of stress-related disease caused by Stress Syndrome and – ultimately - the Adaptation Crisis. Disruptions of Self-Referral interrupt many feedback loops between brain and body. We know that stress affects heart, lungs, and arteries. What happens when stress disrupts Self-Referral between brain and muscle? To answer this question, we must know .more about Self-Referral and movement. How does Self-Referral apply to movement?

Returning to the concept of the Tao, the pair of opposites *contract-relax* are perfect examples of opposing forces, or opposites. When the opposites are perfectly balanced, we have harmony, balance, and perfect Self-Referral. Let's take a closer look at the Tao. Improving our understanding of the philosophy of the Tao will give us greater understanding of the role of Self-Referral in movement.

When we translate the Tao, single word definitions fail. Because of the structure of Chinese language, translating ideas into English is often difficult. Much of written Chinese depends upon complex characters, called pictographs. These symbols are made up of many lines and shapes. Pictographs are symbols that stand for clusters of interrelated ideas.

This is a different approach to language than English, where single letters are of little use. We combine English letters to form words, and words form sentences. We put sentences together to create paragraphs. A single Chinese pictograph, by contrast, may require a phrase or a whole sentence in English to convey the same meaning.

Let's say we want to write the word "bark" in Chinese. We do not write a series of letters to spell the word "bark." Instead, we combine two pictographs - the symbol for "mouth" and the symbol for "dog."

The resulting pictograph means "bark." This is how reading Chinese is different from reading English. Each pictograph is a cluster of ideas that, together, convey meaning. This is why English translations of a pictograph often require complex phrases. [669]

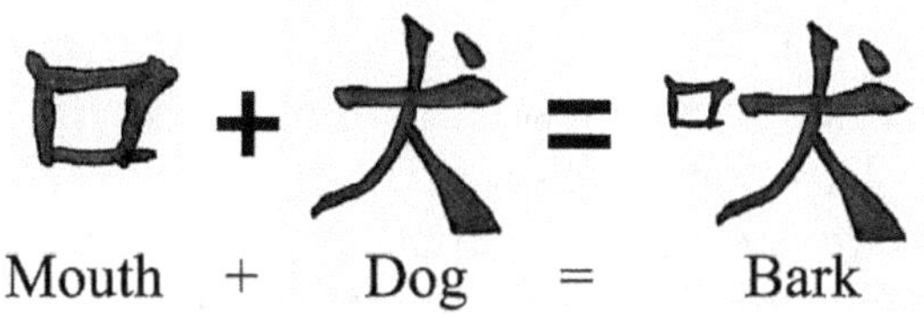

Chinese Pictographs Combine to Make A New Idea

This is why sometimes many words or phrases can be needed to translate complex ideas in pictographs to understandable English equivilent words.

Ignoring language differences, we need many words to define the Tao because deep philosophy lies behind the term. Some English translations of “the Tao” are "the way,” “the channel of a river,” “a road," and "the way to go." [670] My personal interpretation of the Tao is "the flow of the Universe," or “the will of God.”

These ideas point toward the most complete, comprehensive, and beneficial flow - of everything. This implies movement – of things, circumstances, ideas, principles in the physiology, and changes in life. Movement thus is central to the Tao. All these definitions imply movement – but specific movement of exactly what?

Movement Means Life

Through experience, we know that everything alive moves. Babies crawl and older people walk or run. Animals and insects walk, run, slither, climb, hop, or fly. Time-lapse photography reveals that even plants move, too slowly for humans to notice. When a living creature falls and never moves again, we say it is dead. *We thus define life itself - in part - by movement. Self-Referral is intimately related to movement.*

The heart, for example, is a pump. Every heartbeat contracts the heart's muscular walls, shrinking the heart's internal chambers. The force of this movement propels blood through the heart and drives it throughout the body. Between beats, the heart relaxes and fills with blood – preparing for the next beat. Movement drives each heartbeat, and each heartbeat is a balance between contract-relax – perfect balance of a pair of opposites.

Blood circulation is critical to health. Our bodies depend on blood moving through arteries to deliver critical oxygen and nutrients. Blood moving through veins carries off waste products and carbon dioxide.

Muscles in the arteries contract-relax to distribute the blood's flow. Movement of body muscles around veins help blood to return to the heart. This combination of heart, artery, vein, and muscle coordinates circulation throughout the body. Movement drives circulation, and the work of circulation is a balance between *contract-relax*.

The body depends on movement to breathe. Muscles expand and contract the rib cage and diaphragm with every breath. Air moves in and out of the lungs, regulated by bronchial muscle - like the muscles in the arteries. Movement drives breathing, and the work of each breath is a balance between *contract-relax*.

Our ability to eat and digest food depends on movement. Muscles help us bite, chew, and swallow food. The stomach, largely muscle, grinds food to aid digestion. Muscular intestines move food along for more grinding and absorption of nutrients. Muscles of the colon and rectum eliminate waste products. We depend on movement to process water and other fluids. Bladder muscles allow us to eliminate urine. Movement thus drives eating, digestion, and urine and waste disposal. All this is a balance between *contract-relax*.

This is how our bodies are always in some kind of motion, even though we do not notice it. All this internal movement is hidden from view - but our lives depend upon it every day. Movement thus drives the vital activities of the body's many parts, and the work is a balance between *contract-relax*.

Here we see the importance of the Tao-like balance between contract-relax. If all the body's contract-relax is in balance, we have health; an imbalance causes disease. This same mechanism provides health and prevents disease with the heart, the intestine, the muscles of the leg, the lungs, and circulation. *How exactly does the body maintain the ongoing balance between contract-relax?*

The Brain: Why So Complex?

The brain as the Self-Referral Center coordinates information from the outside world with the internal body environment. The senses act as input ports to bring information about the outside world to the brain. The brain also receives information from the body's internal organs and tissue. This is how the brain coordinates what is going on around us – and monitors the internal body environment to optimize health.

When we consider the brain as the Self-Referral Center, we must understand its composition. The brain is made up of nerve cells, or neurons. Each of its nine billion nerve cells has at least 5,000 connections with other nerve cells or body tissues. In scientific notation, each neuron of the cerebral cortex has 10 to the 2,783,000 power possible connections to other parts of the body. [671] The complexity of the human brain thus is unique in nature – and its function as the Self-Referral Center is doubtless why it is so complex.

Self-Referral coordinates the whole body to make life possible. When we consider breathing, circulation, movement, posture, digestion, and management of waste products – all at the same time – we start to see why the brain and nervous system are so complex. Add to all this the additional functions of self-awareness, thought, and emotions common to all human beings and we have a whole new definition of complexity.

Self-Referral regulates all automatic body functions like heart rate, breathing, and blood pressure. None of these functions are unique to human life, however. Many animals rely on these same functions to stay alive. We distinguish humans from animals chiefly by their brains. Most scientists believe that the human brain is the most complex on Earth. This is what separates humans from the so-called lower animals. Why do humans require such a complex brain compared to animals?

One distinction is the human's complex thinking and reasoning abilities. Animals like the whale and dolphin have highly developed brains, rivaling or exceeding the human brain in size and complexity. Despite the structural brain similarities, most scientists still regard them as mere animals. This understanding will remain unless we communicate with these creatures. A dolphin or whale may have profound thoughts or emotions - but until they tell us about them, or we understand them, they are unknown to us. This is why most scientists assume that humans are the only natives of Earth with true intelligence and self-awareness.[672]

Another big difference between humans and animals is the complexity of body structure. The body plan of dogs, horses, cats, and humans has much in common. All have a brain encased by a skull, a spinal cord protected by a bony vertebral column, and similar internal organs.[673] By comparison, the human body has more complicated joints, muscles, and related structures. We do not see the same degree of complexity in animal structure. The human body structure allows body movement that is uniquely human. Why is this so? There are several reasons for this complexity.

One reason is our upright posture. No other creature on Earth exclusively stands and walks upright. The constant pull of gravity requires a different body arrangement than walking on all fours or moving in a stooped posture like a monkey. Humans need a more complex brain to coordinate the body's many muscle groups that makes standing and walking possible. This is why the upright human posture requires a more complex brain.[674]

Another reason is the human use of hands to make and use tools. Bare handed, one human is weak compared to many animals. But allow for technology, and the same human is the most powerful and dangerous life form on the planet.

To illustrate, consider the long-term effects of human actions. Human-created pollution or warfare can destroy the planet. Could any of the so-called lower animals willfully destroy the rain forest of the Amazon basin? Could animals construct devices to go to the moon and back? The use of tools and technology requires brain and hands working together. This behavior is uniquely human. The manual use of tools and technology thus make human civilization possible. They define in large part what being human means. [675]

Bone, Muscle, and Brain

Bones form the skeleton of the human body. Bones are solid and rocklike. They provide protection, as in the skull shielding the brain from head injury or ribs keeping the heart and lungs safe from body blows. The bones also act as a rigid frame for the body to resist the pull of gravity, as in the pelvis, legs, and spinal column. Finally, the bones act as a framework for muscles to anchor and pull, making posture and movement possible.

Bone and muscle form the musculoskeletal system, making up about 60% of a human's lean body mass. The skeleton's bones provide stability for posture and movement. Muscles are bands of tissue that connect one part of the body with another. The ends of a muscle attach to bones, muscles, or connective tissue. Muscles contract, or shorten, following their long axis. When a muscle contracts, it pulls the two attached parts closer together. If the same muscle relaxes, the parts separate, largely due to the constant pull of gravity. This is the practical aspect of contract-relax as it applies to posture and movement.

The brain works with bone and muscle through Self-Referral. The brain receives information from sensory nerves all over the body. These nerves constantly report body position and muscle tension. The brain causes each muscle to contract or relax, compensating for changing conditions. This signaling between brain and muscle involves billions of nerve cells and trillions of nerve pathways. Whether we walk across the room, hold a cup, or ride a bicycle - the brain coordinates our muscles to allow movement. [676] This is how the body balances contact-relax.

Muscles work in groups to carry out body movement. The biceps and triceps muscles connect the forearm with the upper arm and shoulder. If we contract the biceps, the elbow joint closes, bringing the forearm, wrist, and hand toward the shoulder.

If we contract our triceps muscle, the opposite movement occurs, and the elbow joint opens. Muscle groups all over the body work the same way.[677]

How Muscles Work

No matter where muscles are in the body, they all work the same way: Contraction and Relaxation.

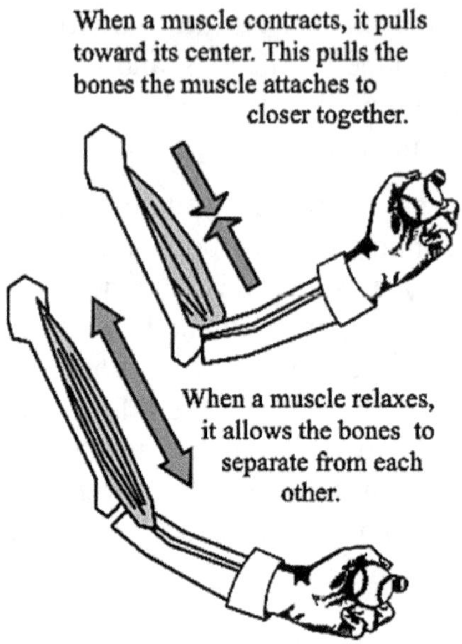

The brain controls individual muscles to coordinate movement. When we move, some muscles contract, but others relax. Why is this? Muscles work in opposing groups – when one muscle contracts, the opposing muscle must relax - or no movement can occur.

To illustrate, think of a weightlifter showing off their arm muscles. They flex both the biceps and the triceps. The result is a stalemate: the arm does not move, but the muscles bulge as they try in vain to move the arm in opposite directions. This same maneuver applied to different parts of the body lies behind the classic poses of body building athletes. [678]

Complex movements like running and jumping require many muscles to work together. One muscle contracts, a second relaxes, and a third muscle partially contracts. In Cybernetic terms, these complex movements require a staggering amount of communication and control between brain and muscle. Whether we type a letter, play basketball, or drive a car - brain and muscles are in full play. We literally see Self-Referral as a speed skater whizzes across the ice. We cannot miss the flow of Self-Referral as we watch a concert pianist translate dots on a page into beautiful music.[679]

Remember that the brain – as the Self-Referral Center for the body – must constantly interact with the environment. Changes in the external environment must be considered when coordinating the body. Different weather conditions make different demands on muscular Self-Referral: an icy sidewalk, for example, demands more focused attention than walking on a dry sidewalk. Why is this true?

Even without hazards, walking requires a lot of Self-Referral between brain and muscle. A slippery sidewalk adds to the stress of life. Brain and muscle work hard as we concentrate on every step to avoid falling. This is how brain and muscle adapt to the constantly changing environment. Self-Referral thus prevents broken bones and similar injuries.[680]

Stress, Brain, and Muscle

We see now that the routine work of the brain is far from simple. It governs automatic activities like breathing and digestion. The brain also coordinates all muscles and makes posture and movement possible. Self-Referral balances the body's opposites; for human movement, Self-Referral balances contract-relax for over 600 muscles - all day, and all night.[681] Coordination of posture and movement thus is one of the brain's major functions. This is why the constant work of coordinating muscles is doubtless a major source of stress.

We have so far focused on stress-related diseases of internal organs. These include the heart, blood vessels, lungs, and intestines. Does stress disrupt the musculoskeletal system?

Hans Selye knew that movement creates stress, and that stress provokes movement. We often call the body's stress reaction the *Fight or Flight Response.* Running from danger demands vigorous movement from major muscle groups. Fighting also employs major muscle groups.[682] What happens in a Fight or Flight Response situation?

When we encounter danger, the brain stimulates the adrenal glands, located above each kidney. These glands pour stress chemicals into the bloodstream that support movement - either to fight or run away. The heart beats faster, blood pressure rises, and muscles prepare for action. These changes redirect blood toward the muscles and make all muscles contract.[683] This is how the Fight or Flight Response prepares us for action.

Hans Selye states that repetitive physical actions cause physical and mental stress. [684] These are exactly the movements required of today's office and factory workers. Whether we work at a desk or on an assembly line, Self-Referral coordinates hundreds of muscles. This balance of opposites makes posture and movement possible.[685] Repetitive physical actions disrupt the Self-Referral of posture and movement. This disruption causes painful muscles, backache, headache, and similar problems.[686]

Musculoskeletal problems cause a lot of misery and work loss. Even ignoring accidental injuries like broken bones and torn ligaments, the toll is enormous. Millions of workers suffer from painful conditions of bone and muscle. Research shows that stress increases muscle spasm, aches, and pains. This is why modern people often suffer from tight muscles and backache.[687]

Modern life causes stress, but is it really that obvious? The constant barrage of television advertisements for pain relievers proves the reality of this problem. Sales of these medications for stress headache and backache number in the billions of dollars every year.[688] In this sense, whole industries exist just to deal with these effects of stress.

Stress causes a multitude of diseases, many of them deadly. Heart attack and stroke, for example, are among the top ten causes of death worldwide. Disruption of Self-Referral also causes muscle spasm and pain. Are aching muscles just as serious as sudden death? How can we compare muscle-related pain with a heart attack or stroke?

The Cost of Aching Muscles

The stress of modern life combines key factors that create more stress than ever before. Modern life features a fast pace of life that gives little time for rest or sleep. Mechanical repetitive movement – either in the office or the factory – constantly strains muscles and bones. Finally, the modern high-tech environment creates endless change. All this piles on more and still more stress. These factors contribute heavily to headache and back pain.

Most doctors consider such muscle pain to be a minor problem, but the facts are otherwise. When we examine work loss, insurance costs, and misery - muscle and bone pain is a major problem. Low back pain is a good example of this situation.

Low back pain is one of the most common problems treated by family doctors. Three out of four people suffer low back pain sometime during their lives. Low back pain lasts from several days to two months - and many people have frequent attacks.[689]

Low back pain affects about 75 million Americans a year. Of these, two million will be out of work due to low back pain.[690] Only a few low back patients - about 300,000 - will need surgery for problems like lumbar disc.[691] The remaining 74.5 million will receive medication, rest, and physical therapy of some kind.[692]

The cost of low back pain is enormous. Low back pain causes 93 million missed workdays per year. It is second only to the common cold in causing missed workdays.[693] Low back pain especially affects young people in the prime of life. It is the most common reason for missed work in people 45 years old or younger. Pain in the low back causes missed work in older people, too. Low back pain ranks third as the cause for missed work in people aged 45 to 64 – second only to heart disease and arthritis.[694]

Missed work causes problems for both employers and workers. Employers lose workers that they need. This disrupts production and causes business losses. Workers suffer pain, inconvenience, and lost wages from missed work. For example, in 1992 Ohio Workers' Compensation low back claims totaled $400,000. Considering lost work and benefits paid out, this added $761,604,000 to the cost of Workers' Compensation patients for that year.[695]

Translating that to 2018 dollars brings the annual total cost to a staggering $1,209,954.[696] That is a lot of money – but this was only for the state of Ohio; adding the other states' costs makes the loss monumental and a very serious problem. Even ignoring these costs, medical care for low back pain is expensive: the average episode of low back pain costs about $4,300.[697] Insurance companies thus pay over $7 billion dollars a year for medical costs and compensation of workers with low back pain.[698]

Workers are not the only victims of low back pain. Many people suffer low back pain unconnected with work. These people seek medical help without the benefit of Workers' Compensation insurance. The total money spent on low back pain every year amounts to roughly 25 dollars for every person in the United States.[699] Low back pain thus has major economic impact.

Many patients with headache also have pain in the neck and low back. Why is this true? Many muscles that move the head connect with the upper back and neck. These also share attachments and nerve connections with muscles of the low back. Walking and working with a sore low back often distorts posture and movement, affecting the head and neck. This is why low back pain causes tight muscles throughout the back, neck, and head.[700]

At any given moment 25 million Americans seek relief from headache.[701] Stress causes migraine headache through vasospasm and muscle spasm. Other stress related headache includes cluster headache and muscle tension headache.[702] Underlining the role of stress, doctors treat vasospasm-related headache with Beta Blocker or Calcium Channel Blocker drugs.[703] Muscle tension headache responds well to muscle relaxants, painkillers, and physical therapy – to reverse the effects of stress.

People with bone and muscle pain are suffering and naturally seek relief. Where do they go for help? Can today's medical care solve their problems and relieve their pain?

Aching Muscles: Seeking a Remedy

The stress of modern life makes tight muscles, backache, and headache common. Since these problems are painful, people often seek relief - both to escape pain and for a speedy return to work. People also want to return to an active life. How do people with stress related pain seek relief?

Many people treat themselves with over-the-counter pain relievers like Aspirin, Acetaminophen, or Ibuprofen. When home remedies do not work, most people seek their family doctor. Most routine aches and pains respond well to prescription painkillers, muscle relaxants, and simple physical therapy.

If obvious measures fail to provide relief, family doctors often refer patients to specialists. The most common referral is to an orthopedic surgeon who specializes in the surgical treatment of bone and muscle disease. They test people via laboratory, X-ray, Ultrasound, and CT or MRI imaging to find the cause of stubborn bone and muscle pain. After diagnosis, some people need medication and physical therapy. Others benefit from injection of painful areas with medication. A few of these people will need surgery to correct a bone or muscle problem.

Many patients get relief with the care described above, but many more fall between these two extremes. These people have severe muscle pain, but they have no clearly defined problem needing orthopedic care. These people seek help with doctor after doctor, only to be disappointed; despite medical care, they still suffer pain. What can we do to help these people?

Today, many professionals use Manipulative Therapy to relieve muscle pain.[704] Manipulate means to work with the hands. Osteopathic physicians use their hands to help people with muscle related pain. This is how Manipulative Therapy integrates with the rest of Modern Medicine. Other professionals who use Manipulative Therapy include Physical Therapists, Occupational Therapists, Kinesiologists, and Chiropractors.

The use of Manipulative Therapy clearly distinguishes between DOs and their MD colleagues. MDs have historically resisted any use of Manipulative Therapy, even to the point of calling such techniques quack medicine.[705] DOs, by contrast, believe that Manipulative Therapy is useful and should be part of every physician's training and practice.

MD and DO medicine were at odds over these issues from the 1890s to the 1970s. The result was ongoing disagreement and frequent political conflict between the professions. This situation has improved since the 1970s. Today MDs and DOs work together as colleagues with mutual respect. The MD side of the medical world has created a new specialty in their profession to deliver Manipulative Therapy: the Physiatrist.[706]

Many MDs are becoming interested in Manipulative Therapy – but there remains a gulf between how MD and DO physicians treat patients with musculoskeletal pain. Today this is less from disagreement about theory and practice and more relating to the history of the two professions.

In my practice, I routinely see improvement using Manipulative Therapy on patients who non-manipulating doctors have dismissed as either baffling or hypochondriacs. Simple Manipulative Therapy often produces immediate relief. This is logical to DOs and patients who are familiar with this kind of diagnosis and treatment - but it seems unusual or even miraculous to people in pain and the non-manipulating doctors who care for them.

The situation for patients seeking relief from musculoskeletal pain strongly parallels that of people seeking relief from stress. People know what the problem is; they just need the best solution to correct it. People want relief, but there are many confusing treatments available. They do not know where to find help - and conflicting advice from different doctors only compounds the confusion. The resulting chaos bewilders patients and doctors alike. How did this situation arise?

Manipulative Therapy: A Short History

From the earliest times, healers used their hands to ease pain. This should not be surprising. If a mother suspects her child is sick, she uses her hand to check for fever. When we visit the sick, we instinctively place a comforting hand on the sufferer; our instinct is to touch someone who is sick or hurting out of compassion.

Manipulative Therapy goes far beyond expressions of sympathy and compassion; it is a system of care that relies on the physician's hands. First a hands-on examination determines what is wrong. Then the physician uses hands to correct the problem.

The therapeutic use of hands is as old as medicine itself.[707] Doctors in India have used Manipulative Therapy for six thousand years.[708] Four-thousand-year-old statues in Thailand display the use of Manipulative Therapy. Ancient Egyptian physicians used Manipulative Therapy in the Nile Valley three thousand years ago.[709]

About 400 BC[710] Hippocrates - the father of Modern Medicine - used traction and leverage techniques to treat spinal disorders in ancient Greece.[711] Ancient Roman physicians used Manipulative Therapy. Galen, Celisies, and Orabasius - notable figures in the history of medicine - wrote about Manipulative Therapy.[712]

The true split between Doctors and Manipulators occurred in seventeenth century England. English Bone-Setters practiced a type of Manipulative Therapy in the 1600s and were members of the Barbers and Surgeons Guild of London. This was an organization like today's American Medical Association. Before 1745, people regarded Bone-Setters as the Orthopedic Surgeons of their day.

The association of doctors and barbers sounds odd until we remember the practice of bleeding patients. Barbers commonly made a small incision in the patient's arm and allowed it to bleed for a time. They believed bleeding allowed ill humors, or poisons, to leave the body. Today's red and white barber pole was originally the symbol of a bandaged arm following a bloodletting session.[713]

The Doctors, Barbers, and Bone-Setters separated in 1745. Doctors formed one professional organization - and barbers and Bone-Setters formed another. The professions separated as Doctors became more scientific.[714] Another cause for the split was the rampant Bubonic Plague of the time. People were reluctant to touch each other - and, fearing the plague, Doctors were unwilling to touch their patients.[715] The Doctors' organization later became the Royal College of Surgeons of England. The Bone-Setters lost respectability with Doctors as the medical profession became more scientific.

England's Bone-Setters still exist today as a separate profession. Bone-Setting is an art passed from father to son. Some experts maintain that a hereditary trait exists that makes learning the art easier for some people. Modern English Bone-Setters are very good at treating many painful conditions; but they are not well schooled in the theory and practice of Modern Medicine. This is why English Doctors regard their theory and practice as out of step with current medicine.[716]

Many physicians have championed Manipulative Therapy despite medical critics. In the early 1800s Dr. Edward Harrison of London gained a sizable reputation using Manipulative Therapy.[717] The famous British surgeon Sir James Paget advocated Manipulative Therapy in the prestigious British Medical Journal. He wrote in 1867 that the use of hands to mobilize joints after injury was valuable and highly advisable. He urged other physicians to stay open minded, writing "Learn what is good and avoid what is bad in the practice of Bone-Setters."[718]

Positive attitudes toward Manipulative Therapy after that were rare. One reason for this is the Manipulators lacked training in scientific medicine; this created poor communication between Manipulators and Doctors. Another problem was that of outrageous claims made by some Manipulators. Overzealous advocates claimed that Manipulative Therapy could cure everything from the common cold to cancer. Some insisted that Manipulative Therapy should replace scientific medicine outright.[719]

Since Paget's time, physician opinion has remained divided. In England, competent and highly respected physicians have spoken favorably of Manipulative Therapy since World War II. Their colleagues later despised these physicians for being open-minded. Unfortunately, this attitude is common across the world today. This is the source of conflict between manipulating and non-manipulating physicians. Some doctors advocate Manipulative Therapy, but others say it is useless.

This leaves the patient in a dilemma. Conventional medicine fails to relieve muscular pain, yet their non-manipulating doctor derides them for seeking relief elsewhere. Most people who seek Manipulative Therapy get genuine relief from pain. In a free society, people hear about what works for an annoying problem. They will seek it out, often in spite of so-called expert advice. It is the consistent success of Manipulative Therapy that has produced such public demand for it.[720]

Modern Manipulative Therapy

Two major schools of Manipulative Therapy now exist in North America. One is the Osteopathic school of medicine. The other is Chiropractic. How did these professions come into being, and what is their role in medicine today?

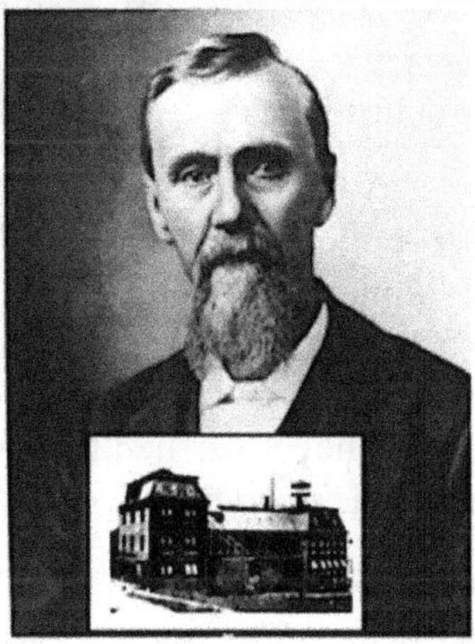

Osteopathic Medicine

Dr. Andrew Taylor Still founded the American School of Osteopathy (inset) at Kirksville, Missouri in 1892. His goal was to add new ideas to medical practice to improve patient outcomes. This set the stage for an American reformation of medicine that continues today.

Andrew Taylor Still, MD founded Osteopathic medicine in 1892 at Kirksville, Missouri. Still was dissatisfied with the medical practice of his time. He proposed Osteopathic Medicine as an improvement to medical practice.[721]

Working over many years, Still created a new system of medicine combining ancient truths with the medical practice of his time. Central to his philosophy was a strong dislike of careless use of medications – which at that time included swallowing mercury and many other toxic substances. He also advocated the use of Manipulative Therapy. Although at first considered a maverick by many, he became known as a great synthesizer of medical thought.[722]

The Osteopathic profession has grown vastly since 1892. There are now 40 colleges of Osteopathic Medicine in the United States[723] graduating over 7,000 students per year.[724] Osteopathic Medicine in the United States is a complete school of medicine and surgery but maintains its unique Osteopathic philosophy and practice.[725] The

Osteopathic profession has grown aggressively through the years, gaining 67% increase in numbers since 2006.[726]

American DO graduates practice the full range of medicine. This includes full medical diagnosis; X-ray, MR, and CT imaging; laboratory testing, prescribing medications, hospital-based patient care, and treatment by surgery. DOs often choose to become Family Physicians.[727] They also can specialize in any area of medicine, including surgery, internal medicine, psychiatry, orthopedic surgery, pediatrics, or any other medical specialty.[728]

Chiropractic was founded by David D. Palmer in 1896 at Davenport, Iowa. Palmer was a self-educated teacher and grocery clerk with no medical training.[729] Palmer practiced what he called magnetic healing and became interested in Manipulative Therapy.[730] He reported an incident in which he manipulated a man's upper back and cured him of deafness.[731] Scientists never verified this cure, but Palmer founded Chiropractic based on the incident.

Many historians contend that Palmer worked with Manipulative Therapy long before that time.[732] It is controversial whether Palmer was ever a patient or a student of Dr. Andrew Taylor Still at Kirksville, Missouri. We do know that Still and Palmer met briefly in Clinton, Iowa in the early 1900s.[733]

David D. Palmer founded Chiropractic, and his son Bartlett J. Palmer worked to create a true Chiropractic profession.[734] The early colleges were in Davenport, Iowa and Oklahoma City, Oklahoma. Palmer taught that alterations in the spinal column caused all disease. Chiropractic adjustment removed such alterations, called subluxations.[735]

Palmer never intended Chiropractic to be a complete school of medicine, instead focusing on musculoskeletal problems and working with Chiropractic to correct them. He did not teach surgery or the use of medications beyond vitamins and simple analgesics.[736] Chiropractic practice in the United States and Canada today is limited to manipulative therapy and X-ray and does not include Modern Medicine, surgery, or prescribing medications.[737]

Today, philosophical differences divide the nine Chiropractic colleges. Many Chiropractors follow the original ideas of Palmer.

Others want to broaden the scope of Chiropractic to include physical therapy machines, diet, and vitamins.[738]

Other health professionals who work to correct musculoskeletal pain and limited function include Physical Therapists, Occupational Therapists, Massage Therapists, and Kinesiologists. All these professions work with patients to reduce pain, restore normal range of motion and function, and normalize tissue. These professionals act on doctor's orders as ancillary personnel in the medical care system.

The Self-Referral of Manipulative Therapy

While the myriad of health professionals who practice Manipulative Therapy do their best to help hurting people regain their health, we need to better understand what they are doing. What do they do that helps people move away from pain and toward normal function? *How does restoration of musculoskeletal function relate to restoring Self-Referral?*

We have examined the body's ability to coordinate posture and movement through Self-Referral. All movement – simple or complex – is made possible by Self-Referral between brain and body. When we watch the movements of a ballet dancer, an athlete, or a jazz musician we literally see the flow of Self-Referral through movement. Skilled coordination of the body's muscles makes the most difficult task look effortless.

We do not usually think of it, but the everyday movements of life are equally complex. When we tie our shoes or eat an apple, the brain coordinates many muscles and muscle groups. Self-Referral between brain and muscle makes these commonplace movements possible. Like the rest of Self-Referral, we take them for granted. We do not usually think of these movements at all unless we suddenly cannot do them.

We lose the ability to move when we break bones and require a cast. Most fractures take four to six weeks to heal - and living with a cast is no fun. Once the cast is removed, we are glad to be free – but there remains some pain and stiffness. This is caused by being immobilized in the cast. We typically receive Physical Therapy – a type of Manipulative Therapy – and soon everything is moving smoothly again.

Anyone confined in a cast knows the frustration of being unable to move as usual. People with muscle-related pain are also confined - by pain. Whether the pain is headache, backache, or other muscle pain, people cannot move the way they want. This interferes with work, income, and enjoyment of life.

Other than pain caused by traumatic injury, most muscle pain is stress related. The stress of life interferes with Self-Referral between brain and muscle. Stress overwhelms the brain and interferes with coordination of muscles. Without Self-Referral between brain and muscle, chaotic muscle function occurs. Tight, painful muscles then further interfere with posture and movement, and more pain results.

When people have stress related muscle pain, they often seek relief with common medicines like aspirin. When this does not work, they seek a doctor. A minority of these people need the services of an Orthopedic Surgeon. Many people with muscle related pain do not need surgery. Many of these people respond to Manipulative Therapy. How does Manipulative Therapy work?

Self-Referral/Maximum Health seeks to restore the body's ability to govern itself. When patients have stress related muscle pain, non-manipulating doctors dismiss the problem as annoying but minor. This problem is anything but minor to the person in pain. Medication masks the pain for a time, but it seldom removes the pain's cause. The pain's cause is yet another stress induced interruption in Self-Referral.

We have examined other interruptions of Self-Referral. Restoring Self-Referral is effective in reversing the negative effects of stress. Manipulative Therapy, when correctly applied, restores Self-Referral. This is a bold assertion. If true, it suggests that Manipulative Therapy may be a widely neglected treatment for a common and costly problem. It also suggests that we should examine Manipulative Therapy more closely.

Chapter 12

Self-Referral and Manipulative Therapy

The brain balances the body's muscles through Self-Referral – creating health. Stress disrupts Self-Referral. Manipulative Therapy restores Self-Referral between brain and muscle.

Self-Referral and Movement

When we study *Self-Referral/Maximum Health*, we seek ways to restore the body's ability to govern itself. We see the flow of Self-Referral through body movement. Brain and muscle work together to orchestrate the complex muscle activity that makes movement possible.

Self-Referral and movement are abstract ideas until we connect them with real life. Many people perform amazing feats through training their bodies. We see Self-Referral at work through accomplished athletes like Olympic skaters or gymnasts. These advanced artists use their bodies to show us poetry in motion.

Olympic athletes are not the only ones who benefit from Self-Referral; ordinary people also depend upon Self-Referral for movement. Whether we change our clothes or peel an orange, Self-Referral between brain and muscle makes it all possible. We seldom think about Self-Referral and movement at all unless we cannot move.

Anyone confined in a cast knows the frustration of being unable to move as usual. People with muscle-related pain are just as confined - by pain. Whether they suffer headache, backache, or other musculoskeletal pain - people are unable to move. This interferes with work and play and has a major economic impact on peoples' lives.

Remember - stress can be physical or mental. Stress is physical when we struggle with repetitive movement or injuries. Stress is mental when we feel strain from work or family pressures. Either way, the stress of life disrupts Self-Referral between brain and muscle.

Doctors who do not use Manipulative Therapy dismiss muscle pain as a minor annoyance. This problem is anything but minor to someone in pain. Pain medication masks the symptoms for a time, but they do not affect the cause of the pain. What can we do about stress related muscle pain?

Painkiller Overuse and the Opioid Epidemic

Overuse of common over-the-counter medications like aspirin, acetaminophen, and ibuprofen is a major problem today. These products are all useful and effective for the relief of common day-to-day pain - if used properly. All these medications carry dosage directions on their labels, but many people either fail to read them or simply ignore them.

This is a predictable situation. Everyone has a need to keep going; parents need to care for their children, working people must do their jobs, and life goes on. People regard even severe pain as little more than an irritation to be brushed out of the way with painkillers.

One critical side effect of painkiller medication is kidney damage. When people overuse these drugs, good medicine becomes toxic. People often take the drug at higher doses to eliminate pain. They also take the drug more often than recommended to keep pain at bay.

The drug then becomes poisonous and causes kidney damage. This can result in kidney failure and the need for dialysis.

Patients have a wide range of body pain depending on what is wrong. Those with severe pain often receive orthopedic care. When the need for surgery or other orthopedic intervention is not a viable answer, the only apparent help is strong pain medicine – which is addictive and causes many negative side effects.

The Opioid drugs include advanced painkillers like Hydrocodone (Vicodin). They contain a far more powerful narcotic (the Opioid ingredient) than older medications like Tylenol # 3 with codeine. These newer drugs are more effective than the older painkillers – but they are also far more addictive.[739]

The synthetic opioid Fentanyl – now the basis for nationwide addiction and overdose death problems – has magnified this problem enormously. This should not be surprising as we know from the manufacture and sale of illegal street drugs. The reason that heroin is sold by drug dealers on the street instead of opium is that heroin is far more addictive, and hence more likely to create a lifetime customer for the pusher – good for business, but bad for addicted people. Fentanyl is far worse.

The fact is, any time opium is refined, it becomes many times more addictive. The very Opioid medications created to relieve severe pain can also quickly make drug addicts out of patients looking for pain relief. The situation has become so serious that national leaders have called for an aggressive campaign to curb the Opioid Epidemic. Many in government and the health professions are doing their best to combat this problem as this book goes to press.[740]

How real is the Opioid Epidemic? The picture in the United States is grim.[741] As many as 80 people a day die from an Opioid overdose.[742] Suicides related to Opioid use increased from 30,000 in 2000 to 44,000 in 2015 – a 25% increase. There is now a suicide related to Opiates every 12 minutes in the United States.[743] Accidental overdose deaths frequently occur among patients using Opioid medications: the number of such deaths jumped from 5,921 to 10,829 between the years 1999 and 2005.[744] As of 2022, the total number of Opioid related deaths totaled 80,411.[745]

A huge part of the addiction problem is overprescribing Opioids by medical caregivers – both too often and at too high a dose. Both create higher risk for Opioid addiction, overdose death, and Opioid-related suicide.[746] As a result, Opioid restrictions have increased across the country.[747] The head of the Food and Drug Administration recently contacted medical insurance companies and physicians to reduce Opioid prescribing.[748]

Government and regulators can only do so much. It is up to physicians to take the lead in fighting the Opioid Epidemic. Doctors control the prescription pad, the pen, and what is prescribed to the patient. They must eliminate lenient prescribing of Opioids that create addicts. They also must take responsibility to get addicted patients into drug treatment rather than perpetuate narcotics dependence.[749]

That is why most Family Physicians like me do not prescribe Opioid painkillers. Whenever someone has pain that requires these medications, I refer them immediately to a specialist physician in Pain Management. These doctors have additional training that makes them appropriate to manage patients with ongoing severe pain.

Manipulative Therapy is Needed

I would clearly state that there are patients who have pain problems that truly need the advanced painkiller drugs. They can get the help they need through the Pain Management physicians. However, there are thousands of people every day who would have immediate relief of musculoskeletal pain by receiving Manipulative Therapy.

I commonly have patients see me who not only have significant pain but also have been to doctor after doctor with little relief. These people have received nothing but muscle relaxant and painkiller drugs. I evaluate and treat them with manipulative therapy and often relieve major pain immediately. They are amazed at how effective Manipulative Therapy is – and how quick and easy it is to receive it.

I seriously wonder how much of the Opioid Epidemic is a direct result of failure to meet the public's need for effective Manipulative Therapy. This is not an idle thought; patients receiving Osteopathic Manipulative Therapy have been shown to have less need for Opioid, non-Opioid, and steroid medications.[750] As these findings are becoming known, the MD world is waking up to Manipulative Therapy as the non-Opioid solution.[751]

We need better alternatives to out-of-control painkiller dependence. The sole answer to musculoskeletal pain is not surgery or addiction. When we understand the principles of *Self-Referral/Maximum Health*, we will have far better answers for these problems.

We know that restoring Self-Referral reverses the negative effects of stress. Manipulative Therapy, when correctly applied, relieves muscle pain caused by stress. The logical conclusion is that Manipulative Therapy somehow restores Self-Referral.

This is a bold assertion; if true, Manipulative Therapy is a neglected treatment for a widespread problem. It also suggests that Manipulative Therapy deserves closer examination. Is there evidence to connect stress and painful muscles? Can Manipulative Therapy restore Self-Referral between brain and muscle?

Osteopathic Medicine Today

When we seek *Self-Referral/Maximum Health* we look for ways to restore the body's ability to govern itself. I suggest that Manipulative Therapy is an important way to restore health - by restoring Self-Referral. How many physicians agree with this idea?

As of 2016, there were 860,939 MD physicians[752] and 108,118 DO physicians[753] in the United States. That means 11% of American doctors are DOs and 89% are MDs. Osteopathic medicine teaches and uses Manipulative Therapy, while MD medicine does not. There are no other schools of medicine that teach Manipulative Therapy as part of Modern Medicine. How did this situation arise? We may learn much through a closer look at the unique philosophy and practice of Osteopathic Medicine.

Andrew Taylor Still, MD did not conceive of Osteopathic Medicine as a non-medical school of medicine. Rather, Still wanted Osteopathic Medicine to improve *all of medicine*. The politics of medicine are like the politics of government: the majority position rules. Organized MD medicine long opposed Manipulative Therapy. Osteopathic Medicine by its very existence functions as a minority party that continues to stand by its distinct philosophy and practice.[754]

Central to Osteopathic Medicine is the use of Manipulative Therapy. Osteopathic physicians thus occupy a unique position in the medical field today. They are fully trained physicians who can specialize and practice in all fields of medicine - but they also advocate and use Manipulative Therapy. Is Osteopathic Medicine unique only in its stand on Manipulative Therapy? We will benefit from a closer look at Osteopathic philosophy.

The term Osteopathy confuses many people - doctors and patients alike. Since only 11% of American physicians are DOs, many confuse "Osteopathic" with "Orthopedic," as in Orthopedic Surgeons. To add to this confusion, some DOs also are Orthopedic Surgeons. What is the origin of the term Osteopathy?

We cannot separate Osteopathic philosophy from its founder: Andrew Taylor Still, MD. Still coined the term Osteopathy from the Greek Osteo meaning “bone” and Pathos meaning "something wrong." Osteopathy thus translates as "something wrong with the bones." Still coined the term Osteopathy because beginners in Manipulative Therapy lack the subtle hands-on skill of trained and experienced Osteopathic Physicians; using the bones as landmarks made Manipulative Therapy easier to explain and teach.

For example: locating the kneecap is something nearly anyone can do with little training. More skill is needed to read the meaning of tissue texture, muscle tone, and fluid dynamics. This is why bones are only landmarks in a vastly more complex system of manipulative diagnosis and therapy.[755] This complexity makes those who are newcomers to it have problems understanding it and doing it.

What does *OSTEOPATHIC* mean?

Dr. A. T. Still used the bones of the skeleton as landmarks in diagnosing and treating the body. OSTEO means "bone." PATHY means "something wrong with."

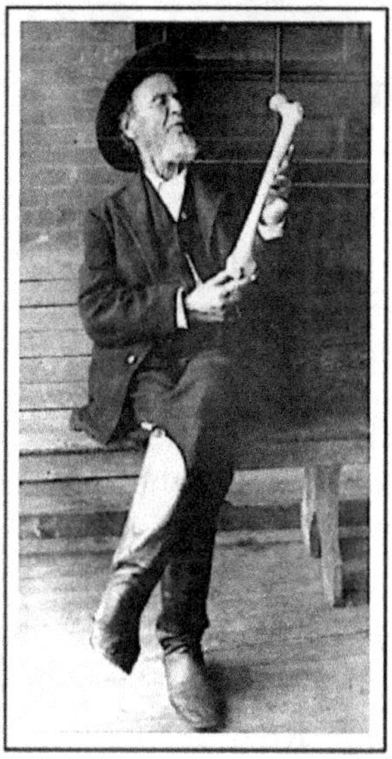

Osteopathic medicine places great importance on the body's bones and muscles. This is the musculoskeletal system. It can fall prey to the effects of stress.

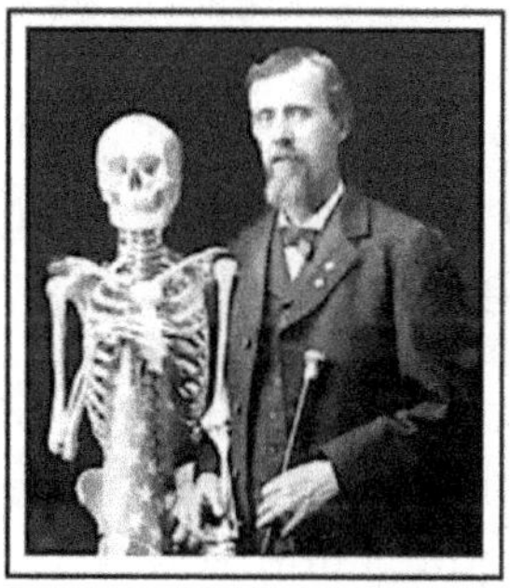

The Ideas of Dr. Andrew Taylor Still

Andrew Taylor Still, MD (1828-1917) was a rough-hewn frontier doctor of the American Midwest. Still was a keen observer of life and studied nature from an early age. He had a strong desire to help others that led him to a career as a physician.

Medicine at that time was primitive by today's standards. There were few reliable pharmaceuticals of any kind. Surgery was limited and hospitals were rudimentary and scarce. That is why medical care outcomes were very poor by today's standards. Like all settlers of the frontier, Still often witnessed advanced disease and death – and developed a strong desire to improve medical practice.

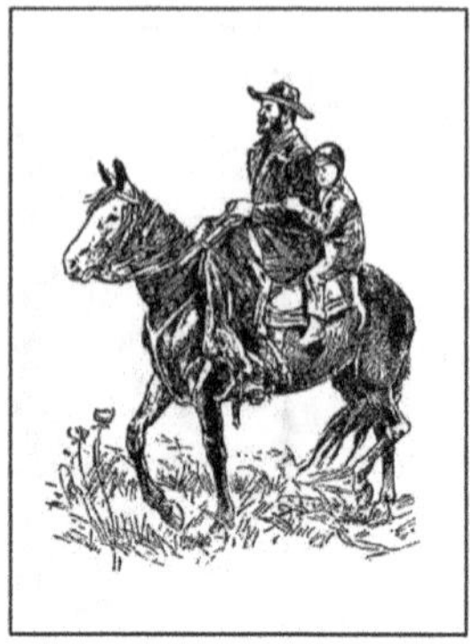

Andrew Taylor Still's father was an MD physician and Methodist minister. He worked as a Circuit Rider for the Methodist Church. He preached and practiced medicine as he travelled through the area by horseback. It is not surprising that Still chose to study medicine, attending the College of Physicians and Surgeons in Kansas City, Missouri before the American Civil War.

Still took a strong stand against slavery. He backed his convictions by leaving medical school to serve in the Union Army - first as a Captain, and later as a Major. As was common in his day, he completed his medical training after the war by studying with doctors already in practice.[756]

In the spring of 1864, Still lost three children to meningitis. This personal tragedy persuaded him to seek a higher order of medicine. Still committed himself to study the structure and function of the human body. He carried out extensive dissection work on human cadavers and experimented on himself with Manipulative Therapy. Still wrote: "A thousand experiments were made with bones, until I became quite familiar with the bony structure."[757]

Dr. Still thus spent a long time thinking and formulating his new ideas. His goal was to better understand how human anatomy and human function were related. He reasoned that normal human function depended upon normal human anatomy. Along with that understanding came the idea that abnormal or distorted human anatomy could be the cause of interruptions in health: disease.

By 1874 his ideas were ready for presentation to the medical world, and he began writing about them. In 1892, Still founded a new school of medicine: the American School of Osteopathy at Kirksville, Missouri.[758] The practical application of Still's original system of medicine focused on Manipulative Therapy to restore health, but his ideas went far beyond hands-on work. A short synopsis of Still's ideas follows:[759]

Self-Referral

Maximum Health

Key Ideas of Dr. Andrew Taylor Still

REMEMBER: Dr. Andrew Taylor Still was a doctor of the late 1800s who worked to improve the medical practice of his time.

The human body is a unit. If one part of the body becomes structurally impaired, all the body suffers.

We can better understand disease if first we understand health.

There is within the human body a capacity for health. We can recognize this capacity and work with it to normalize the body and restore health.

The body's musculoskeletal system forms a structure that – when disordered – disturbs the function of other parts of the body.

The human body is subject to mechanical strain.

The ability of the body to adapt itself to environmental change is the essence of health.

The Disease Approach Vs. the Health Approach

Alert readers will notice immediately that Still's ideas form the basis of *Self-Referral/Maximum Health.* This vision of human structure, function, and health is as new today as when it was first taught in 1892. Just as it was at that time, the call for Osteopathy is the clarion call for the Health Approach to medicine as opposed to the Disease Approach that holds sway today.

Today's medical care acts like the fire department, putting out fires as diseases are discovered and a critical need for action becomes apparent. Today's medical care is stuck and mired in the Disease Approach to medicine.

By contrast, Still's vision of human structure and function sees the body in health as a unity of design and function. That unity naturally produces health and by default prevents disease. This is clearly the Health Approach to medicine. Compare Still's idea of body unity with the wisdom of ancient India's *Upanishads*:

> That is the Whole.
> This is the Whole.
> From Wholeness emerges Wholeness.
> Wholeness coming from Wholeness,
> Wholeness still remains.[760]

Consider Still's idea of first knowing health to understand disease. Still wrote in 1899 "To find health should be the object of the doctor. Anyone can find disease."[761]

Today's medical care does an excellent job of finding disease once it exists; today's medical care also has excellent medical, pharmaceutical, and surgical treatment of disease once discovered. What is sorely lacking is a comprehensive definition of health, ways to quickly and easily identify health, and – most importantly – ways to promote health.

Our own thinking and assumptions create this situation – and that involves patients, doctors, and health professionals of all kinds. By staying focused on what is wrong, there is always plenty to do. We readily identify disease and get to work treating it. And before we know it, all our time and resources have been spent that way.

It requires a real change in thinking to focus on promoting health - and preventing disease. Embedded within these thoughts is the ancient Chinese idea of prevention. We read in the *Tao te Ching*:

> Prevent trouble before it arises. Put things in order before they exist.[762]

I suggest that Still's "capacity for health" is none other than *Self-Referral/Maximum Health*.

The Role of Mechanical Stress and Strain

Still wrote that mechanical stress and strain interrupts Self-Referral. "We say disease when we should say effect," Still wrote. "Disease is the effect of a change in the parts of the physical body. Disease in an abnormal body is just as natural as is health when all parts are in place."[763]

Still identified Future Shock nearly a century before Alvin Toffler, although he did not call it that. He noted that people in primitive cultures seldom fall victim to the stress of life. Still clearly taught that the stress of civilized living wreaks havoc upon the body. He wrote in his 1899 Philosophy of Osteopathy: "If you burst a boiler by high pressure or otherwise, your engine ceases to move. And just the same of an over-worked brain or body."[764]

Finally, Still was firm that Manipulative Therapy could restore Self-Referral. Osteopathic theory assumes that the body has a natural ability to maintain health, and thus avoid disease.[765] Still identified tense muscles - caused by stress - as a major root cause of all disease. Manipulative Therapy, he maintained, simply restored the body's ability to maintain health. Still wrote: "Harmony only dwells where obstructions do not exist."[766]

The Medium of Self-Referral

Here we begin to see Still's understanding of Self-Referral. He clearly knew that Self-Referral created health and maintained health as a default condition. He also knew the key role played by the brain and nervous system in Self-Referral. What else did Still say about the nervous system and Self-Referral?

Still attached great importance to the cerebrospinal fluid, or CSF. The CSF is a clear, colorless fluid that bathes the brain, spinal cord, and nerves. Conventional medicine teaches that this fluid system acts as a shock absorber to protect delicate nervous tissue from injury. It also teaches that CSF bathes and cleanses the brain, spinal cord, and nerves.

Still taught that CSF had a role beyond that of bathing and protecting the nervous system's tissues; he taught that the CSF circulated throughout the body, as blood flows through the arteries and veins. Still wrote in his *Philosophy of Osteopathy:*[767]

> . . . the cerebrospinal fluid [CSF]is the highest known element that is contained in the human body, and unless the brain furnishes it in abundance a disabled condition will continue. He who is able to reason will see that this great river of life must be tapped, and the withered field irrigated at once, or the harvest of health will be lost.

Still here suggests that the CSF has a *trophic* or *nourishing effect* on body tissues; that is, the CSF delivers substances to all tissues that are necessary for health. Still also wrote of the CSF as an active cleanser of tissue. He wrote: [768]

> . . . to withhold the supply from a limb, to wither away would be natural . . . First, for want of supply (hunger), and the burdens of dead deposits along nerve centers...the nerve fiber to its place is king and lord overall.

Still emphasized that CSF is formed in the brain. Then he defined a CSF circulatory system that nourishes and cleanses all body tissues:[769]

> As life finds its general nutrient law in the fascia and the nerves, we must connect them...by a cord running the length of the spine, by which all nerves are supplied by the brain. The cord throws out and supplies millions of nerves by which all organs and parts are supplied . . . [and] all go to terminate in that great system the fascia.

The fascia is a thin, whitish tissue that covers every organ in the body. The fascia also penetrates body tissue, dividing various tissues and organs into sections. It is at the level of the fascia that all nerves from the brain or spinal cord penetrate tissue. For example, the major nerve that connects with the heart's pacemaker enters the tissue at the level of the fascia.[770]

Self-Referral

Maximum Health

Key Assumptions of
Dr. Andrew Taylor Still

REMEMBER: Looking for the medium of Self-Referral, Still tells us the nerve reigns supreme. What is the nerve's purpose that makes it so important to body operations?

The cerebrospinal fluid (CSF) is the highest or most refined element of the human body.

CSF is formed by the brain.

CSF circulates widely in the body, via the nerves to the fascia and tissues.

CSF has 2 functions: 1. CSF acts as a trophic or nourishing factor to all body tissues; 2. CSF acts as a cleansing agent to rid the body's tissues of impurities – especially those found along the nerve pathways.

Disruption of the nervous system in one area of the body can disrupt other areas of the body.

Still also placed great emphasis on the role of arterial, venous, and lymphatic circulation. "The rule of the artery and vein is universal in all living beings," Dr. Still wrote. "Wherever the arterial supply of tissue is compromised disease would surely result."[771] He also pointed out the importance on the venous and lymphatic circulation, stating that toxic buildup from stagnation of tissue fluids also would produce disease.[772]

Remember, however, that the nerve controls all circulation via the arteries and surrounding muscle contraction. This is why Still wrote ". . .the nerve fiber to its place is king and lord over all."[773]

We see in Dr. Andrew Taylor Still's assumptions the medium of Self-Referral. *The physical structure of the nervous system acts as the chief medium of Self-Referral.*

The brain, spinal cord, and nerves are made of neurons. These individual cells are the simplest unit of Self-Referral. These neurons form complex neuronal pathways. The pathways together form the brain, spinal cord, and nerves. It is the successful electrochemical communication and control of the nervous system via Cybernetic feedback loops that makes Self-Referral possible – and creates health. We also see the whole-body nature of Self-Referral in Still's ideas. The nerve reigns supreme because the nerve connects any part of the body with whole body Self-Referral.

We have examined how disruption of Self-Referral in one part of the body affects the body elsewhere. This is particularly true if the disruption of Self-Referral is in the nervous system itself, as in a stroke. *Whether it is a specific brain problem or the chronic effects of stress and Stress Syndrome, interruption of Self-Referral is the basis of all disease and the aging process.*

The Vision of Dr. Andrew Taylor Still

Dr. Andrew Taylor Still was keenly aware of the relationship between stress and disease. He wrote that the high-pressure lifestyle is not healthy. "If you burst a boiler by high pressure . . . your engine ceases to move. And just the same of an overworked brain or body."[774] Please remember that Still was writing in the 1890s; in this context, his vision was truly extraordinary.

How is it that a nineteenth century physician of the American Midwest taught a philosophy of medicine that resonates so clearly with philosophies of the East? How is it that this uniquely American reformation of medical thought so clearly addresses the modern problems described by *Future Shock*? I suggest the reason is that truth is truth - no matter where or when we find it. Still acknowledged this when he wrote:

> . . . our school is young, but the laws that govern life are as old as the hours of all ages. We may find much that has never been written, nor practiced before, but all such discoveries are truths born with the birth of eternity, old as God and as true as life."[775]

Still's idea of a circulating CSF system is truly novel. Before Still's teaching and writing career, conventional medicine taught that CSF was nothing more than a scrubber and shock absorber for the nervous system. Still was a global thinker and writer, and he chose not to go into much detail regarding the CSF circulatory system. It was a later Osteopathic pioneer who applied knowledge of circulating CSF to Manipulative Therapy.

The Ideas of Dr. William Garner Sutherland

When Dr. William Garner Sutherland received his DO degree from the hand of Dr. Andrew Taylor Still, the Old Doctor was 70 years of age.[776] While a student at the American School of Osteopathy at Kirksville, Sutherland carefully studied the joints of the body. He explored how the bones and joints moved based on their anatomy.[777]

When Sutherland studied the skull, he noticed something new that no one had reported before. Students in medical school often study the disarticulated skull. This is a skull that has been taken apart to better see the individual bones.

Most people assume the human skull is one solid bone - but it is actually made up of many smaller bones. We can clearly see this in a skull that has been taken apart and the bones placed on a stand to show their relationships. Examining such a skull, Sutherland had a profound insight.

When we look at the bones that make up the human skull, there are small, jagged edges where the bones meet. In the whole skull, these are the suture lines where the bones fit closely together. While observing the joint edges of the separated skull bones, Sutherland noticed the joints are serrated and beveled in a jagged, saw tooth manner. The question that came to his mind was: What was the purpose of these structures?

The Medium of Self-Referral

Dr. William G. Sutherland proposed that the brain's cerebrospinal fluid (CSF) circulates. CSF is created by the brain's choroid plexus tissue and flows over, under, around, and through the brain. This circulation system extends throughout the body via the nerves and nerve sheaths, which connect with the fascia.

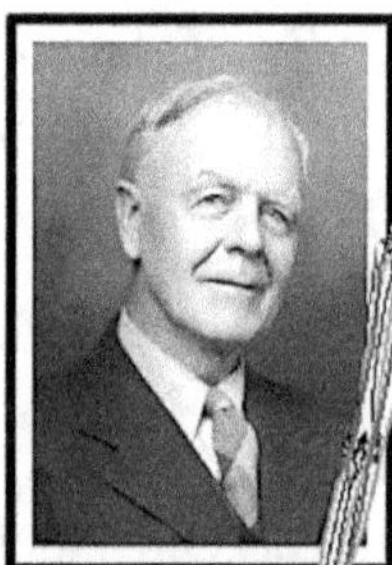

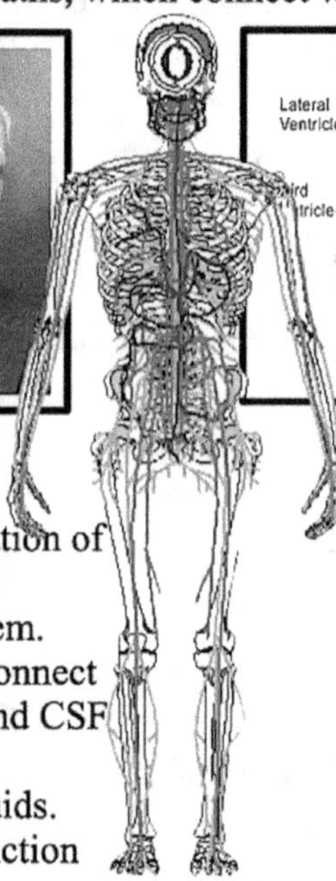

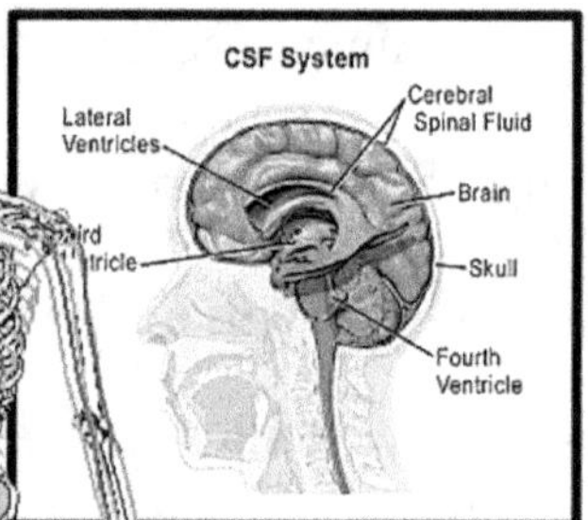

Self-Referral relies upon normal operation of the brain and nervous system. The nerves connect with fascia and CSF mingles with lymphatic fluids. All nerve function takes place in a vast, connected sea of CSF, lymphatic, and related fluids. This cleanses nerves and tissues and delivers nourishing trophic substances to reach tissue everywhere.

Everything in the body is designed for a purpose, Sutherland thought. The question that nagged him was obvious: for what purpose were these skull joints designed?[778] It was then that Sutherland interpreted this anatomy as suggestive of active joint motion. Sutherland wrote in his book *The Cranial Bowl*:

> I contend that in the living skull, normal mobility in the form of expansive and contractile [movement] occurs in the [skull] vault through the specially designed dovetail arrangement of the sutures.[779]

The purpose of this bony movement, he maintained, was to accommodate a rhythmic pulsation of the brain and spinal cord driving an active CSF circulatory system. Sutherland called this rhythmic pulsation the Cranial Respiratory Mechanism or CRM.[780]

Self-Referral

Maximum Health

Common Tissue Rhythms

According to Dr. Harold Magoun

REMEMBER: These are common tissue rhythms felt with the hands through the sense of touch by physicians trained in Cranial theory and practice.

A pulsation synchronous with the heartbeat.

A pulsation that coincides with breathing in and breathing out.

A pulsation not related to heart or lung function that maintains its own cycle.

A pulsation of indeterminate pattern that has not been identified.

While Sutherland identified rhythmic movement in the skull, he also found it about the spinal cord and throughout the body - and anyone can find this movement using their hands.[781] Sutherland thus described a new type of subtle, spontaneous body movement. The purpose of this hidden circulatory system, Sutherland wrote, is to supply the trophic and purifying functions of the CSF to all the body's tissues.[782]

With the patient lying face up on a treatment table, the manipulator sits at the head of the table, cradling the patient's head. Using a light touch with the hands, the manipulating physician works with movement in the skull and related tissues. Sutherland thus discovered a new system of Manipulative Therapy of the skull and the rest of the body.[783]

What do Cranial Manipulators feel and treat with their hands? When Osteopathic physicians interpret what they feel with their hands, descriptions can vary. This is because cranial manipulation is subtle and can produce several common findings. Each is useful to diagnose and treat cranial restrictions. Dr. Harold I. Magoun[784] was an expert in cranial diagnosis and treatment. He described four types of cranial motion:

Of the patterns described by Magoun, we associate the first two with well-known body functions. The fourth pattern is largely unknown, even by trained and experienced cranial manipulators. The third pattern is the most reliable. Most manipulators maintain that this is Sutherland's Cranial Respiratory Mechanism. Averaging about 8-12 cycles per minute, the CRM is readily palpable by trained personnel. Doctors most readily sense the CRM at the head, but they can find it throughout the body.[785]

Health and Body Symmetry

When we look at the human body, we notice that one side looks much the same from right to left. That is, everyone has two arms, two legs, two ears, and so forth. We also readily see that the body is in good vertical alignment.

We call this balanced side-to-side pairing of body parts *body symmetry*. When tight muscles distort posture or restrict movement, body symmetry suffers. This causes a loss of vertical alignment: we look crooked, as opposed to straight.

Disruption of body symmetry causes the aches and pains of sore back and neck, painful shoulders, headache, and so forth. Abnormal body symmetry may be caused by traumatic injury, disease processes, or the chronic effects of stress. This distortion of normal anatomy disrupts Self-Referral; this is the distortion of the body that manipulating physicians treat.

How do doctors decide what Manipulative Therapy to use on a patient? Manual diagnosis is simply the use of hands to diagnose illness. An ongoing controversy is whether manual diagnosis findings are accurate. Those trained in Manipulative Therapy cannot understand why non-manipulating doctors do not recognize what is obvious to them. Non-manipulating doctors scoff at "imaginary" diagnosis and treatment. How can these groups communicate when they apparently have nothing in common?

Research on Manual Diagnosis

Osteopathic researchers have a keen interest in manual diagnosis. These doctors ask the question "how can manipulating doctors show manual findings to non-manipulating doctors?" This is a difficult question to answer. One group has no idea to what the other group is referring. Then there is the problem of communicating manual findings to doctors who do not train to use their hands in this fashion.

Many doctors who do not manipulate are familiar with testing of the muscles and bones. Specialists in orthopedics test the range of motion of the trunk, arms, and legs.[786] They use

these tests[787] to determine disability from injury or disease.[788] Osteopathic examination and diagnosis is far more exact and complex. One article described fifty Osteopathic tests of the spine, pelvis, arms, and legs.[789]

Doctors who manipulate begin with a thorough examination of the patient. This begins with a head-to-toe examination of the patient standing, sitting, and lying on the examination table.[790] What do these doctors find? The most common finding is that one side of the body is not level with the other side. With the patient standing, one side of the pelvis may be higher than the other.[791] Other findings may include one leg appearing shorter than the other. Many less obvious findings are possible; each part of the body has normal and abnormal positioning. More experienced manipulators learn these aspects.

Testing of all body parts for normal movement is important.[792] Another part of examination is noting the texture of muscle, skin, and other tissue.[793] Common landmarks to check include the neck,[794] shoulders,[795] low back, overall curvature of the spine,[796] skull,[797] arms, legs, and feet. It is important to know how the patient compares to normal.[798]

There have been many well-planned studies on manual findings. This research shows that doctors can use their hands to diagnose common body problems. These doctors can study the same patients independently and agree on diagnosis. Other studies prove that doctors can use their hands to examine patients and agree whether they are improving or not.[799]

Do manual findings relate to internal organ disease as manipulating doctors claim? Many researchers have found this to be true. Manual findings are closely associated with lung disease,[800] heart attack,[801] high blood pressure,[802] cancer,[803] congenital hip disease,[804] autistic children,[805] temporomandibular or TMJ syndrome,[806] whiplash injuries,[807] knee injuries,[808] and many other medical problems.

Manipulative Therapy encompasses many individual techniques. No one technique or collection of techniques will solve all problems. That is why Osteopathic physicians train for the full practice of medicine as well as Manipulative Therapy. DOs thus are well prepared to find and treat body problems with comprehensive Manipulative Therapy.

Good Posture and Easy Movement is Critical to Health

We now see the importance of good posture and easy movement. If all nerves are critical for Self-Referral, any distortion in posture will distort Self-Referral. Any restriction in movement will interfere with Self-Referral.

Today's physicians must learn this knowledge of body wholeness. If we treat the patient's internal organs and ignore muscle and bone, we are ignoring 60% of the lean body mass. We also are ignoring the possibility of improving patients' quality of life. Today, we are also allowing untold thousands of patients with painful conditions to go untreated – who often end up as statistics in the Opioid Epidemic. As Lao-Tzu writes:[809]

> The Master views the parts with compassion, because he understands the whole. His constant practice is humility. He doesn't glitter like a jewel but lets himself be shaped by the Tao, as rugged and common as a stone.

Today's doctors need to learn the hands-on methods of Manipulative Therapy. All doctors need this valuable knowledge as a critical tool to diagnose and treat bone and muscle pain. Medical practice will improve as more doctors learn to use Manipulative Therapy.

Osteopathic Physicians: A Closer Look

Osteopathic Medicine now is taught at Osteopathic Medical Schools or through courses taught by other Osteopathic institutions. I am a 1977 graduate of the Des Moines University College of Osteopathic Medicine and Surgery at Des Moines, Iowa. I am Board Certified in Family Practice through the National Board of Examiners in Osteopathic Medicine and Surgery. I have also spent over 40 years studying Still's books and related material to understand his theory of health and disease.

We have examined philosophical differences between Osteopathic physicians – DOs - and their MD colleagues. We have looked deeply into historic Osteopathic philosophy and Manipulative Therapy. Where do Osteopathic physicians stand today - with their philosophy, practice, and the public? Are there other differences in how DOs practice medicine?

One difference is the DO preference for primary care. More DOs than MDs choose to become primary care family doctors instead of specialists. In 2017, 44% of DOs worked in primary care – including Family Practice, Internal Medicine, and Pediatrics.[810] Only 33% of MDs chose these specialties.[811] That means 47,478 DOs chose to become family doctors – *over three times the proportion of MDs*. As of 2023, the DO commitment to primary care has continued to grow

- with 57% of all DOs choosing primary care.[812] These numbers show the Osteopathic profession's dedication to providing comprehensive health care to people of all ages.

The Osteopathic Touch

The Osteopathic profession's commitment to family medicine translates to optimal patient relations. People like to have a family doctor who sees everyone for routine medical care. The DO provides high quality primary care with referral to specialists when needed. People understand and appreciate this comprehensive approach to medical care.

Is Osteopathic care different? Many patients tell me that DOs have a more caring and personal approach to patient care. They also tell me that DOs speak less "medical-ese" and communicate more clearly. Patients say that DOs seem to care more about their patients and are more apt to show it. These are statements of opinion, but - if true - they suggest that DOs promote positive emotions[813] - and positive emotions promote health. Many patients call this *the Osteopathic touch.*

Over 102,000 DOs conduct over 300 million patient visits per year.[814] DOs render this unique Osteopathic care in private offices, any of 143 Osteopathic hospitals, or in mixed MD-DO hospitals and offices.[815] What are the differences between MD and DO care from the patient's standpoint?

Most people see a doctor sometime in their life. Whether the problem is a sore throat or a cough, the ritual is the same.

After some time in the waiting room (often more time than you want!) a nurse takes you into an examination room. The nurse checks your blood pressure and temperature. Then the nurse asks what is wrong and relates the information to the doctor.

Finally, the doctor arrives to listen to the complaint and ask questions. The doctor uses a lighted instrument to look in the ears and throat. He also listens to the heart and lungs. The doctor may examine the abdomen or other parts of the body. When the doctor identifies the problem, he prescribes medications or other therapy. On the way out you schedule a follow-up visit.

Osteopathic physicians carry out the same medical examination, but with important differences. They have additional training in using their hands to diagnose muscular problems. This improves their ability to "read" tissue with their hands.

Improved touch skills help to diagnose painful muscle problems, but they also sharpen the ability to feel subtle tissue changes like infected lymph nodes or soft tissue tumors. This hands-on approach also adds to the personal aspect of the doctor-patient relationship. The laying on of hands in this fashion promotes the positive patient reactions previously described.

I do not criticize non-manipulating physicians as uncaring. Many physicians, DO and MD alike, care deeply for their patients. They often express it by touching their patients, such as placing a caring hand on the shoulder during conversation or during physical examination. The additional training of the Osteopathic physician, however, adds a new dimension to medical care.

Are patients aware of the difference in Osteopathic principles? Do they notice a difference in their medical care as a result? A recent study evaluated 2000 patients seen in an outpatient clinic by DOs. The attitudes and opinions of the DO patients were compared to those of a matched group of patients seen by MDs. The DO patients clearly understood Osteopathic principles and experienced their DO physician's Osteopathic practice of medicine. The DO patients reported that their physician had more empathy – and the patients had more satisfaction with their care. This study makes it clear that Osteopathic ideas and practice strongly impact patient care in a positive way.[816]

Manipulative Therapy: Who Needs It?

Most people know about the Osteopathic physician's use of Manipulative Therapy, but who needs treatment? How did they come to need Manipulative Therapy? We know t people seek Manipulative Therapy due to painful muscles and joints. Why are these structures prone to soreness, and how did they get sore in the first place?

Self-Referral

Maximum Health

Why People Need Manipulative Therapy

REMEMBER: Manipulative Therapy is hands-on therapy to restore normal function and reduce pain in the body's muscles, bones, and joints.

Traumatic injury. Strain and sprain injury from lifting heavy objects and sports injuries not requiring surgery or a cast.

Long term effects of known disease. Severely arthritic joints or muscle spasm due to other chronic disease.

Muscle spasm and pain due to chronic stress.

There is a clear explanation for why the first two categories of patients hurt. Injury or illness causes this pain. Non-manipulating doctors usually treat these patients with medication and rest. DOs also offer medication and rest, but hands-on therapy relieves not only the pain – but also the cause of the pain.

The third category of patients baffles non-manipulating doctors. Because they do not recognize these conditions, non-manipulating doctors ignore them when possible. Without Manipulative Therapy, they can only prescribe painkillers, muscle relaxants, and tranquilizers. Many of these drugs are extremely addictive. This contributes to the accidental addiction fueling the Opioid Epidemic.

Non-manipulating doctors see these people as problem patients. They have no way to understand what is wrong, let alone treat it. The result of this is constant frustration for both doctor and patient. Some patients are misdiagnosed as suffering from psychiatric illness.

These patients easily sense that doctors do not believe them or think they are faking their symptoms. Such patients often fall into a cycle of going from doctor to doctor for relief. Unless they are fortunate enough to find a source of Manipulative Therapy, these people often suffer for years without relief.

Osteopathic Manipulative Therapy

Osteopathic physicians use Manipulative Therapy routinely, along with all the other healing tools of Modern Medicine. DOs use Osteopathic Manipulative Therapy to treat painful bone and muscle conditions. This is how Osteopathic physicians offer people effective relief that non-manipulating doctors do not provide. What does the Osteopathic physician do when they provide Manipulative Therapy?

The first step is a physical examination. This includes checking the temperature, blood pressure, eyes, ears, throat, chest, and abdomen. Osteopathic examination then proceeds to the bones and muscles to determine their structural status. Does the patient stand straight, or do they lean to one side? Is the muscle mass on one side of the body larger than the other side?

These and other signs can point to chronic postural problems that often respond well to Manipulative Therapy.

The next step is usually examination of the body tissue with the hands. Normal tissue should feel warm, supple, and will have good muscle tone. Abnormal tissue often feels cool, clammy, hard, and boggy – in a word, unhealthy.

Many experienced DOs suggest that patterns of abnormal tissue correspond to disease states of other organ systems. This makes sense because all tissue is connected by one or more nerves to the spinal cord and, ultimately, to the brain. Disturbances of normal nervous system function distort the body, and these patterns of distortion are a useful diagnostic aid.

DOs often use range of motion testing. Any joint of the body - such as the knee or ankle - has a normal range of motion. We consider a joint normal if it can move without restriction. If the joint cannot move freely, we say there is restriction in the joint. Restrictions result from tense muscles, bone or cartilage injury, or chronic diseases like arthritis. Whatever the cause, the joint loses its ability to move freely.

Restriction of motion in a major joint like the knee is obvious. All other joints of the body also have a normal range of motion. This includes the pelvis, vertebral joints, and the joints formed by the bones that make up the skull. Restriction of any of these joints also can occur and cause abnormal function.

What Is Manipulative Therapy?

Manipulative Therapy works to normalize all tissue and joint motion in the body. Common methods include:

Self-Referral

Maximum Health

Common Methods of Manipulative Therapy

REMEMBER: Manipulative Therapy is use of the hands to treat painful bones, muscles, and tisseue. All techniques restore side-to-side symmetery and thus restore Self-Referral.

Articulatory Technique identifies joints that are out of alignment. Direct action is taken to correct joints and related structures to normal function. This restores Self-Referral.

Muscle Energy Technique uses the patient's own muscle action to pull out of alignment tissue back to normal. This restores Self-Referral.

Fascial Release Technique identifies abnormal muscle and fascial tone. Working directly with releasing fascial strain restores Self-Referral.

Cranial Technique works directly with restrictions of bone and muscle at a deep level. This restores Self-Referral.

How can we accomplish this? One focus of Manipulative Therapy is to mobilize all joints. Another focus is normalizing muscles and related tissue. A third focus is to work with the body's fluid dynamics. Specific description of all Manipulative Therapy would require another book - but all techniques have the same goal: to normalize body function, remove pain, and restore Self-Referral.

These are broad categories of Manipulative Therapy. There are many variations of Manipulative Therapy within each broad type. Each style of Manipulative Therapy above has its proponents and detractors. Since so many people benefit from it, we will ignore the idea that Manipulative Therapy is of no use whatsoever. Since hands-on therapy benefits so many people, we should examine these techniques for commonalties; perhaps they are restoring Self-Referral from different perspectives.

Considering the variations of Manipulative Therapy, I remember the classic story of three blind men describing an elephant. The first approaches the elephant from the leg; he later describes the elephant as round and enormous, like a tree. The second grabs the elephant's trunk and later describes the elephant as snakelike. The third approaches the elephant broadside and simply describes it as massive, beyond definition.

In this story, three men meet an elephant. However, the blind men were unable to appreciate the whole animal. As a result, they gave a fragmentary report, literally limited to what they could touch with their hands.

Those who practice Manipulative Therapy today are in a similar position. Without adequate understanding of whole-body Self-Referral, we are groping in the dark, blind. Today's manipulating doctors need the comprehensive approach that constitutes *Self-Referral/Maximum Health.*

The medical system needs a better way to equip clinicians to diagnose and treat musculoskeletal problems via Manipulative Therapy. It is unconscionable to withhold this valuable medical tool from so many people who need it. All people of good will must work together to help make Manipulative Therapy available to everyone.

Self-Referral

Maximum Health

Chapter 13

Manipulative Therapy and Health

Self-Referral depends upon free movement of all muscles and joints. The stress of modern life disrupts muscle function. Manipulative Therapy is an important tool to restore Self-Referral.

Restoring Self-Referral

Self-Referral is communication between brain and body. The brain receives information on current body status and then issues commands to each muscle in the body. That is why Self-Referral plays a critical role in coordinating posture and movement; *every muscle is controlled by the brain.* We see the flow of Self-Referral in all body movement because *movement depends on Self-Referral.* Whether we operate a personal computer or chew gum, Self-Referral between brain and muscle makes all movement possible.

We usually do not think about Self-Referral and movement. Movement is so natural and effortless we just take it for granted. Stiff muscles from an injury or stress change everything. Anyone confined to bed with an illness knows the frustration of being unable to work. People suffering from muscle or joint pain are just as confined - by pain. Headache, backache, or other muscle related pain ruins the quality of life and makes work difficult or even impossible.

Today's Adaptation Crisis causes a great deal of muscle and joint pain. This is partly from physical stress – from the repetitive, mechanical movements of the office and assembly line. This physical punishment often pushes muscle and joints beyond tolerance. The mental stress of modern life also disrupts Self-Referral between brain and muscle. All this stress causes tight and painful muscles that interfere with movement. This creates painful muscle and joint conditions that can make normal life nearly impossible.

Doctors who do not use Manipulative Therapy dismiss this pain as a minor annoyance. Those doctors who use Manipulative Therapy report that it relieves muscle and joint pain. We know that restoring Self-Referral reverses the negative effects of stress. Manipulative Therapy, when correctly applied, relieves muscle pain caused by stress. *The logical conclusion is that Manipulative Therapy somehow restores Self-Referral.*

Some readers may find this conclusion too bold to accept. They will agree that Manipulative Therapy relieves back pain, but so does bed rest and medication. Critics demand scientific proof for Manipulative Therapy. They say that other medical therapy must stand the test of science, and Manipulative Therapy should be no different.

From Still to the 21st Century

When we discuss the ideas of Dr. Andrew Taylor Still or Dr. William Garner Sutherland, obstacles arise. Modern readers find these Osteopathic writers difficult to understand. Others find the ideas too abstract and without modern scientific proof. *These are legitimate problems.*

Still wrote in the flowery language of the late nineteenth century. His writing style has much homespun humor, Biblical allusions, and many metaphors. Because of the complexity of his ideas, Still's writing doubtless was confusing to his contemporaries. Modern readers will be even more confused. Considering culture and language drift for nearly two centuries, it is not surprising that Still's books are difficult reading.

Sutherland wrote in the 1930s and 1940s. His idea of cranial bone movement met opposition at the time, even from within the Osteopathic profession. The idea that the skull was not a solid bony case for the brain was more than many doctors – *MD or DO* -could accept. Sutherland also did not write in the scientific style that became the norm following World War II. The ideas lacked the scientific proof that today's doctors demand.

Many of today's harshest critics flatly assume there is no scientific basis for Manipulative Therapy. They say that doctors cannot state the theory of Manipulative Therapy in scientific terms. Critics also charge that there is no proof of the bone, joint, and muscle problems that manipulators claim to treat. They also state that Manipulative Therapy lacks scientific proof.

Strange as it may sound, I share this concern. This seems surprising because I am a strong advocate of Manipulative Therapy. Nevertheless, I believe that Manipulative Therapy must withstand scientific scrutiny to be more widely accepted and grow. This is the same path that every medical therapy has taken. Manipulative Therapy must receive the same scientific scrutiny we give to all other medical therapies.

Harsh criticism has a dampening effect on doctors and patients alike. Manipulating doctors feel unjustly criticized. Patients hear criticism and doubt Manipulative Therapy's value, even when they have benefited from it. Non-manipulating doctors are reluctant to become involved with a controversial therapy. While there is plenty of room for future research, *Manipulative Therapy already has a long history of scientific investigation.*

Early Osteopathic X-ray

Whenever we think of bones, thoughts of an X-ray come to mind. Few imaging techniques are as useful; whenever doctors suspect a broken bone, they take an X-ray. Many people have looked at their own X-rays as the doctor pored over the films, looking for a hidden fracture. X-ray is useful because it is easy to use and shows the bony skeleton so clearly.

The German physicist Wilhelm K. Roentgen discovered X-Ray in 1895. Roentgen received the first Nobel Prize in physics for the discovery. Doctors quickly used the new technology in medical practice. Today, doctors commonly use X-ray.[817]

Dr. Andrew Taylor Still founded The American School of Osteopathy in 1892 at Kirksville, Missouri.[818] Still and the early DOs had a keen interest in imaging the human body. This is why Osteopathic physicians were among the first doctors in the United States to recognize the value of X-ray. The Andrew Taylor Still Infirmary purchased an X-ray machine in 1898, only three years after Roentgen's discovery of X-ray. This was the second X-ray machine west of the Mississippi River.[819]

The earliest Osteopathic X-ray work was in Kirksville. Dr. David Littlejohn of the Andrew Taylor Still Infirmary published a description of X-ray technique in 1898. He used X-ray to locate foreign bodies, to show fractures and dislocations, and to diagnose internal organ disease. He also used X-rays as proof in medicolegal cases.[820]

At a Continuing Medical Education event, remarkably ahead of its time, Dr. H. Robarts, editor of the American X-ray Journal, lectured on X-ray use at the Infirmary in 1898. As is true today, the lecturer stood at a podium and gave a spoken presentation of his work, using projected X-ray views via slide projector to illustrate his work.[821]

DOs used X-ray for many interesting purposes, many of them ahead of their time. Calling his work "Skiography," Dr. W. Smith used X-ray in 1899 to map the arterial system.[822] By that year, doctors from surrounding states brought their patients to Kirksville for X-ray study. Medical writers of the time described Dr. Littlejohn's X-rays as among the finest in the world. The machine used was a ten-plate Van Houston & TenBroeck - the largest sized X-ray machine ever constructed at the time.[823]

Early Structural X-ray

Remember that Osteopathic physicians have a keen interest in body posture. They assume that very small changes in body posture can disrupt health. How small can a postural change be to cause pain or illness?

Dr. Still stated that very small changes from normal anatomy would disrupt health and cause disease. He believed deviations of one one-hundredth of an inch from normal would cause disease.[824] Because of his later work with cranial joints, Dr. Sutherland suggested that deviations of one one-thousandth of an inch from normal could produce disease.

Early Osteopathic researchers wanted to prove Still's theory. They reasoned that X-ray would confirm what Osteopathic physicians found with their hands. They also wanted to improve hands-on diagnosis and Manipulative Therapy. These interests caused Osteopathic researchers to quickly turn to X-ray as an imaging tool.

What did these researchers study? The earliest reports were front and side views of the pelvis and low back. Patients stood on a level surface with their feet shoulder width apart. Workers aimed the X-ray tube at film placed behind the patient. These films showed the bony structure of the pelvis and low back in the standing position. They called the result Standing Pelvis or *Structural X-rays*.[825]

What did researchers look for in these X-rays? Assuming normal anatomy, they reasoned that X-ray should show normal posture. This includes legs of equal length, a straight spine, and a level pelvis. What did they find? The early films often showed unequal leg length, lateral curvature of the spine, and unlevel pelvis. These findings were interpreted as evidence for Still's ideas.[826]

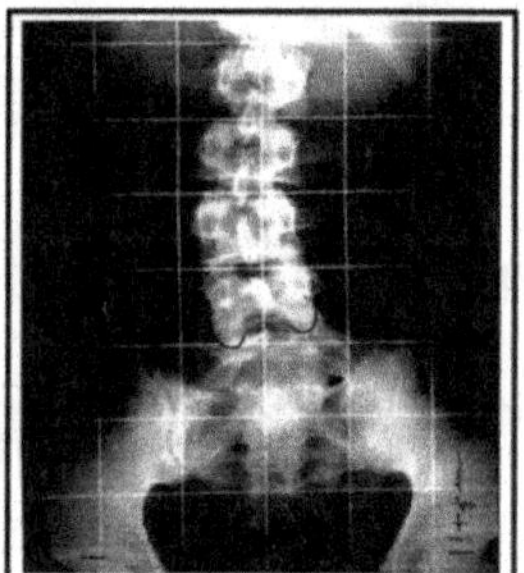

Structural X-Ray showing abnormal spinal curvature

The early films were crude by today's standards, but this use of X-ray was truly original. This is why Structural X-ray and Standing Pelvis technique is a truly original contribution of the Osteopathic profession. Dr. M. C. Beilke made a careful search of the American and European medical literature in 1936. He could find no use of Structural X-ray outside the Osteopathic profession until 1925. That was four years after the publications of Osteopathic researcher Dr. E. R. Hoskins.[827]

DOs saw these findings as vital, but all doctors did not agree. Critics charged the films were made under poorly controlled conditions. They argued that malalignment of equipment, film, or patient caused distortions. They also argued, that no doctor could read such films reliably. They judged leg length difference and other findings to be illusionary.[828]

Modern Structural X-ray

Dr. John Stedman Denslow and colleagues tested these issues in 1955. They tightly controlled the conditions under which they made Structural X-rays. They also constructed an apparatus based on that used by MD researchers Judovich and Bates;[829] they leveled a heavy metal floor plate and aligned the patient's feet with deeply etched lines in the plate's surface. Then they hung an overhead plumb bob behind the patient with piano wire. The plumb bob and wire were later visible on the X-ray film as a vertical reference.[830]

Denslow and colleagues used this apparatus to explore Structural X-ray technique. They tested variations of placement of the patient, film, and X-ray tube. The researchers X-rayed objects at various angles. This was to study distortion and magnification. After exhaustive study, they concluded that standard equipment could make satisfactory Structural X-rays if workers take reasonable care to insure standardized technique.[831]

After a vigorous program of research lasting well over a hundred years, we can safely draw some conclusions. Some patients have obvious X-Ray findings that prove abnormal posture. Structural X-ray clearly shows curvature of the spine, unlevel pelvis, and so forth. These X-ray findings are not the product of mechanical distortions, poor positioning of the patient, or human error. These findings are distinct from congenital problems like scoliosis - a severe and often crippling curvature of the spine. In short, there is ample X-ray evidence to prove that Osteopathic physicians are correct when they report abnormal postural and similar findings.

Anyone using manipulative therapy quickly notices that people with tight and painful muscles and locked joints often also have a lot of stress in their lives. That is why thoughtful people often speculated that there might be a relationship between the stress of life and the distortion of anatomy that causes such problems. What is known about this?

Self-Referral

Maximum Health

Stress Interrupts Self-Referral Between Brain and Muscle

Stress in the brain causes abnormal Self-Referral between brain and body. Osteopathic research proves this breakdown distorts the body through abnormal posture. Tight muscles distort the nervous system and restrict normal movement.

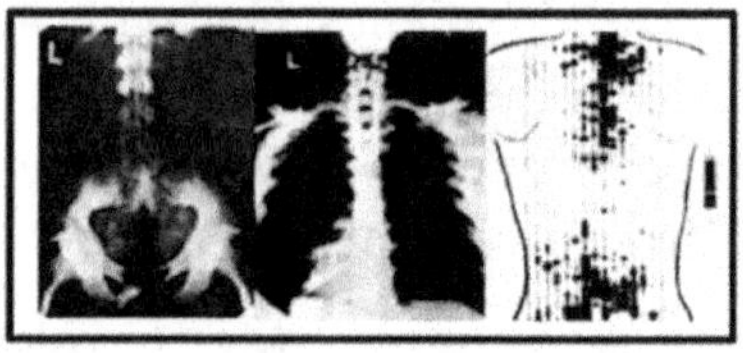

Early Osteopathic research studied posture. Dr. J. S. Denslow proved that X-Ray showed posture imbalance. He also used electronic equipment to study stressed muscles. Dr. I. M. Korr (inset) proved that abnormal posture causes patterns of muscle stress.

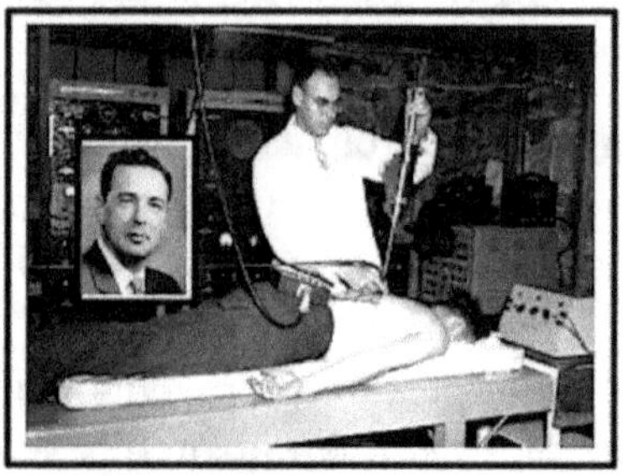

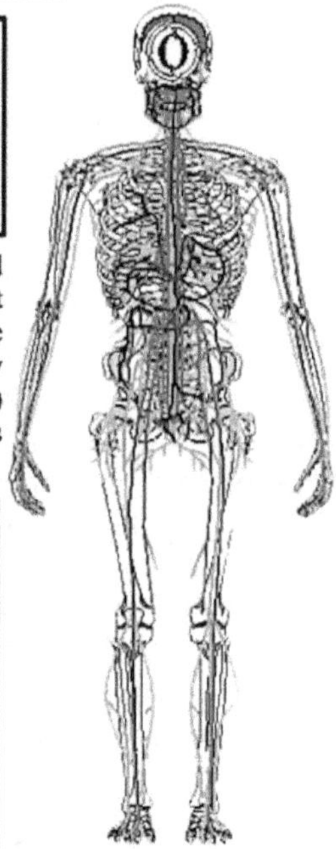

Denslow, Muscles, and Stress

Prior to his well-known X-Ray work, Dr. Denslow was not content to limit his investigations to Structural X-ray. He prepared for his future research career by learning from scientific experts. After attending Kirksville College of Osteopathic Medicine, Denslow worked in the late 1930s with two world-class scientists who trained him in research methods. One was Dr. Detlev W. Bronk of the University of Pennsylvania. A second expert who helped

Denslow prepare for his later work was Dr. George H. Steinhaus of George Williams College in Wisconsin. Bronk and Steinhaus taught Denslow how to use mechanical and electric machines to study muscle function.[832]

Previous to his X-ray work, Denslow used scientific equipment to study patients with painful muscles. These patients suffered from the kind of muscle pain that responds well to Manipulative Therapy. Denslow wanted to know more about why these people hurt and what was causing their pain. He returned to Kirksville to begin his research career.[833]

Working in the early 1940s, Dr. Denslow used instruments to measure the electrical activity of muscles.[834] EMG is short for electromyography. This is a record of the electrical activity of muscle and is similar to the EKG used to study the heart. *He found that patients suffering muscle pain were different from patients who had no muscle pain. Using EMG, Denslow found that sore muscles were tight and had abnormal electrical activity.*[835] What did this mean?

The Facilitated Segment

All muscles have low level electrical activity. This is caused by the muscle's chemical actions. Muscle fibers can either *contract* or *relax*. Muscle control is through nerves that trace back to the spine, and which ultimately communicate with the brain. Thus, when the brain stimulates the muscle, it contracts; if no nerve stimulation occurs, the muscle relaxes.

Normal muscles are pain free and show a low level of EMG electrical activity. Muscles that hurt show abnormally high levels of electrical activity. In other words, the muscles are tight and painful *because they are receiving too much stimulation from the nervous system.* And what causes this over-stimulation? The answer should be quite familiar by now; the cause of painful and tight muscles is *stress.*[836] These nerves in turn trace back and connect to the spinal cord. *This is an exact description of the Self-Referral balance of contract-relax that we previously discussed.* Thus such disturbances of bone and muscles may be defined as interruptions in Self-Referal.

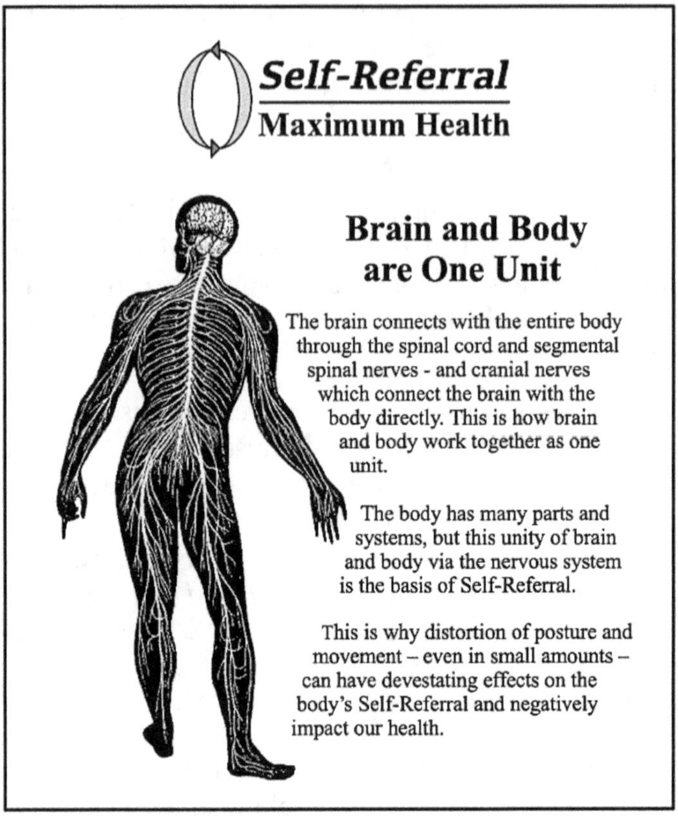

This situation is remarkably like that found in vasospasm, irritable bowel syndrome, high blood pressure, heart attack, stroke, and all the other diseases we have connected to stress. Just as stress can cause a heart attack or a stroke, it can cause cramping bowels, ulcers, or asthma. Dr. Denslow found that the body's many muscles respond to stress the same way as arteries, intestines, and bronchial tubes: they go into spasm. Once spasm occurs, normal function stops, and pain begins.

Denslow's research proved that patients with tight, painful muscles have sustained muscle contraction. That means stress causes muscles to contract excessively – with no purpose. Muscles should only contract to accomplish something – to hold the body in position, as in posture, or to move. Muscles also may contract to do work, as with moving a heavy object or lifting weights at the gym. When muscles contract without cause, they hurt and restrict movement. *This is how stress interrupts Self-Referral between brain and muscle.*

Denslow also found that some muscles become sensitized to over-stimulation as time goes on. That is, instead of relaxing when not in use, chronic stress makes these muscles stay tight - even when they are not being used. These muscles are already tight, sore, and fatigued - and they do not respond correctly to normal stimulation. Instead, they tighten up even more and cause major pain. *This phenomenon is identical to Dr. Robert Eliot's video game driven Hot Reactor: when highly stressed people encounter more stress, they overreact with tight and painful muscles.*[837]

Each nerve branching off the spinal cord has muscles attached to it. This is a spinal segment. *Back pain patients have stressed spinal segments: the nerves fire more easily than normal.* This extra nerve stimulation causes the muscles to be tight and painful – *all the time.* Denslow called such blocks of nerve and muscle *Facilitated Segments.*[838]

Gravity, Muscles and Stress

Denslow later worked with Dr. Olwen Gutensohn to study abnormal posture and EMG findings. They used EMG to study the muscle activity in people with normal posture. Then they took EMG readings of people with abnormal spinal curvature. They found muscles of those with abnormal posture were tighter and had abnormal electrical activity compared to normal posture.[839]

This finding is extremely important in understanding how abnormal posture interferes with Self-Referral. One of the constant physical stresses of life is coping with the downward pull of gravity. Humans can stand and walk upright because our bodies have a strong bony skeleton and muscles to resist the pull of gravity. That is, gravity constantly pulls down. Our bones and muscles constantly work to allow us to sit, stand, and move in an upright position.

Take a jellyfish out of water and place it on land, and it soon becomes a shapeless mass of protoplasm. Why? The jellyfish floats in the ocean, drifting through a watery environment that supports it.

Similarly, placing a human on a high gravity planet like Jupiter would quickly reduce that person to jelly. We thus understand that our bodies are designed to work and live in the conditions found on Earth – and our bones, muscles, and nervous system work together to allow this. We thus see that ongoing disruption between brain and muscles from stress thus profoundly disturbs posture and movement.

Denslow's findings prove that abnormal posture distorts human anatomy. This causes unequal distribution of weight: right to left, up and down. The result is physical stress and strain that causes tight and painful muscles. The result? Muscles get sore and tight; we tense up reacting to more pain; and more pain results. This goes on and on unless the abnormal posture is corrected. Manipulative Therapy works interrupt this vicious cycle.

Korr, Denslow, and Patterns of Stress

Denslow then worked to prove a connection between the location of tight muscles and what underlying diseases are present. This was to prove Dr. Still's claim that stressed spinal segments distribute disease. This is why experienced manipulators can predict what internal disease is present by examining a patient's spinal muscles. Why is this so?

Muscles connect with the spinal cord via nerves, which connect with the brain. Muscles also connect with other parts of the body through shared connecting nerves. That is why patterns of tight muscles correlate with internal organ disease. Denslow found preliminary evidence[840] for these patterns of stress, but the topic needed more work.

Dr. Irvin M. Korr joined the Kirksville College of Osteopathic Medicine in 1945.[841] Korr held a Ph.D. degree in physiology. Soon after joining the Kirksville faculty, he began applying his scientific background to Osteopathic ideas. It was natural that he would meet and join forces with Dr. J. S. Denslow. As they got to know each other, they decided to join forces and study Osteopathic theory. The two men further explored Denslow's work with EMG. Studying patients with muscle pain, they repeated Denslow's work and beyond. They began to see patterns of muscle spasm near the spine.

Over time they proved that stress creates patterns of tight muscles.[842] These are the patterns referred to by experienced DOs who can "read" a patient's health status by examining them with their hands.

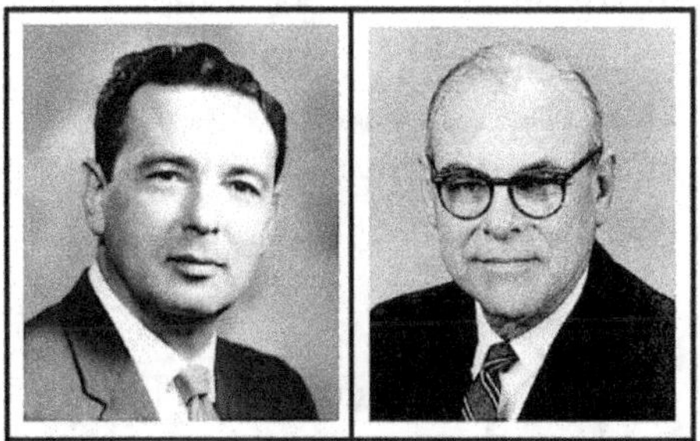

Dr. I. M. Korr (left) and Dr. J. S. Denslow proved Structural X-Ray findings, Somatic Dysfunction, and the undeniable connection between stress and the interruption of Self-Referral between brain and muscle.

Soon after the initial studies, Denslow started his research on posture and Structural X-ray. Korr continued studying the physiology of the muscles and nervous system. His first solo Osteopathic publication was "The Neural Basis of the Osteopathic Lesion."[843] What is an Osteopathic Lesion, and why was this paper important?

Practicing DOs describe the *Osteopathic Lesion* as one or more joints that are restricted in motion. That is, muscles around the joint are tight. These tight muscles prevent the joint from moving normally. These restricted joints are often painful. The tissue around these joints is often hard and swollen. Korr's research showed the physical reality of the Osteopathic Lesion. work also proved what clinical DOs had claimed for nearly a hundred years: that they could identify abnormal body tissue with their hands.

While DOs generally understood that Korr and Denslow had validated much of Osteopathic theory, the world of research is far from the world of practicing physicians. By 1947 many DOs knew of the research of Korr, Denslow, and others, but they lacked a practical understanding of it. Korr wanted all the Osteopathic profession to know there was scientific evidence for Manipulative Therapy. Korr later wrote in 1978:

> A pattern became set with my very first Osteopathic publication. The article was "The Neural Basis for the Osteopathic Lesion," as though it were a final statement! That paper began

> as a personal exercise in verbalizing to myself the exciting new insights that came out of my reading of Sted Denslow's earlier reports, . . . out of our first joint research effort, and out of my beginning studies of segmental variations in sympathetic activity in humans.[844]

What were these segmental variations? Korr continued EMG and related study far past the work that he and Denslow did together. He noted that the spinal cord has nerves at regular intervals. These nerves roughly correspond to the vertebral joints - each joint has one spinal nerve emerging from both sides of the spinal cord nearby. Those nerves in turn fan out like branches on a tree. Each branch ends by connecting with tissue somewhere in the body.

We call all tissue that ultimately connects to the same spinal nerve a *spinal segment*. In many cases the tissue is muscle, but the segmental nerves may connect with any tissue or organ of the body. This is why nerves from the same segment may connect with muscles of the back, the stomach, or heart. It is this series of common connections that make the nervous system so effective. This is also the basis of complex Self-Referral between brain and body through the nerves.

You may remember galvanic skin response, or GSR, from Wallace's early work with TM. We know that GSR is an excellent measurement for stress. A stressed person will have more sweat present at the skin surface. A less stressed person will have drier skin. When we run a low-level electrical current across the skin, we can measure the GSR. If sweat is present, then GSR will be less because salty water conducts electricity better than dry skin.

By 1951 Korr had constructed equipment that could map patterns of electrical activity for the whole spinal column. He accomplished this by creating a light-driven sensor net that recorded a picture of greater and lesser skin resistance. This setup measured the GSR and mapped the results.[845] In 1957 Korr published work using GSR equipment to map these patterns of electrical muscle activity - related to stress.[846]

Stress In and Stress Out

Following the lead of Denslow and others, Korr identified patterns of stress in the patients he studied. These patterns followed the segmental nerves. That means *stress translates via the spinal nerves into tight and painful muscles*. Korr's measurements *proved these changes*.[847]

An important idea that emerged from this work was that *stressed muscles and joints affect internal organs.* That is, if muscles are overstimulated by stress long enough, they pull joints and other bony structures out of alignment. Korr concluded this disruption would cause abnormal nerve discharge that would affect internal organs connected with the same segment.

Another important finding was Korr's discovery that *internal organ disease also creates patterns of stress*. That means someone may have an ulcer in the stomach, and back muscles in the corresponding segment will become tight and painful. The same is true of other internal diseases that have direct link to corresponding muscles of the back.[848]

Korr's work was important because it proved the reciprocal nature of structure and function. Segmental nerve structure allows normal nerve function. Tight muscles distort nerve anatomy and affect internal organs. Likewise, if internal disease is present, this stress will cause external muscle spasm.

We see here a critical explanation of Self-Referral. The body depends on Self-Referral to create health and, by default, to prevent disease. If stress interrupts Self-Referral, we will see internal organ disease like asthma, high blood pressure, heart attack or stroke. We also will see the tight muscles and disrupted joint anatomy described by Korr and Denslow.

This is how stress begets more stress in a circular fashion. If we suffer an external muscle injury like a sprained ankle or a pulled muscle, the resulting pain acts as a source of physical stress. The external injury may be the focus of medical care, but the injury also can transfer stress to the body's interior through segmental nerves.

Likewise, in the opposite direction, internal disease transfers stress out to connected muscles – causing external pain. This creates an ongoing vicious cycle of pain, disrupted function, and more pain. *Manipulative Therapy interrupts this vicious cycle and restores normal function: this is how Manipulative Therapy restores Self-Referral.*

The Circulatory System and Fluid Dynamics

Thus far we have largely thought of the body connected with the brain by nerves like the wiring diagram of a machine. In one sense, that is a perfect description of what goes on, moment to moment. We must now go beyond that idea, but still remember that all Self-Referral is being conducted by the Cybernetic feedback loops we have already examined.

We know that circulation of fluid plays a critical role in Osteopathic thinking – and in how the body works. The obvious reason for this is that circulation of blood and other fluids depends upon freely moving tissue and unobstructed flow through the circulatory system. This idea is so intuitive it seems odd to point it out, but this idea is very important.

If artery circulation to a body part is lost, that body part quickly dies for lack of oxygen and other nutrients. Likewise, if any body part is unable to move venous circulation, that part loses its ability to dispose of waste products. If either of these problems occur, the tissue affected by the loss of circulation is in serious trouble. How does the body balance these functions out so that all runs smoothly?

The Second Circulatory System

Blood circulates throughout the body's arteries and veins, but that is not the whole story of circulation. *There is a second circulatory system called the lymphatic system.* Lymph is a clear, water-like fluid that is found throughout the body. The purpose of lymph fluid is to cleanse body tissue, carry elements of the immune system to fend off infection, and to balance out fluid at the capillary level of blood circulation. How does this system work?

The arteries carry blood from the heart to all the body's tissues. Veins carry the blood from the tissues back to the heart. In the space between these two halves of the circulatory system we find the capillaries. These tiny vessels work to balance out fluid dynamics so that circulation works smoothly.

The circulatory system filters about 20 liters of blood per day via the capillaries. About 17 liters of filtered plasma are reabsorbed directly into the blood vessels. The remaining 3 liters remain in the interstitial fluid – this fills the tiny space between internal organs and tissues of the body.[849] Lymph has its own set of channels like the blood's circulatory system. After lymph circulates and passes through lymph nodes and related structures, it recombines with the blood in the venous system.[850]

This accounts for why the average human adult male is composed of 60% water, and the adult female 50% water.[851] Within this vast sea of fluids lie all the solid organs and tissues that make up the human body. All body fluids connect one way or another; we thus see that over, under, around and through all solid body structures flows a unified sea of fluids. In this sense, we are all literally walking bags of water.

The Third Circulatory System

In addition to the *blood circulatory system* and the *lymphatic circulatory system*, a third circulatory system comes into play – *the CSF circulatory system*. Every nerve that connects the brain with the rest of the body connects with tissue. Many nerves connect directly with muscle. Other nerves connect with body organs like the stomach, intestines, or kidneys.

All nerves – whether carrying signal from the brain to the body, or from the body to the brain – connect with the tissue at the level of the fascia.[852] We are well familiar with the electrical activity of the nervous system; that is the basis of Self-Referral. There is more to these connections than just electrical activity; there is also a connection of body fluids critical to health. This is generally not understood or taught outside the Osteopathic profession – and it opens a whole new range of possibilities for Self-Referral.

Self-Referral
Maximum Health

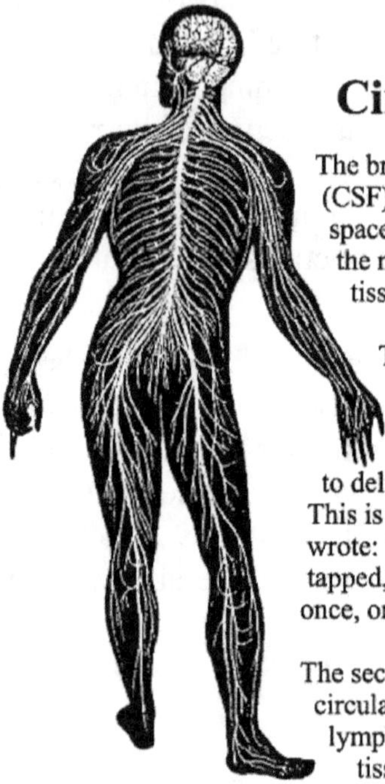

The Third Circulatory System

The brain creates Cerebrospinal Fluid (CSF). This fluid circulates via the space between the nerve sheath and the nerve. This connects with all body tissue at the level of the fascia.

The CSF carries with it substances that have a nourishing or trophic effect on all tissue. One purpose of the third circulatory system is to deliver these nourishing substances. This is what Dr. Still meant when he wrote: "this great river of life must be tapped, and the withered field irrigated at once, or the harvest of health will be lost."

The second function of the third circulatory system is to join with lymphatic and related fluids to cleanse tissue throughout the body.

Both Still and Sutherland taught that the brain's cerebrospinal fluid or CSF is important to all tissues of the body. Every nerve is made up of a series of nerve cells or neurons. Other cells enclose these neurons, creating a nerve sheath. This nerve sheath encases the nerve much as insulation encloses an electrical wire. The structure of nerve and nerve sheath provides a microscopic space that is continuous from the brain's ventricular system to each nerve ending.

What is the purpose of this space? Still and Sutherland taught that *it allows the CSF to circulate from the brain, through the nerves, and ultimately to all tissues of the body through the nerve endings*. The CSF, according to Still, has a nourishing effect on all body tissues. Remember what Still said about CSF:

> The cerebrospinal fluid is the highest known element that is contained in the human body, and unless the brain furnishes it in abundance a disabled condition will continue. He who is able to reason will see that this great river of life must be tapped, and the withered field irrigated at once, or the harvest of health will be lost.[853]

This is a bold assertion, and a departure from conventional medical teaching. Today's medical texts depict the nerves with no circulatory role, and the brain's CSF system is merely a waterbed to protect the brain from blows to the head and spine. What evidence is there to substantiate the Osteopathic claim?

Proving the Trophic Effect of Nerves

Dr. Irvin M. Korr spent the last decades of his career researching the trophic or nourishing function of nerves. Do these ideas line up with known medical thought? The relationship of nerve to muscle is well established; we know that muscles atrophy or wither when we cut their nerves. This is not a new idea - records from ancient Egypt show this to be true. In ancient Greece, Hippocrates wrote of similar problems following nerve damage or injury.[854]

We know today that this is true. For example, polio causes muscle weakness and atrophy; the polio virus damages the muscle's nerves – and muscles wither away, often becoming useless. Polio was a major crippler of people until it was mostly eradicated by polio vaccine.[855, 856]

Osteopathic thinkers note that chronic stress also affects tissue over time. This is much like the effects of the polio virus, but in smaller increments, over a longer period of time. These chronic effects are what DOs report as muscle changes they find with hands-on diagnosis. Those who report such findings describe the muscle tissue as feeling boggy, ropy, or even shrunken and weak. We know interruption in Self-Referral contributes to these findings, but what specifically causes them?[857]

Self-Referral

Maximum Health

Proof of Nourishing Effects of Nerves

Dr. I. M Korr studied the trophic (nourishing) influence of nerves on tissue. He published articles proving that CSF circulates within the nerve sheaths of all nerves - and it delivers chemical substances to the tissue that did not come from other sources. One of his better-known experiments severed the nerve connections to half of a dog's tongue. Once healed, he injected dye into the nerves that terminated in the dog's tongue. What did Korr find?

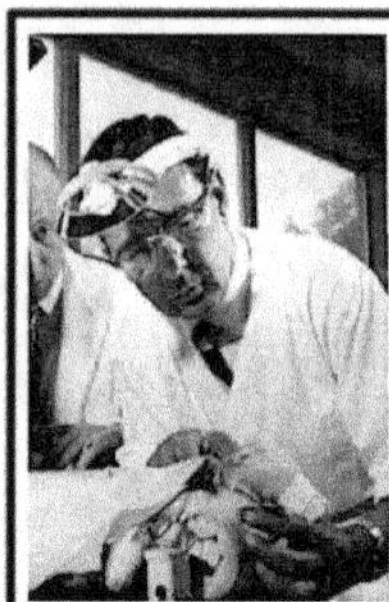

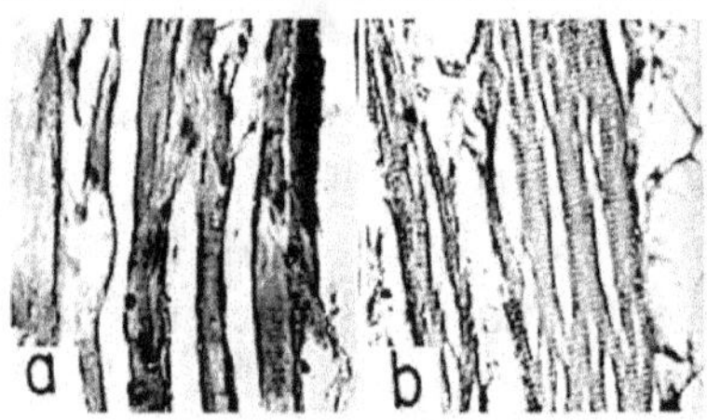

Microscopic study shows the tongue severed from nerves (a) did not receive the chemically tagged substances from the nerves but the tongue with intact nerves continued to receive the tagged substances (b). Korr thus proved that nerves have circulatory function.

When we cut nerves to a muscle – as in animal studies - many argue that the reason that muscle shrinks and shrivels is that the muscle no longer receives stimulation from the nerve. That is a factor, to be sure. But that is not the not the only cause for the withering effect. *The loss of the trophic or nourishing effect of nerves - which brings critical substances to body tissue - also is a major problem.*

For example, if we cut the nerve to an animal's tongue, the taste buds change. After a time, the taste buds lose their specialized structure and function. They no longer taste, and their microscopic appearance changes to that of the surrounding tissue. When we reattach the nerve, however, the taste buds regain their structure, and soon they begin to function again.[858]

How is it that the nerve feeds the tissue with which it connects? What does the nerve feed tissue? Korr's work proved that fluids circulate within the nerve sheath. Further, there are several chemical substances that originate in the brain that move down the nerve sheath toward body tissue.[859] Finally, Korr wrote that compression of the nerve by tight muscles, locked joints, or other tissue stress would prevent the CSF from delivering its trophic substances to the tissues.[860]

Proving the Cranial Concept

We remember that a key element in CSF circulation is the role of the cranial mechanism. Sutherland taught that the skull was not one large bone, but rather made up of many interlocking cranial bones. These bones interlock by means of sawtooth joints. These joints, Sutherland taught, allow tiny movement of the bony skull bones during life. This movement is part of a CSF circulatory system, although its movement is far more minute than that of the heart. What proof can we find for this?

Dr. Philip E. Greenman examined the skull in detail with X-ray to evaluate the cranial concept in 1970. He was able to show clear positional changes of the cranial bones. The bony changes seen with X-ray were the same as those reported by DOs trained in cranial diagnosis.[861] This study proved that DOs report cranial findings accurately, but it did not prove cranial motion.

Key to cranial motion is that the sutures between cranial bones are not solid bone. Rather, they are flexible joints that allow tiny movement within a limited range of motion. Dr. John E. Upledger and Dr. Ernest W. Retzlaff studied cranial sutures by microscope in 1978. They found that *cranial sutures are made of living tissue, and not the expected solid bone*. This living tissue has blood supply and nerves.[862] Follow-up study examined the sutures in cadavers of various ages. The findings indicated that the suture joints were open throughout life, from youth to old age.[863] This was in sharp contrast to today's majority medical opinion that the skull is one solid bone and incapable of movement.

These findings suggest that mobility of the cranial bones is possible, and there is appropriate tissue within the cranial sutures to allow a Self-Referral process between brain and cranial sutures to take place. The external muscles of the skull lie across multiple cranial bones. Each muscle connects with the nervous system and thus has Self-Referral capabilities like the rest of the muscles in the body. We see here a complete system of dynamic positional and pressure monitoring by the skull sutures. The cranial muscles work, by applying alternate subtle external pressure, to create the Cranial Respiratory Mechanism or CSM.

Finally, Upledger used scientific equipment to study cranial motion in 1979. He used strain gauge, EMG, and EKG to measure cranial movement. He found several cranial rhythms easily distinguished from heartbeat, breathing, and other non-cranial movement. Upledger also showed that cranial treatment changed the CRM from a chaotic rhythm to a more coherent rhythm.[864] That showed that cranial treatment was moving the CRM away from the chaos of stress and restoring Self-Referral.

These findings correspond exactly with the EEG research on the Transcendental Meditation technique. The studies of Banquet and others show that TM changes the brainwave patterns of the whole brain. Starting TM, the brainwaves are more random and do not have much coherence. Once we start TM, the brain synchronizes with itself, and brainwaves throughout the brain become more and more alike - front to back, top to bottom, side to side. These findings point toward TM restoring Self-Referral to the brain itself.

Cranial treatment seems to have a similar effect on patients. Cranial manipulators initially report irregular or even chaotic CRM rhythm and asymmetry of movement. As treatment progresses, the CRM settles down into a more coherent rhythm and movement normalizes at the same time. Like the TM research, these findings point toward cranial OMT restoring Self-Referral to the central nervous system – including the brain.

The common good that all Manipulative Therapy accomplishes is removing obstacles to Self-Referral. When we free up locked joints or tight muscles, restore fluid dynamics anywhere in the body, or work with the Cranial Respiratory Mechanism, we are removing blocks to Self-Referral. This is why *all Manipulative Therapy – when done well – restores Self-Referral and is a critical part of medical care that has been lost over time.*

We Know What Plugs the Drain

Dr. Andrew Taylor Still's ideas on CSF circulation thus are proved by scientific research. Dr. William Garner Sutherland's idea of the moving cranium are equally validated. Since these ideas are so effective in explaining health and disease, we should look for some central mechanism for disease based on fluid dynamics. Still wrote concerning the CSF circulation:

> To withhold the supply from a limb, to wither away would be natural. First, for want of supply (hunger), and the burdens of dead deposits along nerve centers.[865]

There is a substance well known to pathologists everywhere. We associate this substance with the aging process and disease. It accumulates in cells as a marker of sick or injured tissue. Following a heart attack, for example, we find much of this substance in heart muscle. If we look at diseased tissue under a microscope, we can see it as a harbinger of aging and death. This substance is *lipofuscin.* What is lipofuscin, and why do we find it in diseased cells and tissue?

We can see lipofuscin on microscopic examination of cells. This is a yellow-brown pigment. Lipofuscin is what remains of vital cell parts after the death of the cell. We commonly see lipofuscin in liver and heart cells of aged individuals. We also see it in muscle tissue of old or sickly people; we then call it brown atrophy. That is why *we call lipofuscin the "wear and tear pigment."*[866]

We now know that CSF flow plays a critical role in cleansing tissue and insures timely removal of waste products. Disruption of CSF flow thus contributes to cell death leading to lipofuscin accumulation. We find abnormal accumulation of lipofuscin in the brain[867] and throughout the body in patients who have Alzheimer's Disease[868] - and *this in part accounts for their mental deterioration.*

A critical idea to understand all this is: *Maharishi referred to nerve blockage as causing disease. He called such blockages "balls of earth" that clog up the nerve channels and prevent normal nerve function.*[869] I state that Lipofuscin or similar deposits thus are the physical basis of Patanjali's Samskaras. These patterns of stored stress likely lie in the brain, along nerve pathways, or in tissue throughout the body. It is these impurities that are the root cause for long term disruption of Self-Referral.

I suggest that such lipofuscin deposits will be proven to be treatable. Use of TM, manipulative therapy, and cranial treatment will likely treat these problems effectively. This could bring an end to the scourge of early aging and abnormally short lifespan. Working from the inside of the physiology via TM and external to the physiology with manipulative therapy, successful treatment of these problems will be possible.

Somatic Dysfunction

Because stress disrupts the body in such a universal fashion, Osteopathic thinkers have coined a term to describe this phenomenon: *somatic dysfunction.* The word somatic refers to the whole body, but especially by segmental nerve distribution. Dysfunction is a word that means abnormal function.

We hear about dysfunctional families or dysfunctional personalities. These are families or individuals who do not function normally. *Somatic dysfunction thus means impaired or altered function of the body.* Through *Self-Referral/Maximum Health* we now know that the basis for all somatic dysfunction is stress. That is, *stress disrupts Self-Referral between brain and body and causes somatic dysfunction.*

Stress causes disease by disrupting Self-Referral between brain and body. The mechanism causing this is disruption of feedback loops between brain and body. Long term effects of stress are aging, disease, and death; but until now the distribution of these effects have been a mystery. Two people may experience stress, but they do not develop the same illnesses. One person may have high blood pressure, the other asthma. What accounts for these differences?

We know from Post-Traumatic Stress Disorder that the brain's cerebral cortex stores abnormally strong memories as *stressful engrams*. Emotionally strong experiences literally burn these disruptive memories into the brain, causing Stress Syndrome. These memories remain in physical existence as patterns in the brain's nerve tissue. These are the *Samskaras* described by Patanjali in ancient India – possibly composed of lipofuscin and related substances. These physical patterns of stress disrupt the brain's Self-Referral, causing abnormal nerve discharge. This discharge further disrupts Self-Referral between brain and body.

The work of Denslow and Korr proves that the spinal cord and nerves distribute the effects of stress.[870] That is, if the brain's Samskaras fire, they cause abnormal nerve impulses. The brain's organization then sends these abnormal impulses to the spinal cord or cranial nerves. The nerves then distribute these abnormal impulses to the body's muscles and internal organs. *This is how stored stress in the brain distributes the negative effects of stress throughout the body.*[871]

Remember that mental and physical stress both cause the same damage to the brain. Thus, we see that either physical injury or mental pressures can burn Samskaras into the brain. This is how a broken leg or a difficult divorce at one point in time may contribute to a heart attack later in life.

The Common Thread

We thus see a common thread of knowledge running from Patanjali's ancient India to Lao-Tzu's ancient China, to Dr. Andrew Taylor Still in the American Midwest of the 1890s, to the present. This thread of knowledge unites the apparently unconnected subjects of health, disease, stress, Modern Medicine, ancient Transcendental Meditation, and now Osteopathic Manipulative Therapy.

These ideas are exciting and offer a more comprehensive vision of what causes disease. These ideas also show us a more complete picture of how to restore health when it has been lost. This is why the musculoskeletal system directly mirrors the full Self-Referral process - or lack of it. *This is why Manipulative Therapy is so important: the musculoskeletal system provides a unique interface that allows physicians to interact directly with the body's Self-Referral process.*

The spinal cord and cranial nerves act as a switchboard of communication. Doctors who manipulate can listen with their hands and intervene to restore Self-Referral. When we place Manipulative Therapy in the greater context of restoring Self-Referral, we begin to appreciate its true comprehensive nature.

Many dismiss Manipulative Therapy as a medical curiosity, but I sharply disagree. When doctors withhold Manipulative Therapy, something critical is missing from medical care. In a humorous mood, Dr. Still once said: "When a cat gets his tail caught in a door, don't say 'poor kitty', or try to appease its pain by petting it. Open the door and turn it loose."[872]

The Opioid Crisis is largely due to ignoring the cat's tail in the door. Every provider in the medical system needs to learn Manipulative Therapy. Then they can solve the mechanical problems that cause pain instead of prescribing drugs to conceal pain symptoms. This will go far to end the Opioid Crisis.

Another aspect of this situation is the role of Manipulative Therapy in whole body healing. When we engage Self-Referral through Manipulative Therapy, we are tapping into the body's ability to fix, heal, and repair itself. When we relieve a painful musculoskeletal problem, we restore Self-Referral. That is why when we fix the pelvis, spine, or other body part, we are restoring Self-Referral in a direct and powerful way that likely gives health benefits way beyond getting rid of the painful problem.

All this harkens back to the Tao. Remember: the Tao is the perfect balance of all opposites. When we restore Self-Referral through Manipulative Therapy, we are doing something profound. We are creating balance in the patient, balance in ourselves, and balance in the universe. When doctors ignore Manipulative Therapy and only give drugs, they are just not giving the best care possible. Lao-Tzu writes:

> Music and the smell of good cooking may make people stop and enjoy. But words that point to the Tao seem monotonous and without flavor. When you look for it, there is nothing to see. When you listen for it, there is nothing to hear. When you use it, it is inexhaustible.[873]

When we look for *Self-Referral/Maximum Health*, we look for ways to restore Self-Referral. This allows the body to govern itself with the perfect balance of opposites. Today's medical practice ignores Manipulative Therapy at its peril – and to the detriment of suffering patients across the world. Tomorrow's medical practice will include Manipulative Therapy as part of comprehensive medicine. No matter what name we give to it, the most effective Manipulative Therapy will always be based on the theories and practice of Osteopathic Manipulative Therapy.

Self-Referral
Maximum Health

Chapter 14

Self-Referral and Lifestyle

Self-Referral creates health and prevents disease. Stress of modern life disrupts Self-Referral. Can we change and find alternative ways of living that promote Self-Referral and prevent disease?

Self-Referral and Lifestyle

We have examined the stress-creating aspects of modern life and found much of it hazardous to human health. Complete withdrawal from life is not an option for most people – and we all have plenty to do. Finding better ways to cope with stress is the logical solution. We know Transcendental Meditation or TM is especially useful to reverse the effects of stress.

We now know that TM is the most effective stress reduction technique available. Scientific research proves that TM works with brain and body that to create a deep state of relaxation that counteracts stress. This deep rest practiced twenty minutes, twice a day, produces a deeper drop in metabolic rate than a whole night's sleep.

Long term effects of TM are well documented. TM provides deep rest that allows the body to heal from the stress of the day. This natural healing restores Self-Referral, reversing the effects of daily stress. It is therefore no surprise that TM improves common stress diseases like high blood pressure, asthma, and angina pectoris. The good effects from TM are not limited to just reversing the stress of the day; research shows that long-term practice of TM over time improves health problems caused by stress.

We know that TM comes from an ancient tradition of knowledge. Since TM is so useful, we may wonder if there is more knowledge available from the same tradition that gave us TM. Are there other techniques or practices that reduce stress and promote health? Are there other ideas available from this tradition that we can use for health promotion?

Apples and Einstein

We can trace the TM tradition back to Northern India. Scholars know that knowledge dates to the Indus Valley civilization of 6,000 years ago. This is a civilization that is legendary in ancient Indian tradition. This is, according to many ancient texts, the last civilization that was based on Vedic Science.

Vedic Science is science based on the Veda. Veda is an ancient Sanskrit word. Maharishi writes: "The word Veda is from the root, 'vid,' to know. Veda means knowledge." What knowledge does Maharishi mean? Veda means more than just knowing a collection of facts. Veda means knowledge of the totality of life, the Universe, and how everyone interacts with everything.[874]

Central to Vedic Science is awareness of consciousness. In the Western view, we define consciousness as a sense of separate, individual identity. That is, "I" am aware that I am typing at the computer right now, writing this book. This sense of individual awareness is the Western view of consciousness. Basic to this idea is a separateness of my individual "I"-ness from everything else, including the consciousness of other people, animals, and the physical environment.[875]

Vedic Science expands the Western definition of consciousness. Western science assumes a separateness of the scientist from the experiment; that is, the scientist is an isolated individual, separate from what the scientist studies. Vedic Science assumes that consciousness simply exists, and the scientist and experiment are somehow portions of it.[876] If this sounds paradoxical, don't be surprised; it is. To understand this idea, we need to talk about quantum physics.

Before we talk about quantum physics, we must understand what came before it. The dominant way of thinking before Einstein was Newtonian physics. This was physics based on the ideas of Sir Isaac Newton. You will remember Newton as the fellow who was hit by a falling apple and discovered gravity as a result.[877]

The apple falling and hitting Newton in the head is a fine example of Newtonian physics. The apple's attachment to the tree becomes weak as it ripens. The force of gravity, which pulls everything toward the center of the earth, pulls steadily at the apple. Finally, the stem weakens, and the apple falls. The apple hits Sir Isaac Newton, who was fortunate enough to be thinking clearly that day. The rest is history.

This is a clear example of cause-and-effect physics. Gravity pulling on the apple is the cause; the apple falling is the effect. Newtonian physics focuses on the cause that produces an effect. The cause is - by definition - separate from the effect. This way of thinking held sway until Albert Einstein offered new ideas some two hundred years later.

Einstein's vision of the universe includes Newtonian cause and effect but adds many new ideas that we now call quantum physics. Rather than being made up of separate, individual objects that act upon each other, Einstein saw the universe as a vast, seamless field of matter, time, and energy. He would not see the apple falling upon Newton as purely a cause-and-effect collision of separate objects. Rather, he would see one vast field that is the universe. To Einstein the apple, Newton, even gravity itself are but local effects of that vast field.[878]

Einstein's view of the universe assumes unity of all things and forces. He thus questions the separateness of things like trees, falling apples, and bruised scientists. At first, this sounds odd but not difficult. Then we realize that our "I"-ness and so-called "objective reality" are parts of the same whole.

And what is that whole? That whole is best summed up by one word: consciousness. Don't be surprised if this seems confusing. The world's finest scientists still struggle with these ideas - though Einstein introduced them in the 1920s. Let's look at some famous experiments that demonstrate the role of consciousness.

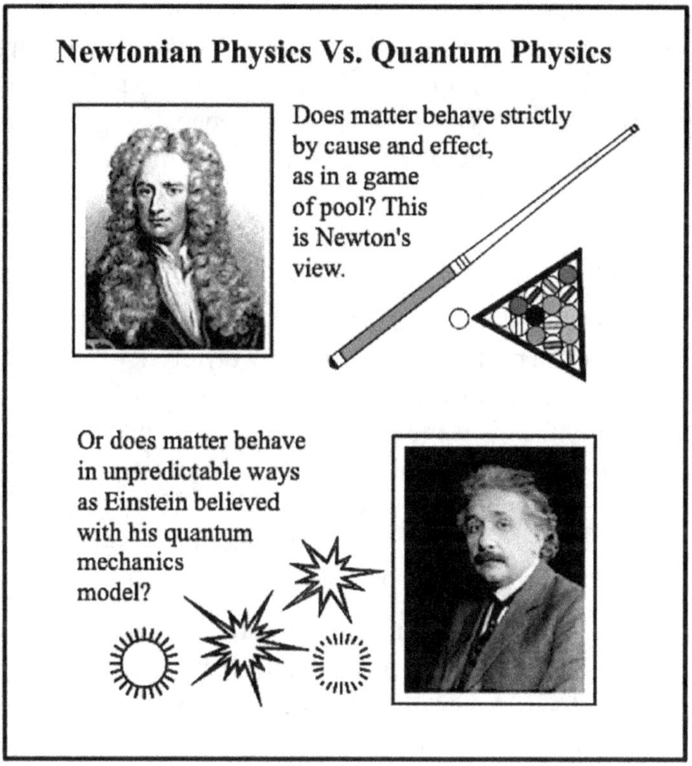

Light Discussions

In 1803 English physicist Thomas Young performed a famous experiment with light. He made a solid screen with two parallel vertical slits cut in it. He then placed the screen between the sun and a dark wall. Young expected the light passing through the slits to form a single lighted area on the dark wall. Something unusual happened: instead of one lighted area, there were five vertical bands of light. The center band was brightest. The two bands on either side were dimmer, and the two on the outside edges were dimmest.

Young was no minor tinkerer. He was a physicist, a physician, university professor, and a specialist in studying artifacts from ancient Egypt. In addition to his light experiments, he identified the visual disorder we now call astigmatism. It will interest readers of this book that he also helped decipher the Rosetta Stone.[879]

What did the five bands of light mean? Let us assume that light truly is waves of energy, each wave with a peak and a trough. This is just like a wave you might see in a pond. The bands of light were proof of what scientists call wave interference. This is like throwing two rocks into a pond at the same time. Each impact causes a circle of waves, but waves from one rock cancel out waves from the other rock. Young's experiment was important because it proved that light is wave-like. This gave important insight into how light works.[880]

Albert Einstein conducted a series of experiments that proved that light behaves as a particle. By measuring different objects as light hit them, Einstein determined that the objects gave off electrons when exposed to light. This is the photovoltaic effect, and we now use this principle to run light-activated switches. These findings prove that light behaves like particles of energy. There was one problem with all this. A particle of light is much different than a wave of light. The question was: how can light be both a wave and a particle?[881]

Many scientists explain this paradox in the following way: Newtonian Physics works very well at the level of day-to-day experience. That is, when we describe throwing a baseball, the moon orbiting the earth, or an automobile driving down the street - the cause-and-effect theory works well.

Things are much different when we examine the behavior of matter and energy at the size of the atom or smaller; Newtonian physics is no longer accurate. Many particles, like the photons in Young's experiment, do not act as expected. It is almost as if they had a mind of their own. *Quantum mechanics thus is the description of the seemingly non-random behavior of subatomic particles like photons*.[882]

The curious wave behavior of light particles suggests that the light particles, or photons, may be behaving in a coherent way. That means that the individual photons, at the subatomic level, may be acting in a coordinated way to move through the slits in Young's experiment. This leads to a startling conclusion. Physicist E. H. Walker writes:

> Consciousness may be associated with all quantum mechanical processes . . since everything that occurs is ultimately the result of one or more quantum mechanical event, the universe is "inhabited" by an almost unlimited number of discrete, conscious, usually non-thinking entities that are responsible for the detailed working of the universe.[883]

Walker clearly suggests that subatomic particles like photons may actually be conscious, although on a very simple level. The obvious conclusion of Walker and many other physicists is that all matter and energy - everything - is made of the same fundamental "stuff" - and that stuff is consciousness. This idea seems surprising, even startling. Changing theories in physics or medicine should not dismay us. Albert Einstein wrote:

> Creating a new theory is not like destroying an old barn and erecting a skyscraper in its place. It is rather like climbing a mountain, gaining new and wider views, discovering unexpected connections between our starting point and its rich environment. But the point from which we started out still exists and can be seen, although it appears smaller and forms a tiny part of our broad view gained by the mastery of our obstacles on our adventurous way up.[884]

I do not think that Einstein's additions to physics would dismay Newton. Rather, I believe Newton would be pleased. Sir Isaac Newton, like Albert Einstein, knew that his was not the final word on physics. He wrote in his memoirs:

> I do not know what I may appear to the world; but to myself I seem to have been only like a boy playing on the seashore, and diverting myself in now and then finding a smoother pebble or a prettier shell than ordinary, whilst the great ocean of truth lay all undiscovered before me.[885]

Great thinkers like Newton and Einstein accepted new and different ideas. Perhaps lesser mortals like us should keep an open mind. This is necessary to learn more about quantum physics and health. While these ideas are new to us, they are actually very old. In fact, many of these ideas have already been expressed - thousands of years ago.

Science Goes East

Over the last four decades, many scientists have become interested in philosophies of the Far East. The nebulous world of quantum physics and a growing need to understand it was the driving force behind many books and articles. What were these scientists saying? There seems to be a nearly astounding correspondence between ancient Eastern philosophy and what modern science calls quantum physics.

Fritjof Capra took his Ph.D. training in physics at the University of Vienna in the late 1960s. He later did research in particle physics at the University of Paris, the University of California at Santa Cruz, Stanford University, and Imperial College in London. After many years of physics research, reading, and thinking he published *The Tao of Physics*[886] in 1976. In it he masterfully outlined the commonalties between the emerging ideas of modern physics and Eastern philosophy. This work stands alongside Alvin Toffler's *Future Shock* as a landmark in scholarship and original insight.

Many authors have followed Capra's lead, producing bestsellers that teach much. Gary Zukav's *The Dancing Wu Li Masters*[887] does an excellent job of explaining fundamental ideas of quantum physics and Taoist philosophy. Bill Moyer's *Healing and the Mind*[888] explores ancient Chinese medical traditions including acupuncture, herbal therapy, meditation, and related ideas. Moyer's *Healing and the Mind* Public Broadcasting Network series explored these ideas in masterful detail.

While not referring to Eastern ideas directly, Kip S. Thorne's *Black Holes & Time Warps*[889] explores ideas of quantum physics and suggests applications to biology. Michio Kaku published *Hyperspace*, an exploration of Einstein's ideas and the emerging new physics.[890] TM researcher Robert Keith Wallace has published *The Neurophysiology of Enlightenment*[891] and *The Physiology of Consciousness*.[892] Both of Wallace's books explore Vedic science and how it can improve medicine and society.

We thus find that interest in the new physics goes far and wide. An article in U.S. News & World Report titled "Alternative Realities" explored the unusual ideas contained in the new physics. The article discussed many of the ideas in Michio Kaku's *Hyperspace*. Author Kaku, a physicist and professor at the City College of New York, offered: "Most people think of physicists as people who wear white smocks and work with tuning forks or study friction. But in fact, we make our living discovering things that blow people's minds."[893]

The search for useful knowledge in ancient Eastern wisdom is something like a modern treasure hunt, except the object of the search is not jewels or gold. Rather, the prize is knowledge itself. Indeed, this book is a product of that search.

Of the various ancient traditions offering current medical applications, those from ancient India seem the most relevant to Modern Medicine. The scientific research done with TM is more thorough and exhaustive than that done on other ancient traditions, such as those of China, Japan, Thailand, and Tibet. While other traditions offer knowledge useful to today's medical practice, research is difficult without access to living experts. Even if we now had a living expert like Maharishi, many years of research could only now begin. The results would be years away.

Further, there is substantial evidence that Vedic Science of India predates other traditions from the area. For example, in the 1990s I saw a display in Chicago's Field Museum of Natural History. The exhibit displayed many medical drawings from ancient Tibet. The museum curator's caption card explained that the four thousand old diagrams were based on medical texts brought to Tibet from India some two thousand years previously.[894]

TM and Vedic Science

TM has benefited from over forty years of dedicated work by Maharishi and the many scientists who studied his teachings. They tirelessly worked to make this ancient knowledge available to Western scientists and physicians since 1958. Despite ongoing skepticism and even hostility, these pioneers forged ahead in quest of knowledge that would help everyone. The result is a rich field of knowledge that is eminently practical. Thousands of years of wisdom thus are validated by decades of scientific theory and research.

It is good to propose grand theories of how the universe works, but theories seldom do much to improve health or the quality of life. TM has proved to be both practical and has stood the test of science. TM is the practical application of Vedic Science to human health. Vedic Science, in turn, comes from a long oral tradition. The Vedic scriptures of India record much of this oral tradition.[895]

Where Does Vedic Knowledge Come From?

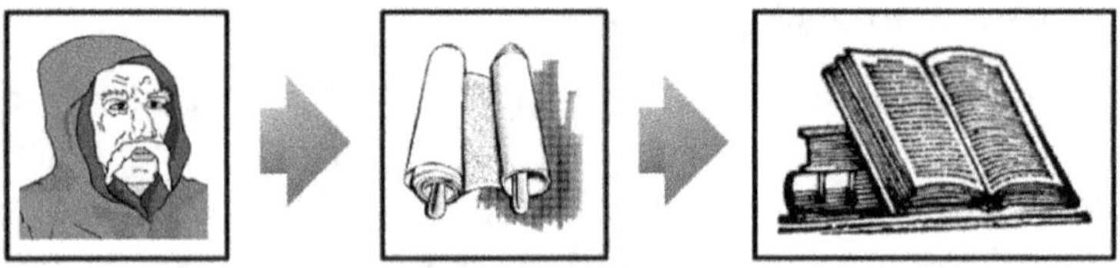

The Vedas have been an oral tradition passed through generations of Vedic Pandits for at least 6,000 years. Eventutally, some of these oral scriptures were written down on scrolls. Only a fraction of those scrolls have been printed as books in Sanskrit with transliteration and English translation. This is why having an expert like Maharishi or Guru Dev is so important to understand and work with the Vedic knowledge.

The Vedic scriptures of ancient India are among the oldest in the world. Masters passed these teachings on to their students, generation after generation. There are many Vedic scriptures; the most central are the *Rig Veda*, *Sama Veda*, *Yajur Veda*, and *Atharva Veda*.[896] While these books contain many words and ideas, the books are not the Veda. The Veda is the field of pure consciousness, the home of all the laws of nature. Veda is pure consciousness, and we cannot know it through the intellect alone. Dr. R. Keith Wallace writes:

> For thousands of years, man has tried to understand the nature of consciousness and its relationship to the laws of nature. Until less than 300 years ago virtually all the methods for gaining knowledge were subjective in nature. At the core of every cultural tradition of mankind can be found specific subjective techniques which attempt to enliven an inner intuitive understanding of natural law. This is particularly true in the Vedic tradition of India, where refined technologies of meditation were developed to probe into one's own nature, into the Self, the state of pure consciousness. Even at the beginning of our Western tradition, in Socrates' famous dictum 'know thyself,' the emphasis was to understand man's essence first . . . by knowing the nature of the inner self the essence of natural law might be realized. As a result, life could be lived more in accord with natural law.[897]

TM, according to Wallace, is the practical application of Vedic Science. That is, we can read about the Veda all day, but until we settle down inside and experience the silence that TM provides, we will not truly know the Veda. Maharishi refers to a verse from the Rig Veda:

> He whose awareness is not open to this field, what can the verses or impulses of pure knowledge accomplish for him? He whose awareness is open to it, he is established in evenness – wholeness of life.[898]

Maharishi refers here to the wholeness of life that medical professionals everywhere seek - perfect health. We know that TM reverses the negative effects of stress by restoring Self-Referral. What other medical knowledge is available from the Vedic tradition?

Ayurveda

Ayurveda is a Sanskrit compound word. Ayus means life, and Veda means knowledge. The root words together (Ayurveda) translate as *knowledge of life*. Ayurveda is the Vedic Science approach to preventing disease and promoting health. The science of Ayurveda, legend has it, is a direct result of Vedic Science as Maharishi describes it.

Legend gives a unique origin to Ayurveda. Four thousand years before Lao-Tzu, an ancient Vedic sage named Bharadwaja wanted to relieve human suffering. Bharadwaja and his fellow sages decided to investigate the basis of human health. They did this not by means of modern experimental methods, but through practicing advanced meditation disciplines. Through individual and group meditation, Bharadwaja and his fellow sages cognized what later became the *Charaka Samhita*. This is the basic textbook of Ayurveda.[899]

Once the knowledge was available, ancient Ayurvedic doctors worked with patients to make Ayurveda practical. They worked with lifestyle changes to avoid disease. They taught TM and other Meditation techniques to reduce stress. Through thousands of years, Ayurveda became a practical health science.

Ayurveda exists today in India as a form of natural medicine. Rather than relying on Western pharmacology, Ayurveda offers lifestyle recommendations on diet, exercise, and daily routines. Instead of treating disease only after it appears,

Ayurveda works to prevent disease before it can take root.[900] This is the basis of a true Health Approach to medical care.

Ayurveda has its own pharmacology, largely based on herbs and other dietary supplements. The herbal preparations often are quite complex and require many rare plants that are difficult to find outside the Indian subcontinent. Preparation of these herbal formulas are complicated and may take as long as a year or more to complete. These herbal preparations may be dispensed as tablets, capsules, powders, liquids, or paste.[901]

An important part of Ayurveda is disease prevention by regular cleansing sessions. These are procedures to clean impurities out of body tissue. These include steam bath, bowel cleansing, purgatives, and similar techniques. The common purpose of all these procedures is to rid the body of waste products created by the stress of life.[902]

Although not widely practiced, Ayurveda has a long surgical tradition. The ancient physician Shushruta pioneered plastic surgery thousands of years before Western doctors performed reliable appendectomies.[903] Today, a Western style medical system has absorbed most surgery in India.

Maharishi AyurVeda

Ironically, traditional Ayurveda as it is presently practiced in India can be mechanistic. Part of this is due to the imposing presence of Western medicine under British colonial rule and modernization after Indian independence. Like Western doctors, Indian physicians turned away from the older traditions of natural medicine as the Western scientific model became more popular.[904]

The TM technique of Meditation was originally a part of Ayurveda. TM is a mental technique to restore Self-Referral. The resulting balanced physiology produces health. How did TM become lost prior to Maharishi's teachings, even to Indians?

One key error that occurred was the incorrect use of mantras. As time went on, at some point the knowledge of the correct mantras was lost. Another reason is that TM requires very specific instruction and practice. The TM technique is so precise that even a small deviation from the correct mental procedure will prevent it from working correctly. As a result, the practice of meditation was far less successful. People eventually abandoned Meditation because it did not work.[905]

This should not be surprising to doctors or patients. Most people know that only the correct medicine will work for a given problem. We do not prescribe diabetes medicine for high blood pressure, or antibiotics for common arthritis. We must apply the correct medicine to any ailment. Likewise, we must use correct mantra and procedure, or TM will not work properly. Using bogus mantras or incorrect technique is extremely unwise.

In the 1980s Maharishi focused on reviving Ayurveda. To begin with, Maharishi contacted many of the current practitioners of Ayurveda in India. The traditional title of Ayurvedic experts is Vaidya (pronounced VIE'-juh). In Ayurveda there are specialists just as there are in Western medicine. Some Vaidyas are specialists in herbal preparations. Other Vaidyas are specialists in purification techniques. Still other Vaidyas are experts at determining the exact combination of Ayurvedic care each person needs.

In 1985, Maharishi met with a group of the leading Vaidyas of Ayurveda in India. Maharishi's purpose was to bring the finest experts together to discuss Ayurveda. Maharishi wanted to apply his revival of Vedic science to Ayurveda to make this knowledge available throughout the world as he had done with TM.

Among those distinguished experts in Ayurveda who were present, three stand out from the rest. Dr. B. D. Triguna was then president of the All-India Ayurvedic Congress and Director of the National Academy for Ayurveda, Government of India. Dr. Triguna's specialty was Pulse Diagnosis, an Ayurvedic examination technique.

The second distinguished expert was Dr. V. M. Dwivedi, Professor Emeritus of Gujarat University and former Vice-Chairman of the Indian Government's Ayurveda Pharmacopoeia Committee. Dr. Dwivedi was one of the last living masters of the procedures for creating Ayurvedic rasayanas, or herbal preparations.

The third distinguished expert was Dr. Balraj Maharshi, an Ayurveda advisor to the India state government of Andrah Pradesh. Dr. Maharshi was the greatest living expert in the identification and use of medicinal plants.[906]

Maharishi and these Ayurvedic experts worked together to hone and refine the knowledge. They sought to create the best combination of ancient wisdom to revive Ayurveda for the world. The resulting revival of Ayurveda was named Maharishi AyurVeda. This is why Maharishi AyurVeda is the best version of Ayurveda available in the world today.

Once Maharishi AyurVeda was formulated, the Vaidyas and TM scientists hosted meetings at important medical institutions around the world. The purpose of these gatherings was to teach the principles of Maharishi AyurVeda. They also encouraged scientific research to study Maharishi AyurVeda.

These experts spoke at the National Institutes of Health, Johns Hopkins Medical School, Yale Medical School, Harvard School of Public Health, and Massachusetts General Hospital. Doctors and scientists welcomed Maharishi AyurVeda and many research projects are now underway to study its various strategies.[907]

Maharishi AyurVeda: A Closer Look

Maharishi AyurVeda is a specific application of Vedic Science to the field of health promotion. We know that TM is the most effective stress reduction technique. The scientific research on TM is very thorough. Because of this solid background, we should carefully examine Maharishi AyurVeda.

Maharishi AyurVeda[908] is a comprehensive approach to total health promotion and disease prevention. Ayurveda is the world's oldest and most complete system of natural medicine. This system promotes lifestyle changes to restore Self-Referral through the approaches of consciousness, physiology, behavior, and environment. The World Health Organization recognizes Ayurveda as an established traditional health science. This world class medical organization declares Maharishi AyurVeda to be effective in the prevention and treatment of disease, health promotion, and life prolongation.[909]

The Maharishi AyurVeda approach to medicine has clear focus on Self-Referral. Consciousness itself is the focus, rather than what body part or process is causing symptoms. How does Maharishi AyurVeda approach medical care?

Ayurvedic diagnosis classifies people into one of ten common body types. This system relies on measures of three characteristics: Vata, Pitta, and Kapha. These characteristics are the *doshas* – fundamental principles of physiology.

Pitta types, for example, may have red or blonde hair, lots of freckles, average body build, and may be easy to anger. Vata types may be thin, nervous, and talkative. Kapha types may have heavier build, dark and thick hair, and may be very easygoing.[910]

A Closer Examination of the Doshas

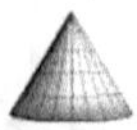 Vata	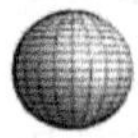 Pitta	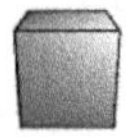 Kapha
Qualities of Vata Dosha include cold, dryness, speed, and lightness. Aggravated Vata Dosha may cause anxiety, constipation, or asthma. Vata Dosha in excess can be balanced by calm surroundings, a hot bath, and anything warm and moist.	Qualities of Pitta Dosha include heat, sharpness, and acidity. Aggravated Pitta Dosha may cause being prone to anger, acid indigestion, or skin conditions. Pitta Dosha in excess can be balanced by anything cooling to the physiology.	Qualities of Kapha Dosha include cold, heaviness, oiliness, and slowness. Aggravated Kapha Dosha may cause dullness, lethargy, obesity, or depression. Kapha Dosha in excess can be balanced by anything warm, sweet, and exercise.

The body types themselves are indicators of a specific style of physiology. The purpose of identifying the body type is to plan the right health intervention for the right person. Diagnosis by body type is simply an aid to determine the patient's type of underlying physiology.

Few people are purely one of these three body types. Doctors trained in Maharishi AyurVeda use a combination of observation and questioning to determine body types. For example, a person could be a combination of Pitta and Kapha - a Pitta-Kapha body type. Another person might be a combination of Vata and Kapha - a Vata-Kapha body type. There is occasionally a three-way body type called Vata-Pitta-Kapha.[911]

How can we use these body types in clinical medicine? Maharishi AyurVeda teaches that needs for diet, exercise, and the like are different for each body type. Maharishi AyurVeda thus provides specific lifestyle advice for people of different body types. Other treatment methods include specific recommendation of herbal dietary supplements and other therapies.[912]

Maharishi AyurVeda advises that different seasons of the year require changes in the daily routine. That is because each season as defined by Maharishi AyurVeda augments or adds to one of the doshas. For example, cold and dry weather adds to Vata dosha. Hot weather adds to Pitta dosha, and cool, wet weather adds to Kapha dosha. Maharishi AyurVeda teaches daily and seasonal routine to better synchronize the individual with the cycles of nature.

For example, let's say that a person has Pitta-Kapha constitution. This person should avoid becoming overheated, especially in hot weather. Heat adds to Pitta dosha, something that this person already has in abundance. The resulting imbalance could contribute to illness or disease. There are similar recommendations for all the other body types.

Maharishi AyurVeda does not compete with Western medicine; rather, Maharishi AyurVeda is a helpful add-on to Modern Medicine. Any doctor can take training in Maharishi AyurVeda and use this knowledge to help patients achieve better health. Nothing changes in our practice - but we have a new set of tools with which to work. The advice we give through this knowledge is far superior and more effective compared to the usual generic pamphlet hand-outs about Risk Factors.

Research on Maharishi AyurVeda

Dr. Hari Sharma is a critical leader in bringing Maharishi AyurVeda into mainstream American medicine. Dr. Sharma long served as Professor of Pathology and was the Director of Cancer Prevention and Natural Products Research at Ohio State University College of Medicine at Columbus, Ohio.

Dr. Sharma's field is Pathology, or the study of the effects of disease. The pathologist's work involves a lot of microscopic study of tissue. Such study examines cells and tissue in great detail, often to determine whether there is cancer present. Pathologists thus are very familiar with the cell changes that lead to tissue disease and death. These changes include the death of cell parts and accumulation of lipofuscin that we examined before. We know that cell damage producing lipofuscin is a common effect of stress.

Dr. Sharma's work led him to ask basic questions about health and disease. He became interested in the subject of free radicals and their role in causing disease. Free radicals are chemical "bad boys" that circulate in our blood. Dr. Sharma calls free radicals "molecular sharks." What do these sharks attack?

The cell membrane is the outside edge of every cell in the body. It protects the cell from damage. Free radicals injure the delicate cell membrane and internal cell parts.[913] Free radicals are caused by stress, environmental pollution, some prescription drugs, tobacco smoke, and alcohol.[914]

We see here another explanation of how stress causes disease. Stress increases the number of free radicals throughout the body, because of interrupted Self-Referral. Free radical researchers believe these deadly substances cause 80 to 90 per cent of all degenerative diseases. Free radicals are strongly implicated as a major cause of heart disease, arthritis, the aging process, and cancer. Clearly, progress in eliminating free radicals will promote health and prevent disease.[915]

Dr. Sharma became familiar with the TM program because of the vast body of research associated with it. He saw the value of TM and learned the technique. Sharma had excellent results from the technique and began learning more about TM.

When Dr. Sharma heard Maharishi talking about Ayurveda, he became interested. One reason for his interest was a longstanding familiarity with the subject. He was born in India and his father-in-law was an Ayurvedic Vaidya. These traditional Ayurvedic doctors spend five years in training and are highly respected. Dr. Sharma reports that his experience with Ayurveda growing up in India left a positive impression on him:

> I was aware, even if only from the experience of my father-in-law, that Ayurveda was practiced by intelligent and sophisticated people who enjoyed

> high levels of success - seemingly without the negative effects [of Western] medicine.[916]

Dr. Sharma was pleased with the results of his TM practice. He heard that Maharishi had organized a physician training program in Maharishi AyurVeda. Sharma attended a preliminary training program at Maharishi University of Management at Fairfield, Iowa - a fully accredited university. He then attended a doctor's conference on Maharishi AyurVeda in Boston. In 1987, Dr. Sharma attended a conference with Maharishi at his headquarters outside New Delhi, India.[917]

While meeting with Maharishi, Dr. Sharma became interested in doing research on Maharishi AyurVeda. One of the research topics discussed was an herbal dietary supplement called Maharishi Amrit Kalash, or MAK. This is a food supplement with a recipe handed down by ancient Ayurvedic Vaidyas.

Most of the 150 doctors at the conference were clinical physicians and had little experience with medical research. After several ideas for research proved inadequate, Dr. Sharma proposed an excellent research program. Maharishi was pleased.

"Good," Maharishi said, smiling. "Now you should do it."[918]

Dr. Sharma returned to Ohio and set about starting a research program to investigate MAK. He contacted colleagues at the University of Kansas Medical Center, South Dakota State University College of Pharmacy, and the Indiana University School of Medicine. These researchers joined forces with Dr. Sharma and colleagues at Ohio State University College of Medicine. Other researchers in India and across the world also began studying MAK. The research that followed produced surprising results.[919]

MAK Research Findings

Medical research showed that MAK is not only effective, but surprisingly so. MAK taken regularly acts as a free radical scavenger. That means MAK works to rid the body of free radicals - no matter what the cause.[920] This makes a strong case that MAK is an excellent dietary supplement to ward off the chronic effects of pollution, stress, and even medication side effects.

MAK also makes platelets less sticky. Platelets are tiny blood cells that are critical in blood clotting. Stress makes platelets abnormally sticky and can cause blood clots to form. These clots can cause heart attack, stroke, or sudden death. MAK taken regularly prevents platelets from being too sticky and thus prevents abnormal clotting.[921] Taking MAK as a dietary supplement thus is likely to prevent heart attack and stroke.[922]

Free radicals often damage the immune system, making people more likely to fall ill. MAK boosts the immune system, thus counteracting this free radical effect. Lymphocytes are some of the body's infection fighting white cells. Lymphocytes are healthier in people who take MAK regularly.[923] MAK also has a beneficial effect on those people who suffer from seasonal allergies, again by improving the immune system.[924]

Preliminary animal studies show that MAK may be useful in the fight against cancer. MAK slowed the rate of metastatic spread of lung cancer in mice.[925] Research with rats suggests that MAK may prevent breast tumors created by cancer-causing chemicals.[926] While these are preliminary findings, the control of free radicals holds great promise as a preventative against cancer.

That one substance would be so effective against so many health problems is surprising. Since Maharishi AyurVeda leaders have consulted with the world's greatest experts in medicinal plants, Dr. Sharma expected that MAK would be effective. The flurry of research that Sharma and his colleagues have produced shows MAK to be medically useful. Ongoing research on MAK and other Ayurvedic preparations continues.

Moving Toward Prevention

The health promotion and disease prevention strategies of TM and Maharishi AyurVeda make several assumptions. One is that doctors can teach people positive lifestyle habits. A second assumption is that patients will adopt the habits and use them effectively. Is it realistic to expect that we can do all this?

Stress expert Dr. Robert Eliot studied the pernicious effects of stress for many years. He verified the Hot Reactor phenomenon as a likely cause of sudden death from heart attack or stroke. Many who are found by testing to be Hot Reactors despair at the news; they feel doomed by their own nature. What if we can't teach people what they need to avoid the effects of stress? What if we teach people and they just fail to carry out what they are taught? Should we feel hopeless about patient education? Dr. Eliot did not think so:

> Emotions and behavior powerfully affect several factors commonly associated with heart disease. A patient's heredity, age, and sex may be unalterable, but other cardiac risk factors, such as hypertension, smoking, high cholesterol level, physical inactivity, obesity, and diabetes are strongly influenced by behavior. Seventy-two percent of risk factors thus are susceptible to change.[927]

And that seventy-two percent risk factor change includes all the risk reduction work we know how to do *before* TM and Maharishi AyurVeda. This is an exciting possibility. Rather than being passive victims, we can work actively to improve our health. *The lifestyle choices we make are pivotal in determining our own future*. This is a wonderful idea, but what scientific proof is there to support this position?

Researchers recently reviewed the literature about patient education for patients with heart failure. They checked medical journal articles from all over the world. What did they find? Heart failure patients who make positive lifestyle changes live longer and improve their quality of life.[928]

Recent research proves that we can effectively prevent heart disease by patient education. Patient education can reduce the risk of heart attack and sudden death by simply teaching patients about risk factors. These risk factors include smoking, obesity, sedentary lifestyle, high cholesterol, high blood pressure, and diabetes.[929]

A third assumption made by Maharishi AyurVeda is that doctors can make the change from the Disease Approach to that of the Health Approach. A recent address to the American Heart Association showed such a change. Dr. Edward S. Cooper told this distinguished group of medical leaders about prevention:

> Prevention is the key to progress in the control of cardiovascular diseases and stroke. This means not only the prevention of disability and death but also the avoidance of risk factors. Although prevention is our most important goal, we are also aware that its close ally is early detection.[930]

Here we see the marriage of ancient wisdom and Modern Medicine. Compare the modern wisdom stated by Dr. Cooper with the ancient wisdom of Lao-Tzu:

> Plan for what is difficult while it is easy, do what is great while it is small. The most difficult things in the world must be done while they are still easy, the greatest things in the world must be done while they are still small. For this reason, sages never do what is great, and this is why they can achieve that greatness.[931]

Many medical experts say that now is the time to emphasize health promotion and disease prevention.[932] The huge baby boomer bulge in the population is reaching middle age. Our healthcare system stands to be stressed beyond tolerance. If doctors and other health care workers - and the public - act now, we may avoid untold suffering and expense.

Adding Maharishi AyurVeda to Modern Medicine will be a huge step toward health promotion and disease prevention. We will continue to enjoy the benefits of Western medicine while adding the best in Eastern medical knowledge. Because all this works so well with Modern Medicine, perhaps there is more we can learn. What do we know about other ideas of Ayurveda?

Timing is Everything

Maharishi AyurVeda teaches daily routines to structure our lifestyle. The goal is to synchronize our behavior with the cycles of nature. Practice of TM morning and evening is part of the daily routine. Some other daily routine practices are going to bed early and getting up early, regular meals, and so on.

Maharishi AyurVeda assumes that the human body has natural cycles, and that these cycles correspond with the cycles of nature. What evidence is there that the human body has natural cycles? Do these cycles have any relationship to cycles of nature outside the body? We will examine some ideas from *chronobiology* - the relationship of biology to time.

There is a natural rhythm to many biological events in the human body. Much of our body chemistry corresponds to the cycle of the 24-hour solar day. The pineal gland, located deep inside the brain, acts as a master timekeeper. This causes changes in hormones and other chemical activities in the brain, nerves, and other parts of the body. These changes, largely chemical, regulate many key processes. These include when we sleep, when we wake up, and how we feel.[933]

We know that there are daily surges in stress chemicals during the early morning hours.[934] For reasons that are unclear, there is a sharp early morning increase in the brain and adrenal gland's output of key stress hormones.[935] If people are already stressed, this surge can cause stroke and heart attack. Both killers[936] commonly occur during early morning hours.[937]

As a result of this knowledge, medical practice is changing to work with chronobiology.[938] Knowing that patients have a 24-hour cycle allows us to better administer medications for high blood pressure,[939] diabetes,[940] high cholesterol, and many other disorders. Giving medications at the time of day when they will be most effective is becoming more and more a part of medical practice.[941]

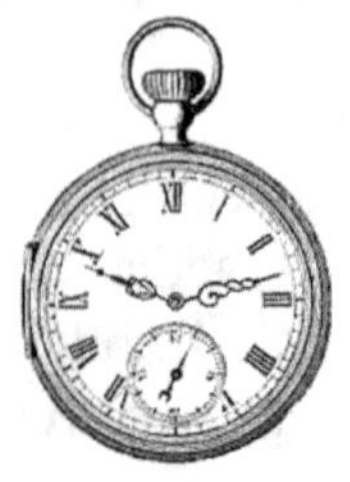

Human physiology runs within cycles of time: the 24 hour cycle and seasonal cycles.

Perhaps the best example of chronobiology is the effect of suddenly changing our environment. This happens to people who travel by airplane across two or more time zones. There may be many hours' difference between local time and the traveler's home time. This changes the day and night cycle, creating a biological conflict. The traveler's body still thinks it is on home time. This conflict causes the sluggish, disoriented sensations of jet lag.[942]

Most of the body's hormonal cycles follow the 24-hour cycle of day and night. This is the natural rhythm for the body, created by an untold number of years of humans living on this planet, in this solar system. When we abruptly change our time frame, as with jet lag, the body has all the reactions associated with stress. These include elevated blood pressure, excess stomach acid, irritable bowel syndrome, and headache.

How do we treat jet lag? Barring some problem requiring medication, simply allowing time to pass does the trick. As days pass with the new cycle of day and night, the body adapts to the new time zone.[943]

Daytime Rhythms

Dr. Michael Smolensky is the Director of the Hermann Center for Chronobiology and Chronotherapeutics in Houston, Texas. Dr. Smolensky studies the natural cycles of patients to help them with time-related health problems. One patient, for example, could not sleep well and suffered from depression. After no improvement with medication, his doctor referred him to the Houston facility. Hermann Center doctors studied the patient's natural rhythms and found a surprise.

"We found that the patient had a rare twenty-six-hour sleep-wake cycle instead of the usual twenty-four-hour cycle," Dr. Smolensky reports. "We recommended a dramatic change in treatment including bright light therapy and other techniques to synchronize him to twenty-four hours." The patient gradually improved and was able to return to normal life.[944]

The importance of the seven-day cycle is being studied. Dr. Erhard Haus, a professor in the department of laboratory medicine and pathology at the University of Minnesota, has a keen interest in the medicine of ancient Egypt. Egyptian physicians of 6,000 years ago thought the processes of life, including diseases, worked on a seven-day cycle. Dr. Haus has found truth in this idea: he reports that transplant patients typically suffer rejection of new organs at day 7, 14, 21, and 28 following surgery.

"In the past," Dr. Haus notes, "we thought societal customs were responsible for the seven-day work week and related behaviors." Dr. Haus adds that "unicellular organisms and rodents also display seven-day rhythms, and they don't care about our weekends."[945]

Dr. Franz Halberg is Director of the Chronobiology Laboratory at the University of Minnesota. He believes that doctors need to consider chronobiology much more. Examining a patient at one point in time, he believes, is inadequate. Dr.

Halberg says this is like "looking at a snapshot of someone on a roller coaster." He is now working on what he calls the Human Chronome Initiative. This is a proposed international effort to map human physiological rhythms.[946]

Seasonal Time Rhythms

The body also changes with the seasons. The months of the year mark changes in weather as the Earth orbits the sun. That is because the Earth's axis of rotation is somewhat tilted, and as the annual orbit around the sun progresses, different parts of the planet's surface get varying amounts of sunlight – causing the annual seasons. During winter the weather gets colder, and the days get shorter - while the nights are longer. This causes winter days to seem gloomy because of fewer hours of daylight.

Seasonal cycles affect the body just as much as the 24-hour and 7-day cycles. People during the darker winter months are more likely to feel gloomy than in the brighter summer months.[947] Winter causes mood changes, and some people become seriously depressed due to imbalances caused by seasonal change. Some people need medication to cope seasonally;[948] this is how doctors know definite differences between summer and winter depression.[949]

Chronobiology has helped with this problem by finding a non-drug way to treat people with Seasonal Affect Disorder (SAD): light therapy.[950] This is carried out by simply adding light fixtures with wavelength close to sunlight to the interior environment. Leaving these lights on later during the long winter nights reverses SAD without medications.[951]

Researchers have found that high blood pressure and cholesterol levels have an annual cycle that varies with the seasons.[952] There are weekly and seasonal variations in sudden death from heart attack. A Mayo Clinic study showed that death within 24 hours following a heart attack occurred more often on Saturday than any other day of the week. One reason for this may be the stress of changing routine from the work week to relaxation. More people died during the winter than the summer; the added stress of coping with cold weather likely takes a toll.[953]

All these findings suggest that our bodies adapt to the environment in all ways. This is Self-Referral in a larger sense. We see here that our bodies not only coordinate our internal environment but also must cope with the ecology in which we live. That is, we seldom think about the number of daylight hours or how our bodies adapt to it. Nevertheless, our bodies sense daily, weekly, and seasonal cycles - and adapt to them.

Coordinating with Nature: Body Types

Clearly the human body adapts with the cycle of the day, week, and season. This matches the ideas of Maharishi AyurVeda perfectly. If we could find ways to coordinate with these changing cycles of nature, many health advantages would arise. Is there evidence for this?

Medications may have different effects, depending on what time of day we take them. It is also clear that people are affected differently by these cycles of time. This is why some arthritis patients find their medicine provides more relief when taken in the morning; others find that an evening dose works better. The reason for these differences is that people have different chemical rhythms, largely related to time.[954]

Medical procedures may need to coordinate with the cycles of time in ways we never considered before. For example, one study found that dialysis for kidney failure was more successful if done more frequently and at night. The change in schedule proved easier on the heart and reduced the need for blood pressure medications.[955]

This opens many issues for debate. If research shows that a medication or a medical procedure does not work, perhaps it is because it only works in the morning. If the researchers gave the medicine or procedure in the evening during the study, the outcome could be different. Future drug and medical procedure research thus will have to take chronobiology into account.

We know body chemistry ebbs and flows in cycles, and researchers know these cycles relate to day and night. Some cycles, however, are independent of environmental factors.

Researcher Michael Menaker studies hamsters to learn about their internal cycles. Studying the timing of hamsters isolated from sunlight, he found a strong pattern. Every 24.1 hours, each of his 400 hamsters wakes up, mounts the exercise wheel, and runs for five hours. Menaker can predict within fifteen minutes when each animal will start running - *30 days from now*.[956]

How do these hamsters stay on a 24.1-hour cycle, even when kept in darkness? These animals have an internal clock that controls the ebb and flow of their chemistry. Even more interesting, evidence is mounting that this internal clock is ultimately controlled by genetics.[957] That means the internal cycles of body chemistry may be controlled at the level of DNA.

We clearly see differences in people based on the cycle of the day. For example, most humans are either morning or evening people; that is, they function best by starting their day early, or they feel better later in the day – or even in the evening. We always assumed these were habits formed over many years. Research on chronobiology shows this is not the case. People are morning or evening persons not by choice or habit, but because their genetics make it inevitable.

Animal and human studies thus prove that chronobiology is real. Considering these factors, the idea that people may have different body types as Maharishi AyurVeda defines them is easy to accept. There are cycles to our biology, and they have internal and external cues.

It thus makes sense that modifying diet and behavior to adapt to changing seasons will improve health. Synchronizing our lifestyle with the rhythms of nature thus makes sense and will add to our ability to promote *Self-Referral/Maximum Health.*

Self-Referral
Maximum Health

Chapter 15

Self-Referral and Medicine's Paradigm Shift

Recognition of Self-Referral will be totally transformative to medical practice. This paradigm shift will optimize the healthcare system – and drive Maximum Health.

A New Vision of the Body

Self-Referral/Maximum Health defines a new vision of the human body. That is an intentionally bold statement. Today's beautifully comprehensive picture of the human body has been slowly learned, one discovery at a time, over thousands of years.

Centuries of human progress in anatomy, physiology, and related sciences have taught us much. We know the body is made up of many parts: from the cell, to tissue, to organs. Organs work together to form organ systems. Organ systems work together to form a fully functional human being. What does this new vision of the human body have to offer that is truly new?

Today's colleges of medicine teach that the human body is largely static and unchanging. That is, following conception, our bodies are created during growth in the womb from a small collection of cells. These cells multiply and differentiate to form all the organs and organ systems that make a human being. Today's medical view suggests that birth is like an automobile rolling out of a factory, fully assembled. Size and proportions change as the newborn becomes an adult. But other than injuries or deformities, doctors consider the human body unchangeable.

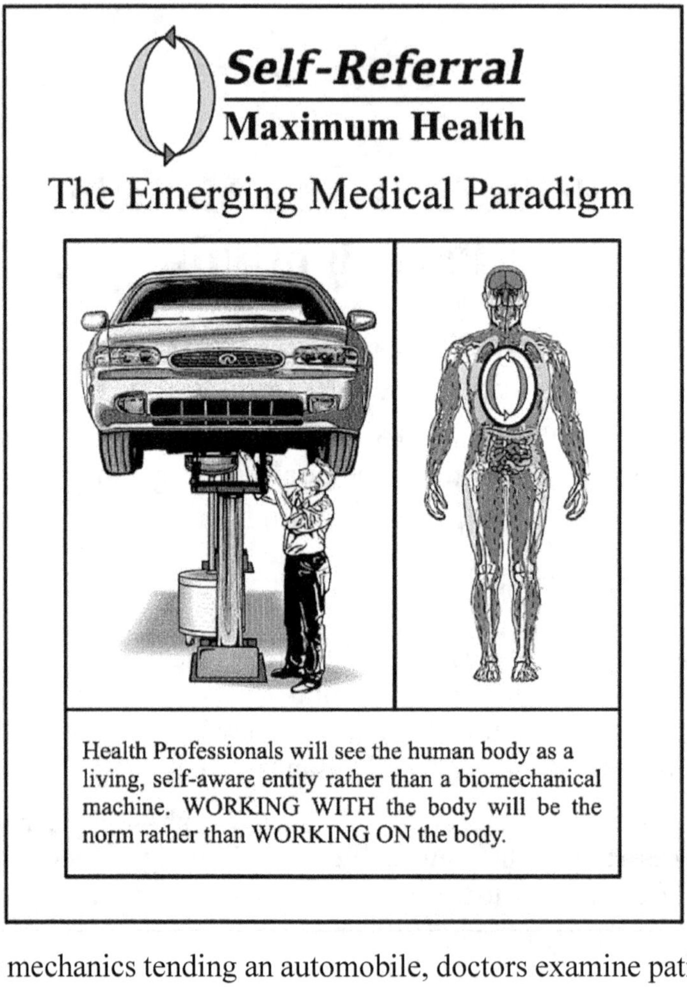

Like mechanics tending an automobile, doctors examine patients and watch laboratory numbers and other test results. When parts fail or wear out, they must be removed or replaced. If some part of the mechanism is malfunctioning, a little wrench work with medication often helps. If we get some rust, antibiotics usually kill off the offending bacteria. Central to all this is the assumption that the body does not change; it stays the same or deteriorates from disease, injury, or the aging process.

Lurking behind this mechanistic approach to the body is the assumption that aging is unavoidable. Why worry too much about side effects, I often hear doctors say, when the patient is only going to live for another five or ten years anyway? Why bother giving lifestyle advice when nobody follows it? After all, many say, nobody gets out of life alive.

I see in this view of the body an obsolete set of assumptions that must change. This whole set of assumptions is central to medicine's current paradigm – medicine's comprehensive set of assumptions. While we do not want to abandon the benefits of Modern Medicine, we need to question many of its basic assumptions. We can now do much more to promote health and do it far more effectively than ever before.

Medicine's Paradigm Shift

Medicine's pending change in attitudes and assumptions is like the paradigm shift that occurred in physics after Albert Einstein. The predominant paradigm in physics before Einstein was Newtonian Physics. This view of the universe is based on cause and effect. For example, on a pool table we use a long, pointed stick to hit the white cue ball. This propels the white cue ball across the table, hitting a colored ball that we have targeted. Hopefully, the targeted ball then moves, dropping into the table's pocket - and we have played a successful shot.

Newtonian Physics is like pool. According to the Newtonian paradigm, everything that happens is caused by one object or force acting upon another. We hit the cue ball, and the cue ball hits the target ball. Then the target ball moves and drops into the pocket. This is all cause and effect. The cause is hitting the cue ball; the effect is the subsequent events that drop the target ball into the pocket.

Albert Einstein, writing in the early twentieth century, proposed a radically different paradigm of the universe. Einstein and others proposed what we now call Quantum Physics. In Einstein's view, rather than being composed of discrete objects, the universe is actually one immense, indivisible field. What we call objects or forces, Einstein would call special local variations of that field.

The ideas of Quantum Physics are slowly spreading through our society. The paradigm shift naturally affected physics first, but it also is changing other fields. For example, one of the hottest topics in mathematics today is Chaos Theory.[958] Chaos Theory looks at mathematical relationships between apparently unrelated events.[959] These relationships show Quantum Physics style interaction between events occurring in the context of a much larger field, as Einstein suggested.

Chaos Theory was discussed in the film *Jurassic Park*, in which a fictional scientist suggested that a butterfly's actions on one side of the world could affect weather elsewhere. This was dialogue in a movie, but the ideas are real. Through elaborate mathematical models, scientists are proving that the Quantum Physics paradigm is true. One field exists, and everything that occurs within the field affects every other part of it.

Innovative medical thinkers are using Chaos Theory to find order in what appears to be chaotic human biology and even human behavior. William F. Allman writes a brilliant description of the role of Chaos Theory in biology:

> The scientific definition of chaos is not the same as the popular notion of something that is wild, random, and unpredictable. Rather, a scientific chaos describes a system whose behavior lies somewhere between complete randomness – the hiss of a radio that is set between two stations, for instance – and the dull, predictable whine of a TV test pattern. In a sense, chaos is more like music; unpredictable in detail, but harboring an order in its overall behavior.[960]

Most of the body functions we have talked about so far fall into the realm of the Newtonian Physics paradigm: they are based on cause and effect. That is, we touch something hot – the cause. Skin sensors send a signal to the brain. The brain recognizes we are touching something hot and damaging. The brain then orders the finger to let go – the effect. All that is cause and effect; all that is within the Newtonian Physics paradigm.

When we look at the finer aspects of Self-Referral, we see there is a lot of deliberation at the brain level between receiving the message that we are touching something hot - and deciding what to do about it. The nerve signals to the brain are easy to understand, as are the nerve signals from brain to finger. But what about the brain activity that makes the decision to move the finger? Many in the scientific world say that pulling the hand back is no more than simple reflex, and no deliberation of the brain takes place. Let's examine this.

Late in World War II, Staff Sergeant Henry R. Erwin was a radio operator aboard the B-29 bomber "The City of Los Angeles." Their aircraft and many others flew from Iwo Jima to bomb the city of Koriyama, Japan. Nearing the target, one of Sergeant Erwin's duties was to drop a twenty-pound phosphorous canister with a six-second fuse. After placing this canister in a mortar-like device that fired down and away from the plane, this marker would explode and create a bright, glowing flare in the sky – showing the other bombers where to join formation for their bombing run.

When Staff Sergeant Erwin fired the canister, something went horribly wrong. Instead of shooting out the bottom of the plane, the flare canister came back up the tube. It exploded in Erwin's face and fell onto the deck of the plane – just feet away from the racked incendiary bombs they were to drop. Caustic smoke filled the aircraft and Erwin's hair caught fire. The skin on Erwin's nose was melting. As the pilot and copilot were temporarily blinded, the plane slipped into a dangerous dive – threatening to kill everyone aboard.

Erwin dropped to a crouch and felt around for the canister, which was burning at 1300 degrees. He picked up that canister, cradling it between his forearm and body and crawled to the front of the plane. With his entire upper body on fire, he yelled to the copilot to open a window – and Erwin threw the burning canister out of the plane.

Erwin fell to the deck, and the pilot pulled the plane out of the dive and leveled out. Erwin's crewmates put out the fires on his body and in his clothing. Without a doubt, Erwin saved the crew and plane through his heroic action – and was awarded the highest decoration for bravery, self-sacrifice, and courage under fire: the Congressional Medal of Honor.[961]

We see through this story how the brain does indeed make decisions about letting go of something hot. In some situations, people may choose to continue holding on instead of letting go - if there is good reason for it. We cannot easily see or understand the complex brain activity that drove this brave man. He chose to hold on and take action to correct the situation instead of letting go to avoid injury.

How do we describe this? Through words like "Valor," "Bravery," or "Heroism?" Here we are truly at the nexus point between physical brain function, thought, and action. One thing we know for sure: something went on in Staff Sergeant Henry R. Erwin's brain, body, and spirit that resulted in an act of extraordinary heroism.

We see here that the greatest external acts of human beings start at the level of thought. This is a much more refined level of body function that is not easily explained by cause and effect; this involves the Quantum Physics paradigm.

When we found that TM – a thought - works so effectively to reverse the physical effects of stress, we realized something important. The use of TM is a whole new level of medical intervention. Acting at the level of effortless thought, the whole physiology is returned to optimum function. This is truly the realm of the Quantum Physics paradigm.

We see here the beginning of a Quantum Physics approach to medicine. The Newtonian Physics model works when we use it to describe everyday experience like the heart beating, the lungs breathing, and so forth. But when we examine areas of biology like brain activity, we approach the scale of submolecular physics – and the Newtonian Physics model fails to accurately predict the behavior of subatomic particles. It is at this level that the Quantum Physics model becomes useful.

Please do not think that I am dismissing Modern Medicine; people are living longer than ever thanks to modern diagnosis, drugs, and therapy. We know that Newtonian Physics-based ideas provide cures for lethal diseases, and we all celebrate the victory. The Newtonian

Physics view has relieved much suffering and has enormously advanced medical care.

But now there is more help to be had beyond all this; *that is what this book is all about*. Now it is time to go farther once again. I propose that we should apply the Quantum Physics paradigm to the human body. This will open undreamed of possibilities for promoting health and preventing disease.

What evidence is there of a Quantum Physics model for the human body? We have examined the Cybernetic view of the body. The basis of body Cybernetics is the feedback loop. The feedback loop is a circular process that allows setting a goal, fulfilling the goal, and monitoring same. The feedback loop responds to the situation as it changes. The feedback loop thus turns goal-seeking activity on or off, based on whether the goal has been met.

We have used the example of a thermostat and furnace working together to heat a room to illustrate the feedback loop. Brain and body work together much as the thermostat and furnace. The goal is to create and maintain health. If all feedback loops work well, people stay healthy. If one or more feedback loops break down, disease will surely follow.

We call these Cybernetic feedback loops working together Self-Referral. *Self-Referral is that perfect set of exceptionless principles that creates and maintains body health. By default, Self-Referral prevents disease.*

Through brilliantly designed feedback loops, Self-Referral succeeds in adapting to an ever-changing environment. Running on automatic, Self-Referral balances out all the imbalances and discrepancies that come up in a demanding environment. When we observe Self-Referral's success throughout a human lifetime, the efficiency is nothing short of amazing.

While the idea of Self-Referral goes far to explain how the body works, at first glance it is still rooted in cause and effect. The brain senses the body, compares the current situation to the ideal, and makes changes. The Quantum Physics aspect of all this lies between when the data reaches the brain, and the brain gives the orders. It is there that Self-Referral works on the level of Quantum Physics.

Emergence of the New Paradigm

I find it very interesting that medicine's emerging new paradigm, as described in this book, resonates so well with ancient Eastern knowledge. This is the same pattern observed with physics; that is, people familiar with both physics and Eastern ideas quickly see the parallels and similarities between the two.

Central to Eastern thought and Quantum Physics is the unity of all things. While each individual person has value and a unique individuality, we are part of a greater whole we call humanity. Western thinkers have often fought this idea, suggesting that the individuality of each person is supreme, and extending that separateness into every field of human endeavor.

Prominent Western thinkers show us a deeper unity of humanity that exists among all individuals. Swiss psychologist Carl Jung worked with Sigmund Freud during the early 1900s. For a time, the men's work coincided, but Jung soon found a great interest in what he called the Collective Unconscious. Jung came to believe in a common pool of memories, ideas, and experiences that made up the Collective Unconscious.

While usually not accessible by ordinary experience, Jung believed that the Collective Unconscious contained much useful information that we glimpse during dreams and visionary experiences. Jung believed that universal human access to the Collective Unconscious explained why so many common myths, ideas, and images appear and reappear throughout history. He also saw the Collective Unconscious as accessible to every human but somehow existing beyond any one human individual.[962]

Joseph Campbell was another advocate of universally shared human experience. Campbell was the world's foremost expert on mythology. He spent his life traveling the world and learning the mythology of world cultures. Most people in the West would find little in common with Buddhist scripture, Bible stories, folk tales of Aborigines, and Native American spirituality. Joseph Campbell found the common threads running through all these apparently disparate histories, legends, and religions.

What were the common threads that Campbell discovered? He found there is a universal nature to mythology; every culture has it, as does every historical period. Through books like *The Hero with A Thousand Faces*,[963] Joseph Campbell shows us in short form what he took a lifetime to learn. The names and places may change, but all mythology serves the same purpose. What is that purpose? Campbell writes:

> People say that what we are seeking is a meaning for life. I don't think that's what we're really seeking. I think that what we're seeking is an experience of being alive, so that our life's experiences on the purely physical plane will have resonances within our innermost being and reality, so that we actually feel the rapture of being alive. That's what it's all finally about, and that's what these clues help us to find within ourselves.[964]

"Resonances within our innermost being?" This is heady talk. While the ideas of Joseph Campbell and Carl Jung are interesting, can we connect these universal human ideas and yearnings with the human body? And more importantly, how does all this apply to clinical medicine?

Jung's Collective Unconscious and Campbell's vision of universal mythology point to a vast body of shared thoughts, ideas, and experiences. This body of knowledge is accessible to all people, at all places in history, up to the present. Could there be a physical basis for this phenomenon? Could all human beings harbor a vast reservoir of common knowledge and experience that is reflected by these ideas? Perhaps we can find a basis for this by applying the Quantum Physics paradigm to the human body.

Today's medicine teaches that the body is made up of many parts that work together to form a human being. We have seen in our examination of *Self-Referral/Maximum Health* that the body is an indivisible unit. That is, if one part of the body is abnormal, disease results. Since the body works together, disease or injury in one part of the body will, ultimately, affect the rest of the body.

The seamless operation of Self-Referral between brain and body uses the brain, spinal cord, and all connecting nerves. The constant communication between brain and body occurs through a nearly infinite series of feedback loops. The speed of Self-Referral between brain and body is virtually faster than thought. This communication is beyond human comprehension: *so much information moves so quickly between brain and body that we cannot possibly track it.* This is clearly in the realm of Quantum Physics.

Emergence of a New Body Vision

That Self-Referral works at all is truly a miracle. The fact that it does work suggests the idea of function transcending form. That is, Self-Referral between brain and body is so fast and the volume of information so enormous that Self-Referral transcends the form of the body. In the living body, Self-Referral goes beyond "a brain," "a spinal cord," or "nerves." There is a functional whole that is far more than the parts.

Strong evidence of a whole that transcends parts is the body in the fluid dimension. While we usually think of our bodies as solid, the human form is only 43% solid; the rest - about 57% - is water. Part of this water is contained in about 4.5 quarts of blood. The rest is distributed about the body in different types of body fluids.[965]

The human being from the beginning leads a somewhat amphibious life. We begin life in our mother's womb, floating in a tranquil sea of fluid. When we think of this fluid, we seldom consider its composition or circulation. It is not a stagnant pool of water but a living, breathing, circulating system of life supporting fluid. Over 95% of the amniotic fluid is water, but one to two per cent is made up of substances like enzymes, urea, sugar, hormones, and fats. There is a small amount of fetal hair and skin cells present from the developing baby. This living fluid constantly circulates through the uterine placenta and is replaced about every three hours.[966]

After we are born, we are highly dependent on water. We need a regular supply of fluids every day, or we become dehydrated. We lose about half a quart of water through the skin every day by sweating. We also lose half a quart of water per day in our breath as air moves in and out of our lungs.[967] Anyone who has the flu with vomiting or diarrhea knows how quickly we become seriously ill through fluid loss.

Perhaps the internal fluid we are most conscious of is the blood. The average human has about 4.5 quarts of blood distributed through the whole body. The heart pumps this blood through the body, beating about 75 times a minute. The heart nourishes itself with blood via the coronary arteries at about two tenths of a quart per minute.[968]

It takes about 60 seconds for the blood to circulate throughout the whole body. It moves somewhat faster during strenuous exercise.[969] When the weather is cool, half a quart a minute flows through the skin. During hot weather, this jumps to three quarts a minute to cool the body through sweat evaporation.[970]

In a minute a quart of blood flows through the brain.[971] The cerebrospinal fluid or CSF is formed from this blood as it passes through specialized brain tissue. The brain produces half a quart of CSF per day.[972] This fluid circulates over, under, around, and through the brain and nerves throughout the body. Elements of the CSF pass into body tissues via the junction between nerves and tissue.[973]

All body organs are constantly awash in a sea of fluids. Other than blood, CSF combined with lymphatic fluid follows the fascia over, under, around and through all body tissue. This fluid cleanses and lubricates tissues down to the level of the individual cell.

This ocean of blood, CSF, and lymphatic fluid provides common ground for many circulating chemical messengers. Many of the endocrine glands like the thyroid and pancreas release hormones into the blood stream. Hormones are chemical messengers that are created by glands at one location, travel by blood stream elsewhere, and finally have their effect at their various destinations.

Roving White Cells and the Body-Mind

Swimming among all the fluids, blood cells, chemicals, and hormones are white blood cells. These cells function as the body's main defense against invaders like bacteria or viruses. White cells have a unique ability: they can move about like amoebas. The white cells can move inside the blood vessels as the blood flows. Even more surprising is their ability to actively crawl outside blood vessels into surrounding tissue. This is how they can actively seek and destroy potential invaders.[974]

Dr. Candace B. Pert was the discoverer of the brain's Opiate Receptors – the area of the brain where Opiate drugs cause their effects.[975] Later, she was a researcher in the Section of Brain Chemistry, National Institutes of Health at Bethesda, Maryland. Dr. Pert had an interest in white blood cells that went far beyond their traditional role as infection fighters.

Pert's research showed that white cells can manufacture a class of chemicals called neuropeptides - like those found in the brain. These chemicals allow one nerve cell to trigger another – and they are the basis of all nerve cell communication.[976] What is interesting is that *the body has neuropeptides receptors everywhere*.

The neuropeptide receptors work as docking ports for the roving white cells. That means that the white cells, as they crawl out of the blood vessels and into tissue, may act as messengers in the same way as hormones. They may receive a message from the brain or elsewhere, and then literally crawl into position to send the message to local tissue.[977]

This creates what Dr. Pert called a psychosomatic network. Psycho refers to mind; somatic refers to body; network implies communication. The term psychosomatic formerly conveyed the Newtonian Physics view that body and mind act separately, one upon the other. Dr. Pert's ideas that body and mind act as one unit are truly the basis of a medical Quantum Physics paradigm.[978] This offers yet another way for rapid Self-Referral to occur between brain and body, body, and brain.

Dr. Pert referred to this new idea as a single, integrated entity called the Body-Mind. In this revolutionary new vision of the body, the mind's thought and emotions have a nearly instantaneous effect throughout the body. If we have emotions of anger or pain, the Body-Mind - in seconds - creates an angry or painful environment in the body's vast ocean. This is clearly the key mechanism for the instant effects of stress throughout the body.[979]

The Body-Mind concept easily explains why the positive ideas of religion are so important. If we constantly encourage thoughts of love, humility, and acceptance of others - we are creating the same environment within ourselves. When we receive treatment from others in this fashion, it also reinforces that internal environment of positivity.

The teaching of Jesus to "Do unto others as you would have done unto you" thus has a clear basis in physical and medical reality; if we are going to create something in ourselves and others, why not go for the best? Why not promote perfect health?

Deeper than the Body-Mind lies the basis of our biological existence. This is the genetic information found in our DNA. These are enormous (by molecular standards) strands of coded information that structure our bodies from conception forward. The DNA code determines everything from our eye color to whether we are fat or thin, short or tall.

I think it interesting that experts in human psychology like Carl Jung and Joseph Campbell refer to "common threads" that run through the dreams, visions, and mythology of humanity. Perhaps the true unity of the Collective Unconscious lies within the threads of DNA - the common genetic heritage of every human being.

The Unified Body

We see now that Self-Referral occurs on many levels – and all at the same time. We have spent most of our time examining Self-Referral between brain and body via the nervous system. That alone explains much of Self-Referral, and it fits the conventional medical background most of us learned in school.

A second level of Self-Referral is that which occurs in that vast ocean of fluid that makes up our body's interior. Hidden from view by our apparently solid bodies, we seldom think of the vast activity literally swimming inside us. Chemicals, blood cells, and hormones move and act in this fluid environment, circulating silently to carry out their tasks.

The vision of Dr. Pert and others shows us that far from being separate from the mind, the body is one with it. Likewise, the mind is not separate from the body; rather, we have a unified structure called the Body-Mind. The rapid-fire interaction of nerve impulses, fluid dynamics, hormones, and white cell messaging boggles the mind. This is clearly where the Newtonian Physics model of cause-and-effect breaks down; there are too many multiple outcome events going on to even track, let alone fit into a cause-and-effect model.

Just as the Newtonian Physics model works in the world at large, we see the Quantum Physics model working to explain the tiny scale interactions of the body at the microscopic level, molecular level, and even smaller levels. This is a comprehensive vision of the body based on Quantum Physics. This vision goes far beyond the separate collection of parts that somehow work together as a human being. This is a far different vision of the human body than that presently taught doctors and other health professionals.

The vast body of TM research clearly shows that when people regularly practice TM, so many body functions move away from disease toward health over time. Again, please remember that this results from a simple mental technique practiced twice a day for twenty minutes. This suggests that the TM technique is literally the key to health – and as we practice it regularly through time, we unlock more and more health.

Acting at deep levels of the physiology, TM offers opportunity for better health. However, given enough time, TM will not just improve Self-Referral but will likely perfect it. That means there is a real possibility for a higher level of health than previously known. There also is a possibility of slowing down the aging process as the body's Self-Referral becomes more and more efficient.

I call the possibility of completely successful Self-Referral a previously undefined physiologic condition: the Unified Body. The Unified Body with perfect health will have seamless Self-Referral between brain and body. The result will be perfect mental and physical functioning without disease. Extension of life span will result, and better quality of life will be a natural product of the Unified Body.

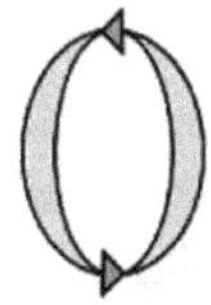

Self-Referral

Maximum Health

Possibility of the Unified Body

Through focused medical care to promote Self-Referral, we work toward Maximum Health. As we achieve Maximum Health, some people will achieve perfect Self-Referral. This is the state of the Unified Body. We will thus see people enjoying better health than any other time in history.

The Stressed Body

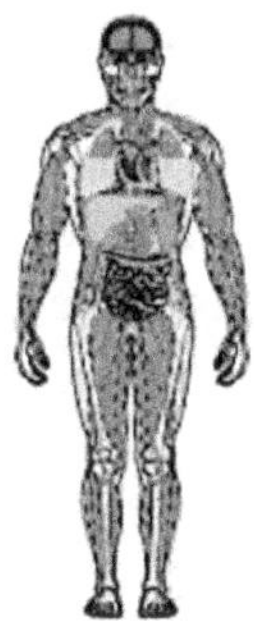

The Stressed Body runs like a collection of poorly integrated parts. Self-Referral is poor and fragmentary. The body is easily overcome by external stress. The result is poor vitality, disease, and early death.

The Unified Body

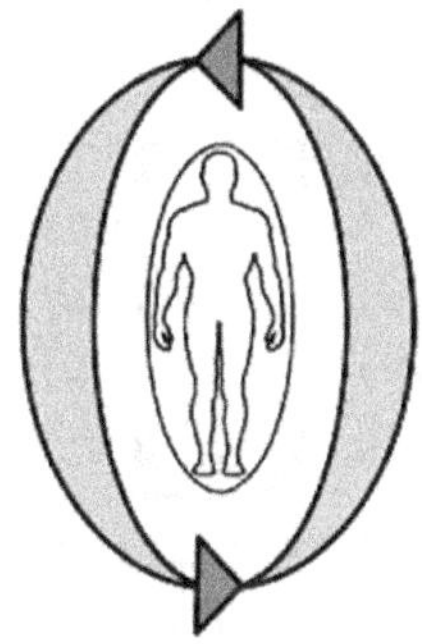

The Unified Body runs as a seamless unity of Self-Referral. Self-Referral is the rule rather than the exception. The body is immune to external stress. The result is great vitality, perfect health, and long life.

Examining all the medical findings of an enormous body of scientific research brings all this home as true. But there is more going on here, more that gives a fuller understanding than that stated here and now. Sometimes we have a moment where we can truly step back from the trees and see the forest more clearly.

What do we know about the relationship between the human body and the universe at large? Throughout history, serious thinkers have tried to explain the body's relationship with the earth, the stars, time, space. While many systems of thought looked initially promising, nearly all the proposed schemas have failed when evaluated by impartial study. Through our discussions so far, we have frequently referred to consciousness as a theoretical construct. Can it be that consciousness – as viewed through the concept of the Unified Body - is more concrete than we have thus far understood? With all that said, we need to consider the work of Dr. Tony Nader.

Dr. Tony Nader, Maharishi, and the Veda

Tony Nader, M.D., Ph.D., and M.A.R.R is a French citizen who was born and raised in Lebanon. In 1975, while still a premedical student, Dr Nader learned Transcendental Meditation. He learned that TM works to unfold full human potential through development of consciousness.[980]

As he continued the practice of TM, he had many profound experiences. As time went on, he grew to understand more about consciousness. Nader stated, "the inner experience is so fulfilling that you just want all your friends, all the people you love, and everyone in the world to have it."[981]

Because of his own experiences, Dr. Nader saw that Maharishi had revolutionized the practice of meditation. Meditation through the centuries had become known as difficult and required meditators to withdraw from society and live a monastic life. This is how the knowledge of TM had been lost for many generations.[982]

Maharishi, on the other hand, taught that the human mind is is naturally drawn to more and more bliss and happiness - and experiencing the full range of consciousness is natural and effortless. Dr. Nader thus soon realized the great possibilities that TM could bring to people everywhere.[983]

Nader finished college and later earned his M.D. from the American University of Beirut. His medical career e started there with a strong background in Internal Medicine and Psychiatry. He then earned a Ph.D. in Brain and Cognitive Science from the Massachusetts Institute of Technology (MIT). At that time, he was also a visiting physician at the Clinical Research Center. He did his post-doctoral work at the Massachusetts General Hospital, Harvard Medical School.[984]

Dr. Nader found himself among Nobel laureates and advanced scientists — people whose work was taught in all medical schools. Working with those great doctors and scientists gave him a thorough understanding of human physiology, especially the nervous system. This was an ideal environment that laid the groundwork for his later research exploring the relationship between brain, mind, and consciousness.[985]

While working at MIT, his interest in natural health care led him to conduct research on Maharishi AyurVeda herbal and mineral preparations to evaluate their safety, effects on memory and behavior, and their ability to prevent ageing and disease, including cancer. He also conducted research on neurochemistry, neuroendocrinology, and the relationship between the factors of diet, age, behavior, mood, seasonal influences, and neurotransmitter and hormonal activity, along with the role of neurotransmitter precursors in medicine. This caused Dr. Nader to want to learn more about consciousness.[986]

As a result of all this, Dr Nader met Maharishi, the founder of the Transcendental Meditation program, at a health conference for doctors and scientists in Switzerland. This was a life-transforming experience. This began a student–teacher relationship that would span nearly 30 years.[987]

Dr. Nader's desire to gain total understanding of the human mind and body led him to study Maharishi's Vedic Science and Technology under the personal guidance of Maharishi. During this time of study with Maharishi, Dr. Nader discovered that there is a one-to-one correspondence between the elements of the Vedic Literature and human physiology, anatomy, cell biology, and DNA. Nader states:

> This correlation reveals that the fluctuations of consciousness as expressed in the Veda are the same as the structure of our body, that the physical is an expression of consciousness. Physiology and intelligence are just different aspects of the same thing.[988]

These discoveries were published initially in his 1995 book *Human Physiology – Expression of Veda and the Vedic Literature*. This book has been reissued in several subsequent editions, each edition revealing deeper and more profound knowledge. As a result of all his work, Dr. Nader has become globally recognized as a profound Vedic scholar in addition to his many Western scientific achievements.[989]

In 1995, Dr Nader became the International President of Maharishi Ayurveda Universities, presiding over the training of over 2000 doctors in Maharishi Ayurveda and thousands of health professionals in Self-Pulse diagnosis — an Ayurvedic diagnostic technique to quickly scan the balance of body processes.

As founder of the Transcendental Meditation® (TM) program, Maharishi planned for the future of the international TM® organizations when he chose Tony Nader, M.D., Ph.D., MARR to be his successor. When Maharishi passed on in 2008, Dr. Tony Nader assumed leadership of the Transcendental Meditation organizations.

The work of Dr Nader now includes advising not-for-profit organizations in over 100 countries that teach the Transcendental Meditation technique and its educational, health, and research programs. Dr. Nader thus guides the Transcendental Meditation program, its advanced practices, and the practical applications of this technology in all areas of national life — education, health, business, defense, agriculture, and more.[990]

Dr. Tony Nader has always been motivated by the desire to understand life — who we are, why are we here, what we can achieve. Thanks to his close association with Maharishi, his understanding of the value of Transcendental Meditation and Vedic knowledge is profound. What lies at the basis of Dr. Nader's work? He states this clearly:

> As soon as I started meditating, I experienced that reality, which is transcendental, which is beyond the sensory level, which is inner, which is more abstract but more full, more peaceful, more blissful.[991]

Dr Nader's vision perfectly matches that of Maharishi Mahesh Yogi: to bring happiness, health, and peace to the minds and hearts of the whole world family. His experiences as a teacher, father, leader, scientist, and doctor inspire renewed dedication to everyone in the world. He has the strongest commitment to bringing consciousness-based health to everyone.

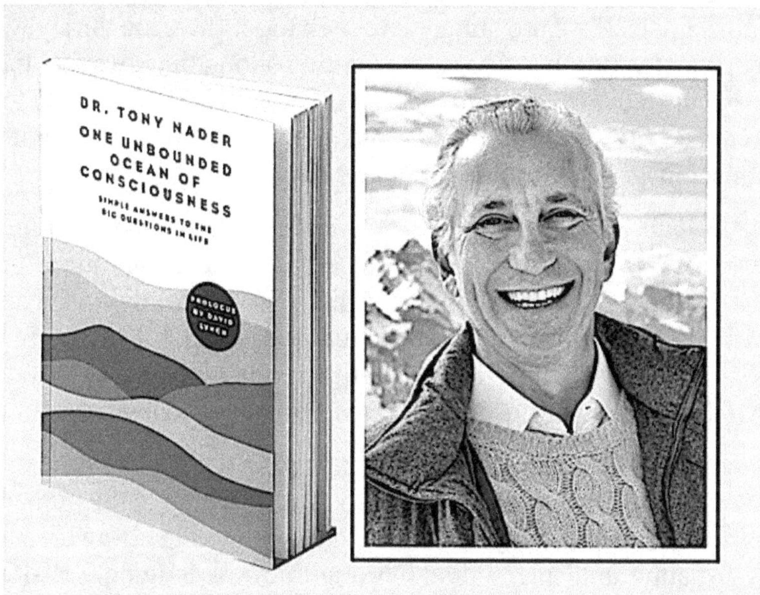

Dr. Tony Nader has brought his latest knowledge and ideas to his top selling book *One Unbounded Ocean of Consciousness.*

Self-Referral is Consciousness

The critical aspect of all this is the concept of consciousness. The term consciousness is defined as "the quality or state of being aware."[992] The medical definition of consciousness is naturally more oriented toward evaluation of the patient. Consciousness in medical care is defined as "arousal accompanied by awareness of one's environment."[993]

Central to this definition is the concept of self-awareness. Anyone who is awake and functioning normally is self-aware; they know that they exist, and they are aware of their surroundings. They know if they are happy or sad; hungry or satisfied; cold or hot - and so forth. Consciousness requires some kind of self-awareness and interaction of that self-awareness with a larger environment.

Any person who is self-aware acts within the environment to fulfill goals. If we are hungry, we seek food. If we are thirsty, we find a drink of water. If we have been sitting a long time, we feel the need to get up and move around. We have the thought that we want to listen to music, so we turn music on and enjoy it. All this is a result of our consciousness – the sum of our self-awareness.

I submit that the concept of Self-Referral as presented in this book is equivalent to consciousness. The body's feedback loops provide the brain with information about distant local conditions. The brain evaluates the information and compares it to physiologic normal. The brain then sends out orders to optimize the distant local conditions. All this clearly falls under the definition of consciousness.

Just as we treat a human being differently than a wooden chair, everyone in the medical profession must wake up to the human body as a wide-awake, fully functional unit with total self-awareness that is dynamic and interactive. Through acknowledging Self-Referral and working with it, we can transform medical care from mechanics working on a machine to physicians working with Self-Referral – through acknowledging the body's consciousness.

Even knowing and understanding Self-Referral, introducing the idea of consciousness into medical practice seems a stretch. Medicine is based on science, logic, and on traditions established through thousands of years of scientific progress. Medical care has recently been discovering more in common with consciousness through studies of the effect of religious practice on health.

Religion is one of those topics that are generally avoided in medical care. All health professionals display respect for people's faith but hesitate to delve any deeper into those matters. What do we know about religion and health?

Religion and Health

Doctors are trained in the tradition of Western science; religion is seldom a subject of discussion at medical school or during training. There are valid reasons for this. Doctors need an objective state of mind to be able to care for patients. This objectivity is important, both to the doctor and the patient.

Maintaining an objective view is important, but this can easily translate into a negative or even hostile attitude toward religion. I believe encouraging people to practice their faith is critical to promoting health and healing. Such encouragement, I believe, is critical to the healing process. Why do I say this?

One obvious reason is that religion teaches healthy moral habits. In today's age of rampant genital herpes, Hepatitis C, and AIDS - religion's insistence on sexual abstinence and monogamy takes on a new urgency. Rather than sounding like hollow advice, this is mandatory behavior in today's world - just to survive. Religion also discourages smoking, alcohol consumption, and drug abuse. These teachings on lifestyle habits, taken together, promote health.

We mentioned before the healing power of the Golden Rule. "Do unto others as you would have them do unto you." That is, treat others as you would want to be treated. If people earnestly try to live this ideal, their quality of life will get better. This improves marriages, families, nations, and - ultimately - the world. The Golden Rule also creates warm human relations and positive emotions – bringing health and healing.

Is addressing the idea of God or religion outside most patient's thoughts or beliefs? One of the most reliable ways to gauge public opinion on anything is the Gallup Poll - which tells us that 89% of Americans believe in God or a universal spirit, and 74% consider religion to have considerable importance.[994] These matters loom large, given that our aging society is likely to face health crises and end-of-life decisions in the near future – and need spiritual support.[995] Such concerns are so prevalent that discussion about medical care requires us to examine these issues. Are religious leaders aware of these concerns?

Leaders in religious circles are keenly aware of the Adaptation Crisis we are addressing in this book. I regularly attend church, and once in the Order of Worship in our Sunday Service Bulletin was the following unison prayer we all said together:

> We are running so fast, God, and we don't know how to slow down. We keep our calendars filled. We carry phones in the car and purse. We constantly check our voice mail, our email, and stay connected by the Internet. We are busy and yet not satisfied. We are moving faster, but we never catch up. We are stressed, God. Is this the way You meant us to be?
>
> Speak to us again your message of peace, of walking beside still waters, of refreshing our souls, of lying down in meadows of green. Speak to our anxious hearts and spinning minds that think if we are not doing, then there is no being. Restore our balance, lighten our drivenness, and make holy our rest. In Jesus' name. Amen.[996]

Finding peace and grounding our thoughts, emotions, and attitudes are central to religious experience. We need to reconnect with the central values taught through religious scripture and practice. One of the most common forms of religion is prayer. Prayer is a conscious mental effort to address God and offer worship. People also use prayer to reach out to God and ask for God's assistance in healing.

Key to this idea is the work of Dr. Larry Dossey. He is the former Chief of Staff at Humana Medical City in Dallas, Texas. He is an internationally renowned educator and lecturer on Body-Mind medicine and related topics. In 1988, he was invited to deliver the annual Mahatma Gandhi Memorial Lecture in New Delhi, India - the only Western physician ever given this honor.

Dr. Dossey's exploration of the relationship between religion and medicine led to a lifelong career bridging the two fields. Dr. Dossey published Healing Words,[997] a doctor's inquiry into the role of prayer in health and healing. He served as co-chairman of the newly established Panel on Mind/Body Interventions of the Office of Alternative Medicine of the National Institutes of Health at Bethesda, Maryland.

Dr. Dossey reports that he left medical school with the impression that prayer was little more than superstition. There was no mention of prayer as having any role in medical practice. No one taught that it might be useful in healing.

After many years in clinical medicine, Dossey was surprised to find scientific evidence for a healing effect of prayer. As a result, he spent over ten years inquiring into the subject of prayer and healing.[998] What did he find? Much to his surprise, Dossey found that prayer works.

Dossey tells the story of Dr. Randolph Byrd, a cardiologist who is also a practicing Christian. Dr. Byrd wanted to study the effects of prayer on sick people. He designed a study to evaluate the role of God in healing. How did he do this?

Byrd studied 393 patients admitted to the coronary care unit at San Francisco General Hospital during a ten-month period. A computer randomly assigned each of the 393 patients to either a group that was prayed for or a control group that was not prayed for. The names of the group that was prayed for were given to home prayer groups.

Each person in the group that was prayed for had between five and seven people praying for them. Those who prayed received no instructions other than to pray for the hospital patient at least once a day. The control group had no prayers from the home prayer groups.[999]

This was a carefully designed scientific study carried out with the same statistical rigor used in more orthodox medical research. The study was published in a mainstream, orthodox medical journal.[1000] What were the results?

Of the 393 patients included in the study, there were 192 patients in the group that were prayed for. There were 201 patients in the control group who were not prayed for. The group that was prayed for differed from the control patients in several important ways.

Those patients who were prayed for were five times less likely to need antibiotics and were three times less likely to suffer fluid in the lungs. No patients in the group that was prayed for needed machine assistance to breathe, while 12 of the control patients required intubation and a ventilator. Fewer people in the group that was prayed for died, although the difference was not statistically significant.[1001] In analysis, Dossey writes:

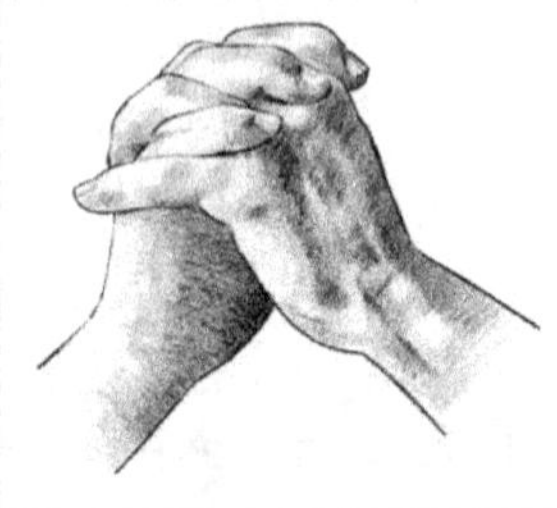

Encouraging patients to pray when facing health problems is proven to help.

> If the technique being studied had been a new drug or a surgical procedure instead of prayer, it would almost certainly have been heralded as some sort of "breakthrough."

Even some hard-boiled skeptics agreed on the significance of Byrd's findings.[1002] Dr. William Nolan, author of The Making of a Surgeon and a highly respected medical authority, was impressed by Byrd's findings. Nolan, who wrote a book debunking faith healing, noted the strength of Byrd's data. "Is sounds like this study will stand up to scrutiny . . . maybe doctors ought to write orders 'Pray three times a day.' If it works, it works."[1003]

Does this mean that prayer is a substitute for Modern Medicine? No, of course not. What this *does* mean is that doctors and patients alike need to take prayer seriously. Doctors can encourage their patients to pray for themselves and others who are sick or injured.

What about the overall health effects of being religious? One study examined a large group of people facing health challenges including amputation of a limb, polio, breast cancer, prostate cancer, and spinal cord injury. Religious patients reported comfort and strength from their faith and believed they would be fine despite their illness. They were also less stressed about the future. The non-religious group had a significantly poorer quality of life and less life satisfaction than the religious group. Their social, functional, and emotional well-being were considerably worse than the religious patients.[1004]

Another study examined a large group of residents in an extended living facility. Attendance at weekly religious services was followed for six years. Health was monitored as was religious service attendance. After six years, 22.9% of the religious service attenders had died versus 37.4% of the non-attenders. Survival rate of the religious residents thus was 14.5% better for the six-year period. This indicates a survival advantage over time for the religious service attenders. Again, religion was shown to have a beneficial effect on health.[1005]

The positive effects of religion and prayer on healing should be no surprise. We have detailed the unity of body and mind on so many levels - nervous system feedback loops, the vast fluidic interior, the body's vast chemistry, and roving white cells. When people make the choice to fill their thoughts and actions with love, should we not expect to create an internal environment of love? And would not that love create health?

I believe doctors should encourage their patients to practice their faith. Regular attendance at church, synagogue, or temple is a good idea. There we hear our bedrock beliefs and rules for positive, life supporting behavior. These reminders create harmony, happiness, and successful living. Encouraging prayer is a good idea for the same reason. In this sense, I know that medicine and religion can work together effectively.

Achieving the Unified Body

How do we achieve the Unified Body? We must restore Self-Referral. This sounds like mouthing a truism, but at this time in history restoring Self-Referral is completely ignored by Modern Medicine. And where is the blame for this? The blame falls on the lapse of time – wherein all truth, no matter how well stated, becomes forgotten. The purpose of *Self-Referral/Maximum Health* is to revive these ideas and make them practical again.

When we look for ways to restore Self-Referral, we seek ways to help the body govern itself. Modern medical practice focuses on disease. Doctors identify disease through physical diagnosis, laboratory testing, or imaging. Once the disease is identified, doctors prescribe medicine, therapy, or surgery.

This system of medical practice often restores patients to health, but in piecemeal fashion. When we remove the appendix, we solve the immediate problem. Once the patient recovers from surgery, doctors seldom offer lifestyle follow-up. Most doctors are too busy with the next surgery to consider major lifestyle counseling.

We must stop assuming that the human body is static and unchangeable. That way of thinking confines medical care to a mechanistic, cause and effect Newtonian Physics model of body operation. We must move toward the Quantum Mechanical model: the body is alive, aware, and changeable for the better.

When disease is found, both doctor and patient share a sense of doom and inevitability of future problems. Medical personnel must offer encouragement. Teaching the patient that better choices bring better future results is critical. We must actively engage the patient and encourage lifestyle changes for the better.

Will we dramatically transform every patient? Maybe not, but even a few small steps toward improvement will have a powerful effect. As it says in the *Bhagavad Gita*:[1006]

> No step is lost on this path, and no dangers are found. And even a little progress is freedom from fear.

Everyone living today's lifestyle needs the stress relief that comes from regular practice of TM. They must take time to calm down and reverse the stressful effects of modern life. We now know that TM is the most effective stress reduction technique. We must work to get as many patients taught TM as possible, the sooner the better. This will reverse the pernicious effects of stress. This will move patients toward health and away from disease.

Many patients suffer from bone and muscle pain that would obviously benefit from Manipulative Therapy. Over 89% of all doctors do not identify or treat those problems. Doctors treat such patients with rest and medications. The ongoing muscle related problems go untreated, resulting in many patients being misdiagnosed or ignored as drug seekers. Many of these patients are prescribed painkiller drugs, creating a huge part of the Opioid Crisis.

The precise lifestyle guidance available from Maharishi AyurVeda will be of great benefit. Identifying specific patient types and specifying for them precisely how to optimize their daily routine, diet, and other aspects of daily life will promote Self-Referral and move them toward health. Working at the healthiest habits will reap the reward of Maximum Health.

Along with those good ideas, we must encourage patients to practice their faith through regular attendance at church, temple, or synagogue. Patients benefit from practicing their religion, thereby being reminded of healing truths. They also help themselves and others through an active prayer life – bringing about healing in themselves and healing in others.

The common theme here is: we must create a truly comprehensive approach to medical care. Today's medical practice focuses too much on technology and too little on the human beings we treat. Too many doctors are specialists and cannot offer the kind of broad family medicine that most people need. There is too much focus on disease instead of restoring and promoting health – which is what every human being seeks.

Many of today's most tenacious diseases will nearly disappear with proper treatment of stress. The incidence of ulcers, high blood pressure, heart attack, stroke, asthma, and many other diseases will drop drastically with proper stress reduction.

What today's medical professionals and patients need is to learn about Self-Referral - and to begin restoring it. Self-Referral maintains health and prevents disease. This is the vision for an expanded and improved medical practice. This is why restoring Self-Referral is the goal of medicine.

Chapter 16

Maximum Health: The Goal of Medicine

Self-Referral maintains health and prevents disease. Optimizing Self-Referral creates Maximum Health: The Goal of Medicine.

We Have Completed a Long Journey

We have completed a long journey, you and me. We have travelled the road of learning about Self-Referral and its critical role in body operations. We learned how the body works via brain, nervous system, and Cybernetic feedback loops. We learned of control systems that switch body operations on and off. We know about the vast fluidic system that unifies the body. We know how the brain works through this vast system of Self-Referral to create health and prevent disease.

We examined Modern Medicine's Disease Approach and contrasted it with the Health Approach. We know that medical practice needs to expand its focus from identifying and fighting disease to include promoting health and preventing disease. This is a big change, and one that will require focus and determination.

We identified stress as the major disruptor of Self-Referral. We know stress is the underlying cause of disease and the aging process. We found that modern life creates more stress per unit time now than any other time in history. This creates chronic stress that repeats over and over, creating Stress Syndrome – an endless cascade of stress response, causing stress related disease. So many people under so much stress cannot cope – and this creates the Adaptation Crisis that we find ourselves in today.

The Adaptation Crisis is the basis of declining health in modern populations. It also is the cause of social disintegration on all levels: individuals, families, social structure – even our ability to maintain peace and avoid war. We need to overcome stress for better health – but *we also need to overcome stress and its pernicious effects to survive as a species.*

Thus, finding an effective way to reverse the effects of stress goes far beyond the ideas of improving health or lowering Healthcare Expenditures. Reversing the effects of stress is the only way humans can navigate successfully through the Adaptation Crisis. The same work we do to restore Self-Referral in our bodies will – in the long run – help to reverse the Adaptation Crisis and insure humanity's survival.

We now know that Transcendental Meditation or TM is the most effective way to reverse the effects of stress. We can use Maharishi AyurVeda to optimize diet, exercise, and lifestyle to promote health and avoid stress. We know to use Manipulative Therapy to correct bone and muscle problems caused by stress. We know to encourage patients to exercise their faith and prayer for healing. *In short, we have learned a whole new set of tools to optimize patient health.*

But how does all of this integrate with the way we practice medicine today? How do we work with these ideas to make them practical and useful in everyday medical practice? *What is the specific goal of all this?*

Maximum Health

The goal of all this is the stated and assumed goal of all of medicine. That goal is best stated through the term *Maximum Health.* We have spent a great deal of time - through many long chapters - talking about Self-Referral, but very little time talking about Maximum Health. What is Maximum Health? How can such a nebulous term be put next to the term Self-Referral – which has been explained until we can all now doubtless define it in an instant?

Health is simply the normal state of the human body. The heart beats, the lungs breathe, digestion is carried out – life goes on unhindered by disease. All the body's organ systems run in harmony, there are no malfunctions of any kind, and there are no disease problems to identify or fix. To say that health is the opposite of disease is only partially accurate; health in the fullest sense is the *complete absence of disease*.

Now, anyone who practices medicine - or is a patient - knows this is unrealistic. Sure, you can use diet discipline to cut pounds and get to your ideal weight. You can apply the finest custom workout program to get you into the best shape ever. You can optimize everything you can think of - but nearly always something comes between you and perfect health.

It may be a tendency to put on weight. You may have high blood pressure or prostate problems. A skin condition may plague you with itching or less than perfect complexion. Perhaps you have asthma problems when weather conditions are just right. Or maybe you have a chronic tendency to depression. These or any other health problem may disrupt your quest for perfect health.

This is where we come to the idea of Maximum Health. Our assumption is that few people – if any – have absolutely perfect health and no need for medical care. We know that few people have spotless good health – but through excellent Self-Referral based medical care *people can make better choices*. Through diligently working toward ideal habits, people can move toward the best health possible – Maximum Health. This is a goal truly worth pursuing.

Maximum Health: Getting from Here to There

Now we are where the rubber meets the road; that is, all this theory is great. All the ideas we have covered so far have been truly informative. It is good to get a fresh look at health, disease, and related thoughts. But the central question to answer is this: How do we move real people with a list of real health problems from where they are - to Maximum Health?

Self-Referral
Maximum Health

Learning from 42 Years of Medical Practice

Practicing medicine over 42 years teaches you many things if you are amenable to learning. What did it teach me about helping patients move toward Maximum Health?

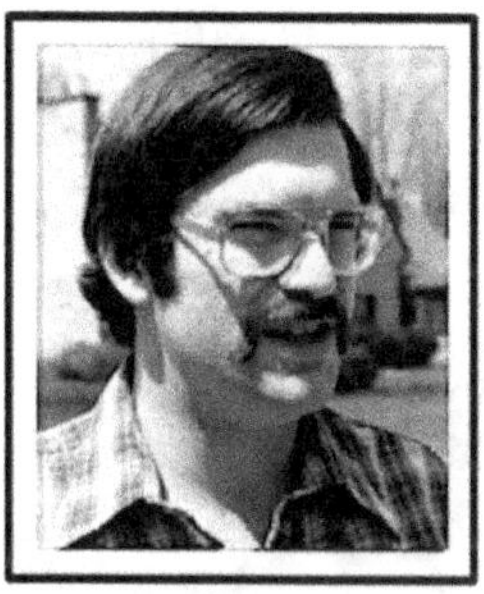

Dr. Michael Borger 1978

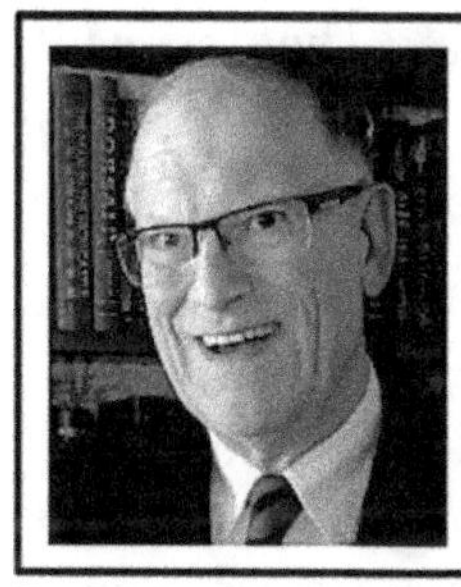

Dr. Michael Borger 2020

Teaching patients is just as important as *treating patients.*

The human body is far more *plastic* or *changeable* than most people understand.

We are not passive victims losing our health to unknown forces; we can take an active part in combating disease and returning to health – Maximum Health.

A key challenge is getting those who render medical care to change. Many will say we already have a successful medical system in place. Doctors and patients alike are used to patterns of thinking that are many generations old. Many say that doctors and patients do not know how to change. How can we move from where we presently are to embrace these new aspects of medical practice?

I began medical practice in 1978. My training and Board Certification are in Family Practice and Osteopathic Manipulative Treatment. I was trained to think and practice in the Disease

Approach. As time went on, I decided there had to be a better way to render medical care.

While I worked to help my patients over the years, I came to clear conclusions about medical practice: we must change. What do I mean by this? As time passed, I found that *teaching patients is just as important as treating patients.*

People commonly come to see the doctor with a sense of dread. They fear the doctor will find something is wrong or - worse yet – that what is wrong will be major and fatal. Central to all this is the idea that the body is in a fixed, immovable state and unable to change in any way. That means if you get diagnosed with high cholesterol, diabetes, or other problem - you are just stuck with it. The only recourse is to take medicine and do your best to dodge the bullet of suffering and death.

There is a critical truth that people need to hear. This whole set of assumptions is false. *The human body is far more plastic or changeable than most people understand.* That is, if we improve our diet, reduce stress, and get fit through reasonable and measured changes in our habits, the body can and will change for the better. *We are not passive victims losing our health to unknown forces; we can take an active part in combating disease and returning to health – Maximum Health.*

This teaching always brings a remarkable change in every patient I have seen. They typically come in hopeless, scared, and intimidated. When they hear the good news that they can fight back, improve, and often actually win - they are transformed.

Those who are able learn everything they can, put it to good purpose, and regain their health. Those who cannot understand or lack motivation to change *still improve* because they invariably learn some part of the whole. They take even a small part of knowledge and put it to work, improving their health. *Over time, they see progress and will want to learn the rest.*

That is how I work with people every day who come to see me for one reason or another. I meet them where they are, hear their complaints and stories, and then get to work moving them from where they are toward a state of Maximum Health. It is a process of education, coaching, and encouraging.

Every health professional works with the same situation every day. We meet people, who come in with health problems that need help. The way most healthcare goes, tests will be run to identify likely problems. Once the problems are known, the patient gets the logical medication, advice, surgery, or therapy that is needed. Then the patient gets follow-up appointments to monitor progress.

To help those with health problems, we need to understand the people AND the health problems. Other people are no different than you and me; we all have more in common than at variance. We all want to move from a less happy, less content state to one of more happiness and more contentment. As a doctor, one thing I can always count on is that people want to get out of the misery zone and into the happiness zone. What that takes depends on what health problems are present.

Whether the health problem is high blood pressure, too much weight, arthritis, heart disease, aches and pains, or any other disorder - one thing is clear. People have changed from the perfect health they used to have to a less than perfect state of health. They have suffered a *health decline*, and their present condition is what brings them into the healthcare system. They want to reverse the situation and return to their former state of health. Why didn't the person just stay healthy? How did this health decline happen?

The Origins of Health Decline

Nearly everyone coming in for medical care has one or more problem that needs assistance. Perhaps they have a sore throat, or a strained low back. Others may come in for help with obesity. All these people have one thing in common: they need help with health problems.

A good question is: how did these people get this way? Since most babies and children are overall in close to perfect health already, what happens that causes our health to fade away and health problems to crop up? *What causes health decline?*

Self-Referral
Maximum Health

What Causes Health Decline?

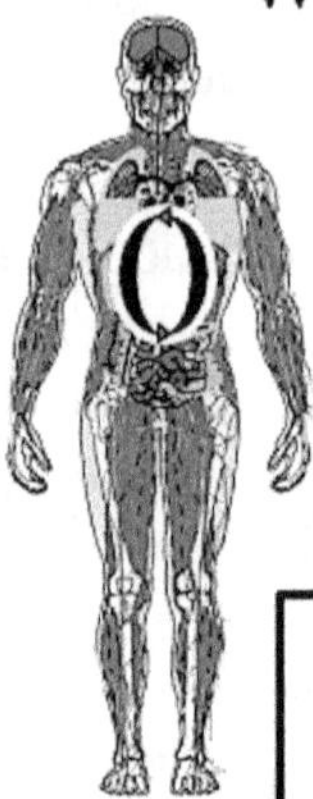

Everyone starts out with the same health possibilities. Health Decline occurs because of several factors.

We may have genetic tendencies beyond our control. These can negatively impact our health.

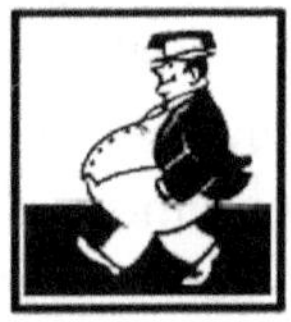

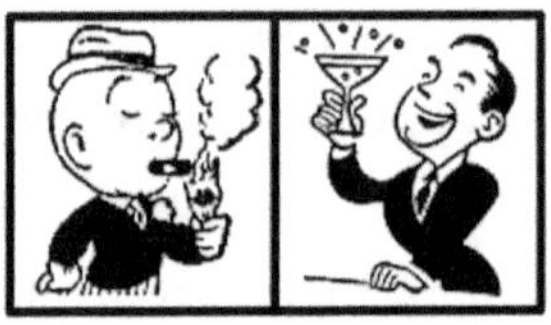

We may make poor choices such as smoking and alcohol consumption that impacts our health.

We may live with some very difficult situations in our lives. This stress negatively impacts our health.

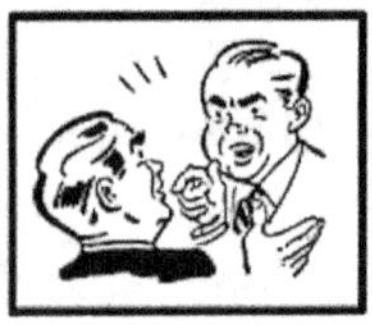

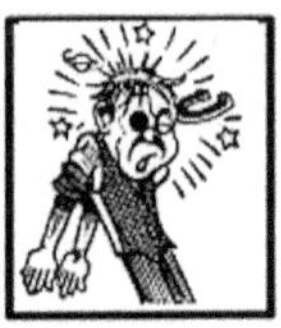

Many health problems arise from physical injuries. Chronic pain is common, and some injuries create long-term disturbances in the physiology that impacts our health.

We must deal effectively with Health Decline to move toward Maximum Health.

Some health problems are essentially genetic tendencies. Individuals just have high blood sugar, high blood pressure, or high cholesterol. These problems are often found in the person's parents or extended family; they inherited the tendencies through family genetics. These problems come up even when the person is doing all they can to stay healthy. This is an inherent weakness in their physiology that causes health decline. No one should lose hope if they have genetic tendencies to health decline; if they follow good advice, the situation can usually be remedied.

A major source of health problems is making bad decisions that affect health. Poor lifestyle choices like smoking, alcohol use, illicit drug use, poor diet, or lack of exercise take a significant toll. These problems all stem from poor lifestyle choices that have known negative health effects. When we make poor choices over time, they have a snowballing negative effect. For example, someone has a sedentary lifestyle and develops high blood pressure. Another person puts on a lot of weight; over time, they develop diabetes. Fortunately, our choices can change, and such health decline can be turned around for the better.

As we have discussed in detail, stress is a major source of health problems. If anyone comes under sufficient stress, they will become ill with infectious disease or develop any of the long-term stress diseases like high blood pressure, ulcers, or depression. Stress also pushes people into bad habits as they seek relief through alcohol, drugs, or sedentary life with endless television watching. Like other causes of health problems, stress untreated will certainly cause health decline. Combating stress via TM and lifestyle choices will reverse this health decline.

Another major source of health problems are the circumstances of life. If someone is in military service or otherwise subject to extreme stress, they may develop Post Traumatic Stress Disorder. Someone else may be subject to physical strain stemming from job demands. Another person may have anxiety, insomnia, or depression from difficult circumstances in life. While life challenges must be faced and dealt with, all of them can be worked with to improve people's quality of life and reverse health decline.

Finally, many health problems are direct results of physical injuries that cause long-term problems. These include chronic pain or disability from old injuries. Old injuries also can create long-term disturbances in the physiology that create disease. We may not be able to make these long-term effects go away entirely, but we certainly can do a lot to alleviate the problems caused by them, reversing health decline.

Moving Patients Toward Maximum Health

People that I meet and care for as patients have one or more health problem that needs help to correct. They may have one clearly defined problem, they may have a short list, or they may have a bewildering roster of difficulties. One might ask: where do we begin to sort all this out?

Despite the complex and often bewildering presentations, one principle we can rely on is the logic of body function. The complaints nearly always line up with the known functions of the body. By matching the complaints with the corresponding body part or function, we quickly get an idea of where the trouble is and what to do about it.

Another factor that helps is that human physiology is the same from person to person. This is why we use the same laboratory tests to evaluate anyone's health - no matter what the specific complaints are. A major help is to obtain the basic laboratory tests that check for blood diseases, cholesterol, sugar, kidney function, and so forth. Other common tests include Chest X-Ray and EKG. These studies identify health problems we can work with to move the patient toward Maximum Health.

Introducing Transcendental Meditation to people is very simple. TM restores Self-Referral directly and is critical to success in reaching Maximum Health. *That is why TM treats and improves nearly every health problem* – nearly anything we encounter in medical practice. Advising patients of the benefit of TM is quite easy and successful. Learning TM thus is a key part of moving toward Maximum Health.

Maharishi AyurVeda offers a whole new way to categorize and diagnose patients according to their physiology. Through Ayurvedic methods of asking questions and learning about the patient, we can determine their Ayurvedic body type. That guides us in making recommendations in lifestyle, diet, exercise, herbal supplements, and behavioral changes – all of which restore health through balancing the physiology. In this way, we can move the patient toward Maximum Health.

Manipulative Therapy works wonders when properly applied to the right patients. Diagnostic examination reveals the basis of painful bone and muscle problems. X-Ray or other imaging – when needed - helps determine the root cause of pain and related problems. Immediate treatment often is the answer and is effective when rendered by trained and experienced manipulators. One to three treatment sessions are typical to resolve most common problems – and moves the patient toward Maximum Health.

Working with patients to provide Manipulative Therapy is easy if the doctor already knows how to do it. Otherwise, it is simple to network with area providers of Manipulative Therapy to get what the patient needs. Using Manipulative Therapy thus is a key part of moving toward Maximum Health - and all healthcare providers can employ it.

A very important part of patient care is determining the quality of their lifestyle. Do they get enough exercise? Is their diet healthy? Do they drink too much alcohol? Do they use drugs? Have they exposed themselves to sexually transmitted diseases? Is their job a good fit? Are their family relationships good? Are they generally happy or troubled?

Whenever people are open to the subject, I always ask about their faith background.[1007] Nearly everyone tells me they grew up in this or that faith. Then I ask them where they are with their faith now.[1008] Some people tell me they are strong in their faith; others say they had faith a long time ago but fell away from it. Some people say they have never had faith of any kind.

Part of bringing people to Maximum Health is *encouraging their faith*. No matter where people are in their faith experience, health problems can be a major life crisis. People want to know where to turn for the kind of help that medical care alone will not provide. Nearly everyone appreciates bringing this subject into discussion; no matter what your background, praying for healing is the right thing to do.

As I work with people, I get to know them as individuals. Everyone has their style of communication, their likes and dislikes, their way of going about life. As Ralph Waldo Emerson said, *"the secret to education lies in respecting the pupil."* Everyone I meet as a patient is me in a different set of circumstances. What all that means is I love and respect everyone and do my best to treat them as I would want to be treated in the circumstances at hand.

A truly critical point is introducing the idea that whatever their health status is, *we can change direction away from disease - and move toward Maximum Health.* Remember – Maximum Health is not perfect health; rather, it is *the best possible health for the patient.* If all this is done well, doctor and patient forge a true alliance to improve health based on mutual respect. Common cause to conquer health problems, moving toward health and happiness, drives patients toward Maximum Health.

Move Forward, One Step at a Time

To help people move toward Maximum Health, we must start somewhere – but we also must take a measured approach. Giving all possible advice, we can send patients home with a book-length list of recommendations. That accomplishes nothing; it only paralyzes the patient like a deer in the headlights. Patients toss the handouts into the trash, and we have lost them as allies to improve their health.

An important principle in this process is that of *baby steps.* Baby steps means we know that change itself is tough enough – and the easier we make it to change, the more likely people will be willing to change.[1009] Let's say someone has high cholesterol in the range that makes control via diet and exercise possible. Rather than slam-dunking them on toxic statin drugs, I always take a lifestyle change approach.

Instead of an extremely complicated diet plan, I give a very short list of items to favor and items to reduce. I add that to an easy walking program. Neither set of changes is particularly difficult, and I build bridges with the patient by explaining everything in terms they will understand. But the principle is baby steps – just get them started in the right direction.

A critical part of this process is prompt follow-up. Whenever I evaluate someone's health, I always plan follow-up that tracks progress and accountability. With elevated cholesterol, I have them return for laboratory testing in 90 days and meet with me two weeks later. At that visit, we review results.

Nearly everyone tries to improve their health once we identify what is needed. If they make any effort, and nearly everyone does, their laboratory numbers will improve. That gives the patient a wonderful sense of taking control of their own health. This is how we establish good habits that will improve health over time. The same principles apply to nearly every health problem.

It is a critical part of medical care to give the patient positive feedback and encouragement. When one of my patients improve their numbers, I report the good news. Then I put down whatever is in my hands and make a point of shaking their hand. I tell them how proud I am of their efforts and success, followed by high fives and a fist bump. We all need encouragement, and it means so much when we get it. This has enormous positive effects on the patient, who then redoubles their efforts to improve.

Most patients respond well to these principles. If we fail to achieve recommended results, this is not a defeat. All efforts still move the patient toward Maximum Health. If the patient needs to be on medication to solve the problem, so be it. The improved habits will still advance them toward Maximum Health.

Remember - the goal of all medical care is Maximum Health. We want to identify and combat known health problems defined by Modern Medicine. We use TM for stress reduction, Maharishi AyurVeda to optimize lifestyle, and Manipulative Therapy to remedy bone, joint, and muscle problems.

Bringing all these strategies to bear is promising – but will everyone achieve perfect health? Perhaps some will achieve perfect health but remember - *Maximum Health is not necessarily perfect health; rather, it is the best possible health for each patient*. No matter what health challenges people face, moving toward Maximum Health helps them achieve the best health possible.

Current Attempts at Health Promotion

We have given a plan for comprehensive health promotion. But is all this new, or have those in the medical field been looking at these ideas? Ignoring TM, Maharishi AyurVeda, and Manipulative Therapy, healthcare professionals have always been looking at ways to promote health. Today, nearly all these ideas are focused on the goal of reducing Healthcare Expenditures.

One popular idea is the *Patient-Centered Medical Home.* The idea of the Medical Home is for each medical practice to organize itself to better serve patients. This is done working with a computer based Electronic Health Record. The goal is for every patient to receive complete medical care. This requires written standards of practice that outline an elaborate system to do all this – and a dogged determination to make it happen.

What does the Medical Home model accomplish? All patients are tracked via the medical record. The list of immunizations from childhood forward is a good example, as is tracking growth and development. Risk Factors like smoking and obesity are identified and remedied. Medications get careful monitoring. Regular checkups promote early detection of disease and better care of known health problems.[1010]

The Medical Home model is used in physician practices across the United States. It has reduced diagnostic errors;[1011] improved teamwork among doctors and staff;[1012] improved care of chronic conditions;[1013] improved cancer screening;[1014] and reduced medical costs for high-risk (and high cost) patients.[1015] The increased efficiency of the Medical Home model can make money for the practices as well: the insurance companies are willing to pay for better run practices that also save them money.

The Medical Home model is well known through the *Quality Movement* in healthcare.[1016] The Quality Movement champions scorecard-style care like that of the Medical Home – including completion of immunizations, regular health evaluation, key preventative tests like mammography and colonoscopy, and meaningful use of the Electronic Health Record.[1017] The Quality Movement got regulatory teeth when it became part of Medicare requirements. Fulfilling the Quality standards are rapidly becoming mandatory to get fully paid for medical services.[1018]

Have these measures improved medical care? Medical practices following the Medical Home and the Quality Movement plans are working harder to provide better medical services.[1019] That means more patients are getting more evaluation and treatment as a result. But does all this produce healthcare savings?

Those who advocate the Medicare Quality and Medical Home have published articles showing savings in the 5-18% range in selected limited studies[1020] - but those in the medical economics field doubt that significant savings will result over time.[1021]

Why are healthcare costs so hard to reduce? This is due to the medical system's dedication to the Disease Model. If nothing can be done to reduce the rate of disease, guess what? The annual cost of medical care cannot change. We can work our brains and fingers to the bone to reduce healthcare costs with little effect. Unless we can find a way to reduce the rate of disease – *the need for care* - no matter how we shuffle the deck it comes out the same. What can we do about the high cost of medical care?

Defining the Healthcare Crisis

Few problems in public policy can compare to the massive cost of medical care and how to pay for it. Everyone needs medical care at some point in their lives. Many factors contribute to the high cost of medical care, but few truly effective ideas have emerged on how to effectively deal with this issue.

Efforts to improve the economic side of medical care has been an ongoing struggle for decades. The central problems are holding down the cost of medical care and determining who pays for medical care. Broad efforts to control the cost of medical care seem to help somewhat, but beyond that nearly every attempted remedy fails in the long run. Healthcare costs keep going up no matter what anyone does.

The subtitle of this book is "Solving the Healthcare Crisis." This is a bold statement. What exactly is the Healthcare Crisis? Can we make a practical definition of the Healthcare Crisis? And once we define the Healthcare Crisis what can we do to solve it? We will switch to a more visual presentation for a while and return to a detailed text discussion afterward.

Self-Referral

Maximum Health

Defining the Healthcare Crisis

Why is medical care costing more than ever and delivering less and less?

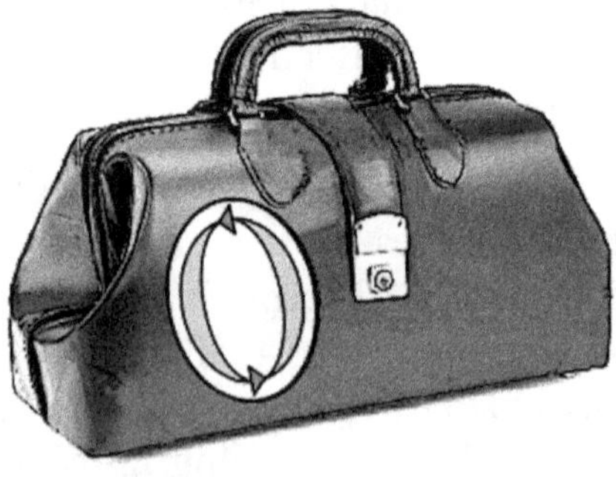

Self-Referral
Maximum Health

United States Healthcare Spending Has Increased Dramatically Since 1960

United States Healthcare Spending increased sharply from $27 billion in 1960 to $3.5 trillion in 2017.

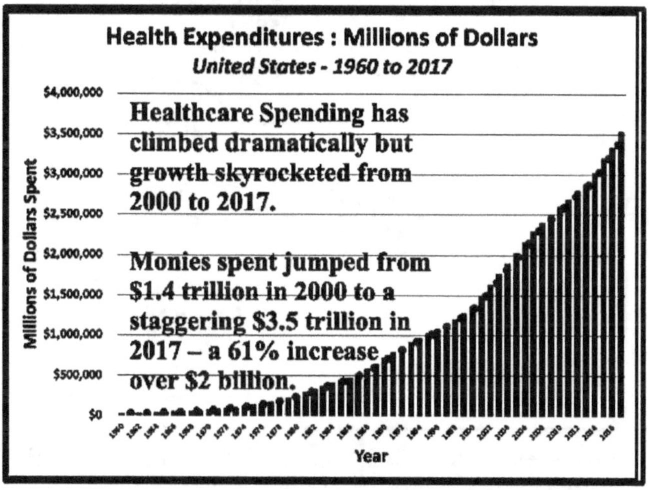

Healthcare Spending increased dramaticially between 1960 and 2017. Everyone needs medical care in every country. Comparing United States Healthcare Expenditures to other countries will be useful.

Self-Referral
Maximum Health

United States Healthcare Spending Compared to the Rest of the World

How does United States Healthcare Spending compare to that of other countries?

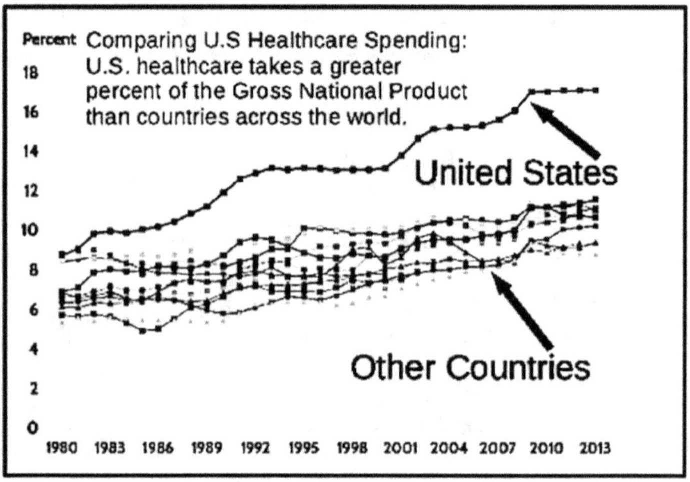

From 1980 to 2013, the countries of Great Britain, Austria, Germany, Canada, France, Sweden, New Zeland, Japan, and Austria spent an average 9.3% of the GNP on healthcare. In the same period the United States spent an average of 15.3% of the GNP. Healthcare spending is also rising much faster in the United States than in the other countries for the same time period.

Self-Referral

Maximum Health

Does Higher United States Healthcare Spending Increase Life Expectancy?

Length of the average life is important to everyone. How does the United States compare to the populations of other countries?

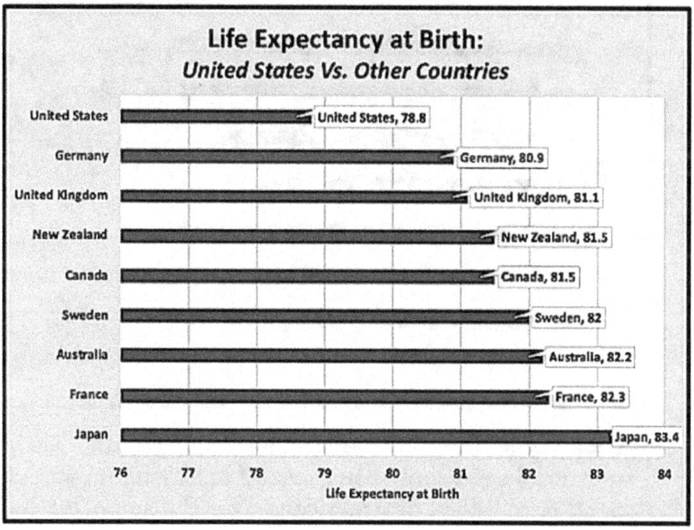

After paying more than any other country in the world, statistics do not show better health justifying the money spent. Life expectancy at birth – the expected length of life in the US – is lower than that of other countries.

Self-Referral
Maximum Health

Does Higher United States Healthcare Spending Affect Chronic Conditions?

Better healthcare should decrease the number of chronic conditions in older people. How does the United States population compare to the populations of other countries?

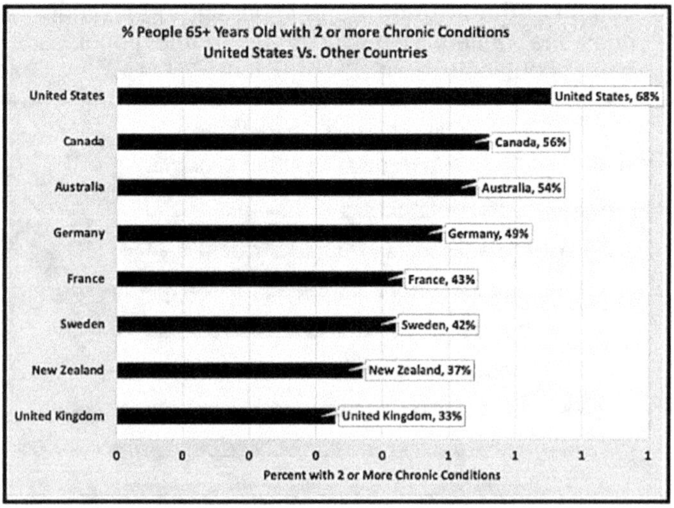

After paying more than any other country in the world, statistics do not show better health justifying the money spent. A full 68% of Americans over the age of 65 had two or more chronic conditions.

The High Cost of Medical Care

The cost of medical care today is staggering. In 1960, the cost of medical care in the United States was $27 billion dollars.[1022] That was a lot of money in those days, but it has gotten much worse. The cost of medical care has increased dramatically from then until 2016 when it was $3.3 TRILLION dollars.[1023] In 2018, the bone-crushing cost of medical care totaled about $3.7 trillion dollars.[1024] When we look at these numbers, they are difficult to comprehend. Looking at a graph of these Healthcare Expenditures makes things much easier to understand.

Growth in healthcare spending has climbed dramatically since 1960, but numbers from 2000 to the present have been truly alarming. There was a 61% increase in Healthcare Expenditures between the years 2000 and 2017. In that time frame, the monies spent jumped from $1.4 trillion dollars in 2000 to a staggering $3.5 trillion dollars in 2017. That is an increase of over $2 billion dollars.[1025] *It is this rapid increase in Healthcare Expenditures that many suggest endangers the United States' ability to ever balance the national budget.*

We know the need for medical care is universal; all human beings need it. A logical question to ask is: how do we manage the cost of it? That is, no matter where people live, they need medical care. That is why every country has a healthcare system to meet the needs of their citizens. An important question is: how does the United States compare with other countries regarding healthcare spending? Do other countries face the same cost problems? Comparing the United States to other countries will offer some helpful insights.

The Gross National Product is the sum of all economic activity in any country, typically figured by the year.[1026] The GNP is one of the most widely recognized and understood measures of any country's economic performance.[1027] Perhaps the best way to compare healthcare costs is to show what percentage of the country's Gross National Product or GNP gets spent on healthcare. This provides a true side-by-side comparison.

From 1980 to 2013 the countries of Great Britain, Austria, Germany, Canada, France, Sweden, New Zealand, Japan and Australia spent an average of 9.3% of their GNP on Healthcare Expenditures. During the same period, the United States spent an average of 15.3% of its GNP on Healthcare Expenditures.

Looking at the graph showing all this at once, two points are clear. One point is that the other countries are moving up and down in the same tight range, while United States healthcare spending is far above that of any of the other countries. The other point is that United

States Healthcare Expenditures are rising at a much faster rate than those of the other countries in this period. Thus, the United States is both higher in costs, AND those costs are rising faster than those of the other countries.[1028]

Since the United States is spending so much more on healthcare, one would assume the American population would show much greater health than the other countries - who spent far less. Figures comparing population statistics show that just the opposite is true. Looking at life expectancy at birth, the American population ranks dead last compared to the other countries. In other words, the United States is spending far more on healthcare than other countries - and Americans are living fewer years compared with countries who spend far less.[1029]

Another finding is that, as the aging process proceeds, people develop chronic conditions like hypertension, heart disease, or prostate problems. Looking at the health of these countries' older population, 68% of Americans aged 65+ had two or more chronic conditions – and the other countries? Their average rate was 45%. The United States ranked worst in this category as well – 25% worse than the other countries – who, again, spent far less on healthcare.

The United States thus is spending far more than other countries on healthcare - and Americans are ending up in poorer health at the end of life compared with countries who spend far less.[1030] This should cause everyone – healthcare providers, patients, and leaders at all levels of our country – to seriously examine this situation. We cannot ignore these facts.

What Causes Rising Healthcare Expenditures?

What causes skyrocketing costs and poor results? One major cause is the increasing number of older people as the American baby boomer generation ages. The tremendous number of children born in the years following World War II are reaching age sixty and

beyond. This is the largest segment of the American population – and major health problems begin after age forty. The baby boomers are now straining the American medical system past tolerance – and this causes high Healthcare Expenditures.[1031]

A second cause is the progressively high-tech nature of medical care in the United States. Everyone in the world loves American medical advances, but there is a caveat; these innovations demand the ultimate in evolving technology – and this drives healthcare costs up. Devices like CT scanners, kidney dialysis machines, and the like save lives but are very costly.[1032]

Dr. William Schwartz was a physician, economist, and Professor of Medicine at the University of Southern California. He was keenly aware of the costly nature of Modern Medicine. "We are the victims of our own success as a biomedical research community," said Dr. Schwartz. "Most of the new things we do add enormously to expenses." For example, he tells us, doctors used to prescribe aspirin and a walker for people with diseased hip joints. "Now we do a hip replacement operation costing $25,000," Schwartz explained. "We have wonderful new things that are both effective and expensive replacing old treatments that were both ineffective and cheap."[1033]

A third cause for skyrocketing costs is the crisis in litigation. Fear of medical malpractice suits forces doctors to order every possible diagnostic test, whether needed or not. For example, a common problem that brings people to the Emergency Room is a blow to the head. Whether the blow was major or minor, these patients routinely get X-ray, CT, or MRI imaging - whether they logically need it or not. Why does this go on? Today, every doctor in America constantly must look over their shoulder for spurious lawsuits. This causes many tests to be ordered far more often than needed - adding more and more cost to medical care.

A fourth factor in high medical costs is too many doctors specializing rather than becoming family doctors. We can quickly see this proven by examining office call charges. In northern Indiana in 2018, family doctors charged about $128 to see a patient for most common problems. That includes a health history, physical examination to diagnose the problem, and planning a treatment strategy with referrals or prescriptions. A specialist in Pediatrics charged $150 for the same services. A specialist in Internal Medicine charged $166, a General Surgeon $208, an Orthopedic Surgeon $250, and a Neurosurgeon $522. We quickly see that the more specialized the doctor, the higher the cost of medical care.[1034]

Clearly, we need more family doctors. Leaders in the American Medical Association are working toward providing more family doctors through their training programs. Likewise, the leaders of the American Osteopathic Association are working to emphasize training family doctors. As time goes on, this imbalance will be corrected.

We Must Reduce the Need for Medical Care

Looking at the skyrocketing cost of medical care, it is easy to blame population pressures, technology-driven costs, medicolegal concerns, or distribution of Family Physicians. It is my opinion - after examining all these factors - that we are truly missing the point by focusing on one, two, three, or more broad factors that impact healthcare costs. We cannot wave a wand over any of these problems through regulation, legislation, or how we practice medicine. Those costs are going to be there no matter what we do.

It is clear to me that we need to focus on *how we can practice medicine* to reduce the cost of medicine. What will truly reduce the cost of medicine is to have less healthcare to provide. I am not talking about rationing or limiting medical care; *I am talking about reducing the need for medical care.*

Until now, the assumption has always been that disease is unavoidable. We have so many years of good health, the aging process occurs, and we start having inevitable chronic conditions like high blood pressure, heart disease, and the like. But what if we are wrong about these assumptions?

The main purpose of this book is to bring to light the fact that we have new ways to seriously reduce the likelihood of chronic conditions developing. We also have new ways to get chronic conditions under control or even eliminate them altogether. Assuming this is true, and I believe the evidence presented in this book proves it, we can truly focus on serious health promotion and disease prevention. *These actions will make serious reductions in healthcare spending possible*. Let's review the evidence:

Self-Referral

Maximum Health

Solving the Healthcare Crisis

These are the measures we must take to solve the Healthcare Crisis.

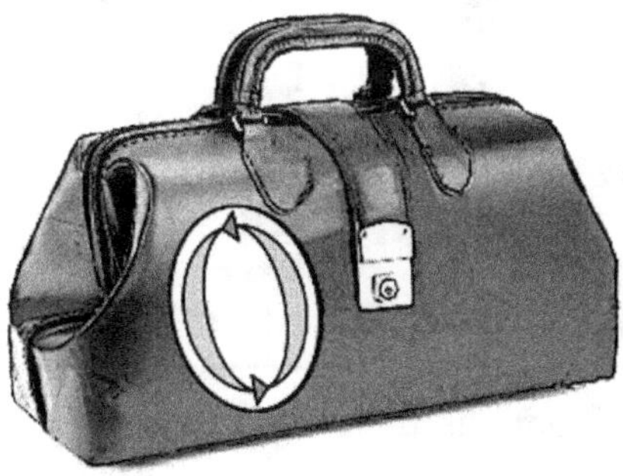

Self-Referral
Maximum Health

We Can Cut Healthcare Spending by Tackling Known Health Risk Factors

Health Risk Factors are habits people have that make them more likely to develop disease that results in more medical care. Health Risk Factors are behaviors that people can change to improve their health..

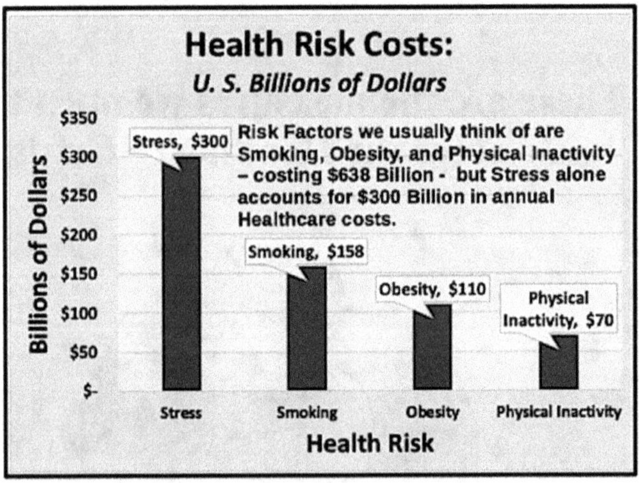

Stress looms as the largest single Health Risk Factor that causes higher Healthcare Spending. In the past, there was no treatment for stress. Transcendental Meditation or TM is the cure for stress and clearly promotes better health – reducing Healthcare Spending.

One question we must ask is: can we find evidence connecting high medical costs with Health Risk Factors that we can hope to improve? What do we know about poor lifestyle choices – Health Risk Factors - and the cost of medical care? Studies have shown that among the top predictors of future poor health – and hence higher healthcare costs – are Smoking, Obesity, and Physical Inactivity. What do we know about the cost of these Health Risk Factors?

Targeting Health Risk Factors

Studies prove that Smoking, Obesity, and Physical Inactivity are among the Health Risk Factors that strongly predict poor future health – and hence are major causes of rising Healthcare Expenditures.[1035] A critical fact is when we compare these to the Health Risk Factor of Stress, these known culprits causing rising medical costs pale by comparison.[1036]

Smoking increases healthcare spending by $158 billion dollars a year. Obesity increases spending by $110 billion a year, and Physical Inactivity increases spending by $70 billion a year.[1037] But the big surprise is that Stress as a Health Risk Factor dwarfs these three threats; *Stress increases healthcare spending by $300 billion dollars a year.*[1038]

This might seem surprising if you had not read the previous chapters of this book. This finding underlines the critical need to better identify and treat stress in our patient population. Recognized as a separate Health Risk Factor, stress clearly costs a lot per year – but *when we know that stress causes nearly every known disease it changes everything.*

This is how stress runs up the cost of medical care. We see here a better understanding that *stress is the clear and present danger of our current place in history*. And now we understand that *stress is driving the sharp increases in Healthcare Expenditures*. The way forward is clear: if we want a healthier population and we want to reduce Healthcare Expenditures, we need serious work to combat stress.

We have seen plenty of proof that TM is the answer to solving Stress Syndrome and the Adaptational Crisis. But what do we know about TM's ability to truly reduce healthcare costs?

Dr. Robert E. Herron and colleagues[1039] conducted an experiment to see whether TM could reduce medical costs. They studied patients 65 years or older – the group known to use more medical care because of chronic conditions. They taught TM to 163 patients and kept records of payments to their doctors for services rendered. They also kept track of 163 matched patients who did not know TM as controls to compare with the TM patients. What did they find?

Self-Referral

Maximum Health

We Can Cut Healthcare Spending by Teaching Patients TM

When patients over Age 65 – those most likely to need medical care – learned TM, they needed less healthcare than those who did not learn TM. Teaching people TM thus is a major tool to reduce Healthcare Spending.

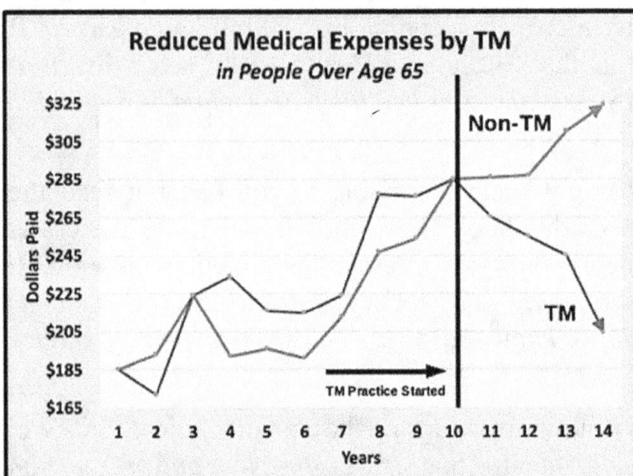

By treating stress with TM, we have a cure for the biggest single Risk Factor and the underlying cause of nearly every disease. We can now seriously reduce the *NEED FOR HEALTHCARE* – reducing Healthcare Spending. *This is a tremendous advance in healthcare.*

Both patient groups were tracked for 14 years total. The TM Group and the Non-TM groups had nearly identical medical expenses from year 1 through year 10. Both groups had the same trend of increase in medical expenses. This is what we expect, all things being equal; the older we get, our health deteriorates, and we need more medical care.

A remarkable thing happened after year ten when the TM group was taught to meditate. At that point the TM and Non-TM groups had markedly different directions in medical expenses. The Non-TM group did what we would expect them to do: they got older, and as time went on, they needed even more medical care, and their medical expenses continued going up.

The TM group, however, did something unique. Their medical expenses went down in year 11, 12, 13, and 14. By year 14 their level of medical expenses had dropped nearly to where they were at year 1. *This proves that learning TM not only improves your health but also radically reduces Healthcare Spending.*[1040]

Do these benefits continue over time, or are they only a short-term improvement? Dr. Herron continued his studies and found that TM practicing patients had reduced medical costs for six consecutive years after starting TM.[1041]

In a separate study, Herron found that TM also reduced medical costs for high-cost patients. These are patients with severe chronic disease that makes their healthcare extraordinarily expensive.[1042] *Trimming costs on these high-cost patients will bring even more Healthcare Expenditure savings because it is well known that high-cost patients account for most of all annual medical expenses.*[1043]

The Critical Role of Transcendental Meditation

Enormous healthcare savings can be had by simply teaching people the TM technique. A 1987 study published in the journal Psychosomatic Medicine compared healthcare utilization of a large group of patients who practiced TM versus control patients. This study examined the medical care statistics of the TM group for a five-year period and compared it to a matched control group.

The study found that use of healthcare services for the TM group was far below that of the control. That means that TM radically reduced use of healthcare services for those patients who practiced TM. The reduction was 50.2% for children aged 0-18, 50.1% for young adults aged 19-39, and 69.4% for older adults aged 40 and above.[1044]

Self-Referral
Maximum Health

Widespread Use of TM Can Make Massive Cuts in Healthcare Spending

When patient populations use the TM Technique regularly, massive healthcare savings become possible. Reducing Stress - the chief cause of disease - will cut the *NEED FOR HEALTHCARE.*

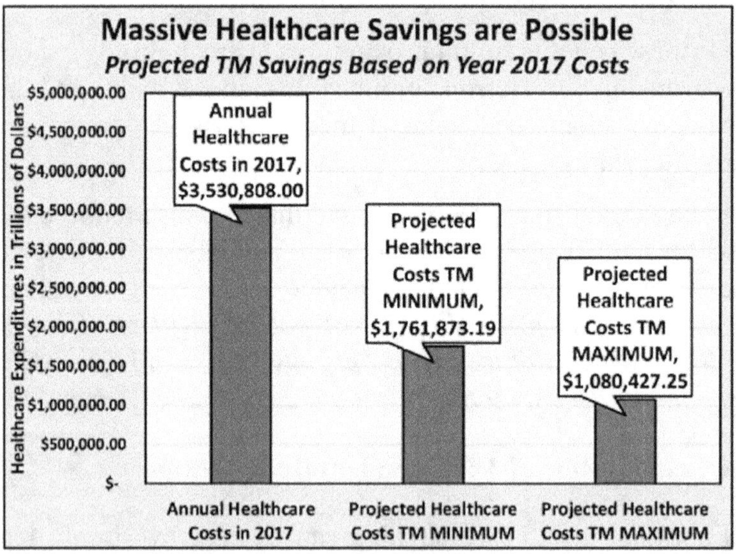

The ONLY way to cut the cost of healthcare is to reduce the *NEED FOR HEALTHCARE.* TM is the cure for Stress and will slash healthcare costs.

In 2017 the annual expenditure for healthcare totaled $3.5 trillion dollars.[1045] Applying this study's reduction rates to the total Healthcare Expenditures of that year is impressive. The minimum predicted reduction in healthcare utilization would be 50.1% and the maximum reduction predicted would be 69.4%. Those percentages mean little until you translate them into real dollars. The minimum predicted savings in Healthcare Expenditures would be $1.8 trillion dollars. The maximum predicted savings would be $2.45 trillion dollars.

A critical point is that the TM Technique is the only meditation technique that will provide these kind of healthcare savings. When I discuss TM with people, the first thing I hear is "Oh yes – I meditate." I ask them what they are doing, and *it has nothing to do with TM, and it will not produce the kind of profound changes in the physiology needed to combat stress and create health*. This is an important point and is likely to be a pivotal understanding for true healthcare cost reduction to take place. What proof is there to support these ideas?

A Meta-Analysis uses statistics to measure conclusions from multiple published research papers. The idea is to find out if the various research findings agree with each other, and how strong that agreement is. This is how we can see if multiple research findings add up. If they do, it makes a very strong case for research conclusions in question – and underlines the findings.

TM was studied by Dr. David Orme-Johnson using Meta-Analysis in 1998. His findings were quite decisive.[1046] 543 research study publications were reviewed, and TM was found more effective than other meditation and relaxation procedures in decreasing hypertension, reducing anxiety, improving psychological health, and reducing use of alcohol, tobacco, and illegal drugs. Review of 146 studies found that TM was far more effective than placebo or other meditation or relaxation techniques in reducing stress.

What all this means is *while many claim that other meditation techniques are equivalent to TM, none of them truly are equivalent to TM*. This is why we should not waste time or money on other techniques as they will not work as expected.

The Critical Role of Osteopathic Manipulative Therapy

Research shows that Osteopathic Manipulative Treatment can provide a major reduction in Healthcare Spending. The Colorado Board of Workers Compensation studied which healthcare provider gave the most cost-effective Manipulative Therapy care. This body commissioned a firm of Certified Public Accountants to compare the cost per claim by various healthcare providers - MDs, DOs, Chiropractors, and Physical Therapists.

The results showed the DO physician cost per case of low back pain for six years running was $1,007. The MD physician cost was $2,895, Chiropractor $2,775, and Physical Therapy was $2,457. The DOs were consistently the lowest cost Manipulative Therapy providers for all six years.[1047] These figures are impressive, but we only see their true impact by applying them to annual numbers for the entire United States.

Projected Cost per Year by Healthcare Provider

Provider:	Cost/Case:	Cost/74.5 Million:
Non-Surgical DO	$ 1,007	$ 75,021,500
Non-Surgical MD	$ 2,895	$ 15,677,500
Chiropractor	$ 2,775	$ 206,737,500
Physical Therapy	$ 2,457	$ 183,046,500
DO Osteopathic Savings/Year		$ 140,656,000

We know that low back pain is one of the most common health problems and affects 75 million Americans a year.[1048] Only a few low back patients - about 300,000 - will need surgery for problems like lumbar disc.[1049] The remaining 74.5 million will receive medication, rest, and physical therapy of some kind.[1050] Applying the cost per case numbers from the Colorado study we can see the potential Osteopathic impact on lowering Healthcare Expenditures:

Self-Referral

Maximum Health

We Can Cut Healthcare Spending Using Osteopathic Manipulative Treatment

DOs are able to reduce Healthcare Spending compared to non-surgical MDs Chiropractors, and Physical Therapists. Why is this the case?

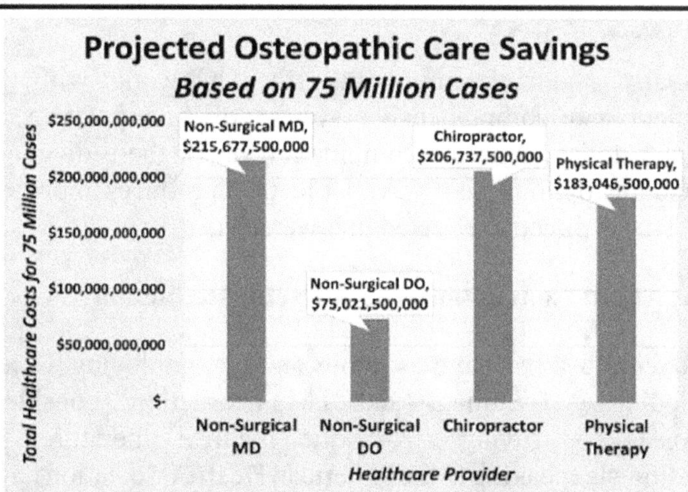

These savings are possible because the DOs alone brings the full range of medical care AND Manipulative Therapy to treat musculoskeletal problems. The result is less cost per case and huge reductions in Healthcare Spending.

Why do DOs provide dramatically lower Healthcare Spending? The DO physician is the only listed healthcare professional who brings all of today's medical diagnosis and therapy together in one format. The MD physician relies on prescription medications, rest, and referral elsewhere for therapy. Chiropractic and Physical Therapy, by contrast, offer manipulative and physical therapy but do not include full medical diagnosis and therapy, especially trained use of advanced imaging and use of prescription medications.

We thus see that the combination of a fully functioning physician that also knows how to diagnose and treat musculoskeletal problems is critical to meeting patient needs. The addition of manipulative therapy to medical care is likely to better serve patients' medical needs – but can it save money?

Most patients need more relief than simple over the counter, non-prescription medicines can provide. These medications may be anti-inflammatory, painkillers, or muscle relaxants. The DO can write prescriptions for these medications as they are needed and oversee their use.

Finally, and most importantly, the DO works with the most complete and comprehensive system of Manipulative Therapy available today. It is the combination of all these diagnostic and therapeutic options being available that produces more effective care. This is directly reflected in lower costs.

What About Conventional Risk Factor Reduction?

To contrast the savings projected by employing Osteopathic Manipulative Treatment and TM instruction, consider other proposals for savings from the medical literature. Leading cardiologists speaking to the American Heart Association have urged doctors to be more aggressive in lifestyle intervention. This includes encouraging exercise, reduction of fats in the diet, and stopping smoking.

These are good ideas that are well supported in the medical literature. Getting people to exercise lowers the rates of all causes of death by 44% - by coached training on a treadmill.[1051] Similar improvements can be expected from quitting smoking and lowering cholesterol. But how does this translate into savings in Healthcare Expenditures? The American Heart Association estimated $10-20 billion in Healthcare Expenditures could be saved by encouraging people to develop better habits.[1052]

Yes, conventional Risk Factor reduction will reduce Healthcare Expenditures – but on a different order of magnitude that that of TM use and Osteopathic Manipulative Treatment care. Widespread TM instruction could save as much as $656.3 billion. Osteopathic approach to low back pain could save $140.7 billion.

Compared to these savings, $20 billion saved through teaching better habits looks very thin.

Comparing these savings in Healthcare Expenditures is striking. But these are estimated figures. Can anyone guarantee these absolute numbers will result if we implement these changes? No one can enforce absolute change, whether in the healthcare system or elsewhere in our culture; but *this information does convey one very important message: it shows us a direction to take that will yield positive results.*

We Must Marshal Forces and Change

Whenever we hear of a good idea that works better than what we are already doing, it is wise to reexamine our efforts. Albert Einstein observed, "The definition of insanity is doing the same thing over and over and expecting different results." All of us in medical care today are faced with considering this assertion quite seriously.

Teaching TM to as many people as possible is not a difficult problem to solve. There are many TM Instructors across the country and across the world. People can even learn TM online. We need to get serious and network with them to aggressively teach TM to as many people as we can. That is perhaps the most important single thing to do to reduce Healthcare Expenditures.

The next task is to make Manipulative Therapy available throughout the medical system, as quickly as possible. Not only will this meet the needs of many patients in pain, but it will make a huge dent in the Opioid Crisis by removing the untreated misery that is largely causing it. Inevitable savings in lost work and income alone justify this action. Finally, widespread use of the DO model of medical practice will reduce Healthcare Expenditures.

Generalized suggestions to reduce Health Risk Factors are bound to help, but we can be far more specific and effective using Maharishi AyurVeda. Matching specific lifestyle recommendations to the correct people will be far more effective than imprecise pamphlet-based instruction. Maharishi AyurVeda also will reduce Healthcare Expenditures.

Encouraging patients to practice their faith and pray is a good idea, but there is far less hard evidence to demonstrate specific Healthcare Savings. Nonetheless, such encouragement is easy to add alongside the other health promoting measures we have discussed. Asking for help and healing from God should doubtless be first on our list of improving medical care rather than last - and is quite likely to reduce Healthcare Expenditures along with the rest of these strategies.

A major problem remains, however. Learning all this new material is truly challenging. Figuring out how to integrate all these strategies with how we practice now is a formidable challenge. We see that adopting these new ideas and practices will improve medical care – but the question remains: How do we move from where we are toward the *Self-Referral/Maximum Health* approach to medical care?

Chapter 17

The Self-Referral Medicine Initiative: Bring Maximum Health to Everyone

There is Nothing Wrong with Modern Medicine

This sounds like an odd statement to make after many chapters of critical talk, but this is the truth. There is nothing wrong with Modern Medicine - *if it is practiced well.* As we have discussed over many chapters throughout this book, a lot can go wrong - misdiagnosis, surgical mistakes, and medication side effects. All that can be easily avoided by practicing medicine well – *which the vast majority of healthcare professionals do every day.* That makes Modern Medicine the safest medical system in history.

Let's make one thing clear: *Self-Referral/Maximum Health* does not seek to dismantle Modern Medicine. There has been far too much progress in Modern Medicine to abandon it. Today's medical and surgical techniques are miraculous blends of technology with the best in pure human compassion. The same is true of the ready supply of the most advanced medications in history that are critical to maintain health and fight disease.

Modern Medicine uses diagnostic tools that would have been science fiction forty years ago. For example, today's imaging technology uses X-ray, Ultrasound, Nuclear Magnetic Resonance, and computers. These technologies produce images that look like anatomy photographs. This is doubly amazing when you realize that these images are of living people – and creating the images causes negligible discomfort. This sophisticated imaging allows doctors to identify tiny abnormalities that would have gone unnoticed in previous times.

Mammography is an excellent example of these advances. Doctors used to be limited to manual diagnosis during annual breast examination. If doctors found a suspicious area, they referred the patient to a surgeon to remove and biopsy the tissue in question. By contrast, today's mammography spots microscopic tumors too small for doctors to feel. This early detection saves lives.

Modern Medicine supplies superior therapeutic tools as well. We reviewed progress in high blood pressure medications. There were just a few medications for high blood pressure in the 1960s. Now there are many *classes of medications*, and research adds more every year. The same is true for other prescription items: antibiotics, diabetes, cancer-fighting drugs, and nearly every other class of prescription medications.

Modern surgery has made amazing advances. Older patients used to suffer crippling arthritis of the hips that confined them to wheelchairs. Today's orthopedic joint replacements allow older patients to stay active for most of their lives. Surgery with fiberoptic instruments allows surgery through very small incisions. This reduces pain, complications, expense, and length of hospital stays.

All these advances are the result of thousands of years of human progress. We need to incorporate the ideas and practices of *Self-Referral/Maximum Health*, but we should never belittle the progress that Modern Medicine has made. Neither should we turn our backs on the advantages that Modern Medicine offers. Rather, we should expand and add to what is already the best single system of medical care in the world today.

Simple Actions Will Improve Modern Medicine

Despite all that is good about medical care in the United States, we still face the serious problems of containing costs and delivering better healthcare outcomes to the American people. Considering all these facts, it is clear to me: *we have got to change*.

Self-Referral
Maximum Health

We Have Asked Questions and Sought Answers . . .

. . . and found exactly what is needed to improve today's system of medical care. To clarify what we have learned, consider what we have found:

WHAT WE NEED:	WHAT WE HAVE FOUND:
We must find a practical solution for the intense stress of modern life - that causes the Adaptation Crisis and punishingly high disease rates and Healthcare Spending.	Transcendental Meditation or TM provides the best technique for deep rest and relief from the stress of modern life. No other technique works like TM.
We need a system of more precise and accurate lifestyle recommendations for all patients and their medical conditions. This will simplify health promotion and bring better help to patients.	Maharishi AyurVeda provides a quick and easy system to accurately evaluate patients and quickly assign specific lifestyle changes to promote health and prevent disease.
We must find a simple and effective system of manual treatment for routine musculoskeletal care.	Self-Referral Manual Therapy can be quickly taught and learned and is gentle and harmless.

The course we now follow is moving us toward more fragmented and less effective healthcare. The course we are on is preventing effective health promotion and disease prevention. The course that we are on is causing the dangerous upward spiral of medical costs that is crippling our economy, our country, and our world. What should we do about all this?

We must move toward the Health Approach – not as a *replacement* for the Disease Approach – *but as a supplement to it.* We must maintain the aggressive stance to identify and treat disease as it is detected – but now we have new tools to promote health and prevent disease. *We must commit to promoting health and preventing disease just as aggressively as we work to identify and treat disease*.

Why Do Efforts to Improve Medical Care Fail?

Our present situation demands action – but it must be *effective action*. We do not need another round of add-on programs that eat up time and destroy morale among both healthcare providers and patients. We need an effective action model to meet well-defined needs. We need specific enhancements to improve Modern Medicine - and we need effective ways to move these good ideas into medical practice.

Moving toward the Health Approach often fails because it seems so complicated and daunting. The routine practice of medicine already consumes a lot of time and energy. It is both intense and fast paced. Anything that comes along as a so-called "improvement" to medical practice is nearly always greeted as "another boat anchor to slow us down." I know these attitudes in health professionals after spending over forty years in medical practice. And I *also* know that response is *more often accurate than not*.

Why do so many attempts at Health Promotion and Disease Prevention fail? Nearly all such efforts are variations of *renewing focus on what we are already doing*. We do our best to pay more attention to laboratory values to better control diabetes or cholesterol. We might focus on encouraging patients to lose weight or exercise. *What all these attempts have in common is doing MORE of the same thing we already do every day.* The idea that simply increasing our intensity of attention on something seldom accomplishes anything except harassing healthcare providers and patients alike.

How We Can Succeed at Improving Medical Care

Throughout this book I have demonstrated the value of the three additions that Modern Medicine needs. Using these new tools is not just another unfocused attempt at making things better, doomed to fail. *Research from all over the world proves that Transcendental Meditation, Maharishi AyurVeda, and Manipulative Therapy are effective. They have proven their ability to improve health AND radically cut Healthcare Spending*. What are the practical steps we must take to move into action?

We can move toward the Health Approach by teaching healthcare providers a set of easily learned skills. These new skills easily integrate with what we are already doing. These services can be billed for as they are delivered to justify the time commitment. And a critical imperative: *there must be resulting patient health improvements that show measurable savings in Healthcare Spending.*

We can take a simple modular approach to make quick progress toward reforming the medical system. This will be easy to design and implement. Doctors and all other health professionals are thoroughly familiar with taking short courses to learn new techniques or services. These modular segments can be organized and taught either live or online.

Health professionals can easily take the courses, demonstrate their competence, and obtain certification in the respective modular areas of study. In this way, health professionals can quickly learn the new knowledge, become competent in it, and deliver the new services to their patients.

There will be no economic or professional barriers to participating in these programs. Additional services that are learned can easily be coded and billed right along with all the rest of medical services. Having additional services to offer makes all professional practices more profitable and adds to services they provide, increasing their ability to successfully compete in their respective medical marketplaces.

All patients will benefit by having access to additional health promoting services, actively participating in their own health promotion, and *improving their health.* Health insurance carriers will benefit through decreasing need for healthcare in their covered patients, *resulting in large savings in Healthcare Expenditures.*

We can think of Modern Medicine as a firm, dependable stool that everyone in medical care relies on. It is strong, sturdy, and reliable. We have come to take it for granted, and any suggestions to change it are nearly always met with opposition. This is as it should be; opposition to ill-advised changes to medical care keeps Modern Medicine safe and effective. But when better options for medical care arrive, they can be met with wide acceptance and will be of great assistance to patients.

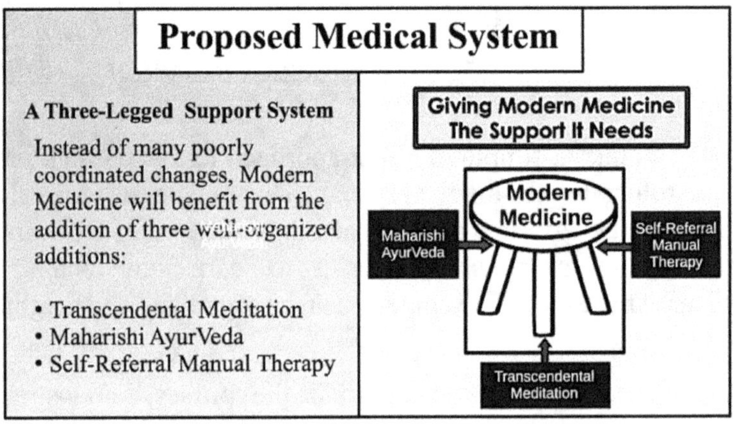

The Firm, Dependable Stool of Modern Medicine Simply Needs Three Additional Supports

That means there will be no changes to the practice of Modern Medicine. No healthcare providers must reinvent the wheel or dodge obnoxious new regulations. Patients will have no new and unfamiliar medical system to navigate. Billing departments will not be harassed by new coding demands. And health insurers will have no need for action of any kind – except for welcome reductions in Healthcare Expenditure payouts.

What do we see as incentives to adopt these three additions to the medical system? We will examine each of the three additions one at a time. Their value will become obvious

Transcendental Meditation (TM)

Modern life causes more stress than the human body can tolerate. The result is the Adaptational Crisis that causes today's epidemic of stress related diseases. *Key to improving medical care is to provide effective treatment to neutralize stress.* We know that stress drives high Healthcare Spending and underlies all disease and the aging process. Our present moment in history absolutely clarifies this problem as never before.

TM offers the solution to today's Adaptation Crisis. Adding two sessions of TM to each day provides dramatic and health building relief from the onslaught of stress. TM allows the human mind and body to settle down and get relief from the crush of modern life. TM also improves the body's ability to cope with future stress.

TM is the only stress reduction technique that has had the full scrutiny of scientific research. No stress reduction technique has been studied as extensively as TM. Many stress-reduction techniques claim to be as effective as TM, but not one of them has objective research findings to prove it. TM is thus scientifically proven – and can be relied on - to improve health and cut Healthcare Expenditures. *Other techniques will fail to produce the desired results*.

Incorporating TM into today's medical practice will be simple. The only necessary action will be to recommend TM to the patient. Each practice can set up easy directions for patients to follow to obtain TM instruction. There are many TM Instructors worldwide and they are well-trained professionals who will be welcome additions to today's medical team. There are also ways to learn TM remotely online.

Providing TM - *the only proven effective stress reduction technique* - will be well received. Rather than offering temporary relief through drugs, patients can learn to reduce their own stress through TM. Regular practice of TM will reduce the incidence of many stress-related problems like anxiety and depression – as well as promote general health. *The best stress reduction technique proven by science will move patients toward Maximum Health - while reducing Healthcare Expenditures by moving them away from disease*.

Self-Referral

Maximum Health

Transcendental Meditation Restores *Self-Referral*

TM provides two sessions a day of profoundly deep rest. This allows the body to rejuvinate itself by normalizing brain and body function. Modern science has proven TM's unique effects.

TM is the one and only meditation technique to restore *Self-Referral* and create *Maximum Health.*

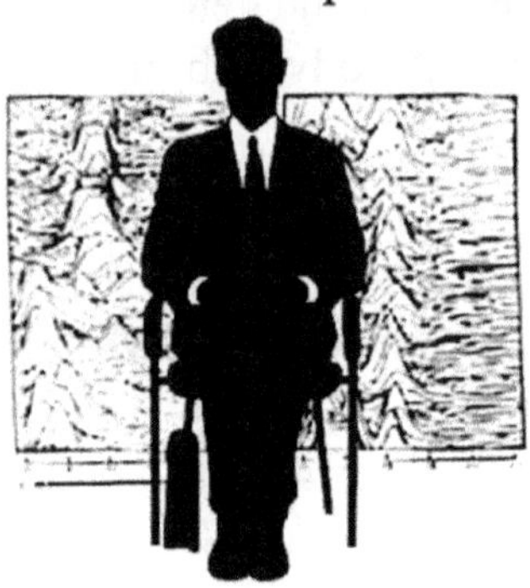

Maharishi AyurVeda

In today's world, giving lifestyle pointers and advice is more and more expected – by patients and by insurance carriers. Imprecise lifestyle and diet advice often yields unreliable results. Maharishi AyurVeda uses an exact, accurate, and effective system of categorizing patients – and specific advice for each patient type.

Maharishi AyurVeda makes it possible to identify patient body types quickly through an easily learned pulse diagnosis technique. Matching the right advice to the right patient yields superior results.

This helps patients get the quickest and most effective health benefit using lifestyle, diet, and exercise.

Self-Referral
Maximum Health

Maharishi AyurVeda Restores *Self-Referral*

By identifying the patient body type, MAV moves the patient into synchronization with the cycles of Nature.

The patient can create an ideal daily routine and diet, and balance their physiology toward Maximum Health.

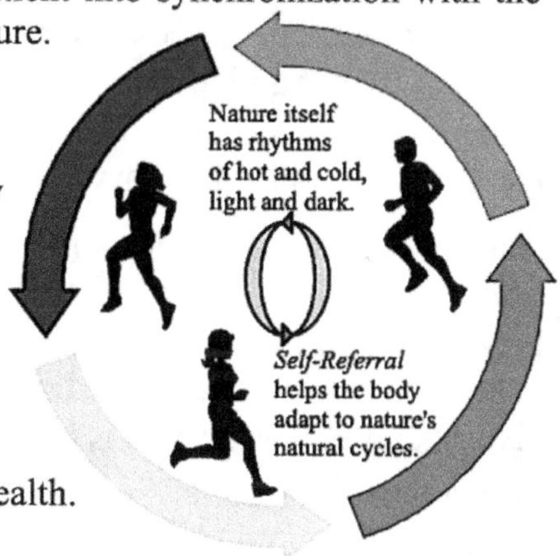

Modern Medicine fights disease effectively - and *Maharishi AyurVeda provides a new opportunity to promote health.* Any doctor can easily add these Ayurvedic skills to their medical practice. The services can be delivered quickly to avoid disruption of schedule. These will be billable services that fall within routine medical care. In this way, patients will retain all the advantages of Modern Medicine – while benefiting from the new services.

Doctors can readily learn Ayurvedic diagnosis of body type and offer practical advice on daily routines to prevent disease and promote health. Timely advice on diet, behavior, and lifestyle will help all people to synchronize with the natural cycles of nature. None of these approaches conflict with Modern Medicine. And, most importantly, they supply avenues of healing that Modern Medicine does not currently offer.

This will help reduce the need for medical care – and contribute to reductions in Healthcare Expenditures. When we work to restore balance of the physiology, we are directly working to optimize Self-Referral throughout the body. *The healthcare provider will easily move patients toward Maximum Health – while reducing Healthcare Expenditures by moving them away from disease.*

Self-Referral Manual Therapy

Chronic stress causes tight and painful muscles, and joints may become restricted or even locked. These prevent normal body posture and movement. These stress related problems are painful and interfere with both work and leisure. The economic impact of these problems is enormous. Lost wages for workers and lost productivity for employers cost millions of dollars every year.

Manipulative Therapy identifies and treats the long-term effects of stress on the body's bones, joints, and muscles. Patients seek it because it relieves their muscle and joint related problems. But how can healthcare professionals without training in that field provide Manipulative Therapy? The answer is to obtain training and add it to their medical practice.

Some health professionals want no part of Manipulative Therapy because of concern about hurting the patient. Many schools of Manipulative Therapy use vigorous force to treat patients, causing many health professionals to avoid learning it. I agree with these concerns. I would quote Isaac Asimov who wrote: "Violence is the last refuge of the incompetent." To remedy these concerns, I have created a violence-free and totally gentle system of Manipulative Therapy that any healthcare professional can learn and use.

Self-Referral Manual Therapy is a new revision of Manipulative Therapy specifically created by Dr. Michael Borger as part of the Self-Referral Medicine Initiative.

Self-Referral Manual Therapy (SRMT) is based on merely touching muscles and applying a gentle traction that can harm no one. This is a simple procedure that is easily taught and easily learned.

Once mastered through one-on-one instruction, SRMT is universally applicable everywhere in the musculoskeletal system. And because there is no violence or force of any kind, any healthcare professional can readily learn SRMT and use it within the boundaries of their training and license.

Self-Referral
Maximum Health

Self-Referral Manual Therapy Restores Self-Referral

SRMT is a system of gentle manual therapy. Easily learned, this therapy only requires gentle pressing and traction to treat deep-seated muscle and bone tissue stress that blocks Self-Referral.

SRMT is a new revision of manual therapy that eliminates all violent snapping and cracking. SRMT is the new universal manual therapy.

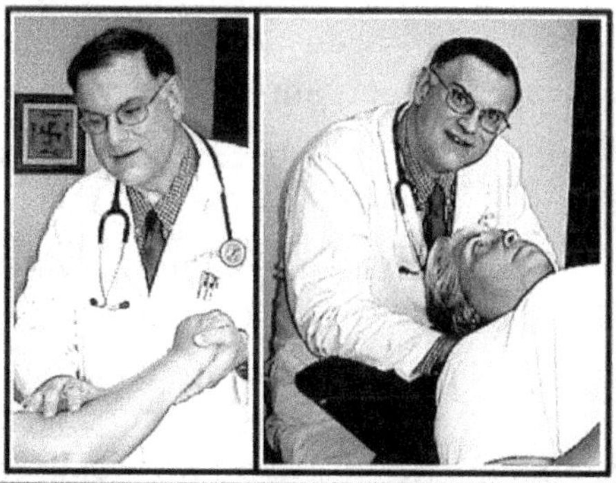

SRMT effortlessly removes painful musculoskeletal roadblocks to health. These are the acute and chronic disorders that send patients from one doctor to another seeking pain relief.

This new approach to manual medicine works so well because it identifies and treats the exact physical blocks to Self-Referral that need resolved. That is because *SRMT directly restores Self-Referral*.

While SRMT is not a cure-all, *it is critical to restoring Self-Referral in people suffering from stress related musculoskeletal problems*. Such patients may obtain all the help they can from

Modern Medicine, TM, and Maharishi AyurVeda - and still fail to achieve Maximum Health. *Cure of many painful muscle and bone problems will remain elusive without proper SRMT diagnosis and treatment.*

SRMT will fill a unique niche in medical care. Because it is simple yet so effective, healthcare professionals will want to learn it. Patients will love it because it solves their pain and mobility problems. *SRMT will move patients away from bone and muscle pain and toward Maximum Health – while moving them away from disease and reducing Healthcare Expenditures.*

The Self-Referral Medicine Initiative

Any theory is interesting, but until it is made practical, it is only an abstract subject in discussion. If we are to bring these three additions to Modern Medicine, we must take practical action. *The Self-Referral Medicine Initiative is the effort to take action to bring the three-legged support system to Modern Medicine.* To accomplish this, we will need cooperation between many healthcare professionals and organizations. Many ask how anyone can get this started, let alone reform all medical practice? Where do we begin to achieve these things?

Many doctors will agree immediately with these suggestions, but others may be slower to change. How can we achieve tomorrow's medicine without all doctors agreeing to change at once? *The answer is: we must create a coalition of the willing*. That is, we do not have to assume that Self-Referral Medicine cannot happen without an act of Congress or some kind of approval from the AMA, the AOA, or specialty colleges.

We can start by simply making small scale tests to evaluate the ideas and skills – and their outcomes. No one should adopt an untested program, particularly in patient care. We will begin with pilot projects that test all parts of the Self-Referral Medicine Initiative.

Work is now underway to create training modules to teach the three additions to Modern Medicine. Actual training of groups of healthcare professionals will soon take place. Once trained professionals demonstrate their proficiency, we will start a pilot program to implement and study results of the three additions

Self-Referral
Maximum Health

Three Proposed Training Modules

1. Transcendental Meditation: Teaches healthcare providers about the TM Technique and opportunity to learn TM. Integrating TM with medical practice.
2. Maharishi AyurVeda: Teaches healthcare providers theory, pulse diagnosis, and patient advice to improve diet, exercise, and lifestyle.
3. Self-Referral Manual Therapy: Teaches healthcare providers practical SRMT including clear and specific skills and how-to-treat patients.

All training modules will be offered live or online. All Training Modules will be short and to the point. Health providers will quickly learn the material and use the practical applications immediately. You may bill for services using existing ICDS and CPT codes.

Contact Dr. Michael Borger:

Email: Dr.Michael.Borger@gmail.com
Website: www.MaximumHealthInstitute.com
Substack: www.Substack.com/@DrMichaelBorger
Twitter: www.Twitter.com/@DrMichaelBorger
Facebook: www.Facebook.com/Dr.Michael.Borger

Training programs will be short to minimize lost work time for health professionals. The courses will teach both the principles and practical skills. There will be three modular courses: one each for Transcendental Meditation, Maharishi AyurVeda, and for Self-Referral Manual Therapy.

We Must Proactively Study Results

Finally, it is the specific plan of the Self-Referral Medicine Initiative to put in place effective data gathering arrangements to objectively evaluate results. We must specifically quantify the performance of these three additions to Modern Medicine.

The goal in implementing these measures is to promote health AND reduce Healthcare Expenses.

We previously examined improving sterile conditions in the surgery room. Those improvements resulted from the work of Dr. Louis Pasteur and Dr. James Lister. Those who ran surgery rooms did not adopt the sterile techniques when Pasteur's microbe theories were published, or even when Dr. Lister proposed adopting sterile procedures to reduce infection. It was when Dr. Lister's post-operative infection rate dropped like a rock that the medical profession took notice.

Looking back across history, it is easy to criticize those who resisted the ideas of Pasteur and Lister. But, as I have stated many times, *keeping medical care conservative is usually the best course*. That is why anyone who plans to implement the three additions to Modern Medicine must get involved evaluating their effectiveness.

It is not enough to say relevant past research or anecdotal evidence automatically justifies making these three additions to Modern Medicine. Through training programs, we will know that healthcare providers have gained the knowledge and skills to make these additions to their medical practice. We must then obtain data to monitor health status and billing for medical services. Thus, *at the same time we implement the Self-Referral Medicine Initiative, we also will put in place means to measure results.* We must determine the Initiative's effect on patient health and Healthcare Expenditures. This is mandatory to validate moving forward with the program.

All stakeholders will work together to start data gathering and evaluation as *Self-Referral/Maximum Health* skills are taught and put into place. The goal will be to know at the end of the study

(1) whether the new measures are improving patient health and (2) whether there are reductions in Healthcare Expenditures. *These*

arrangements will be set up so as NOT to cause more work for healthcare providers, nursing personnel, or office personnel.

Self-Referral
Maximum Health

We Must Proactively Study Results Of the Self-Referral Initiative

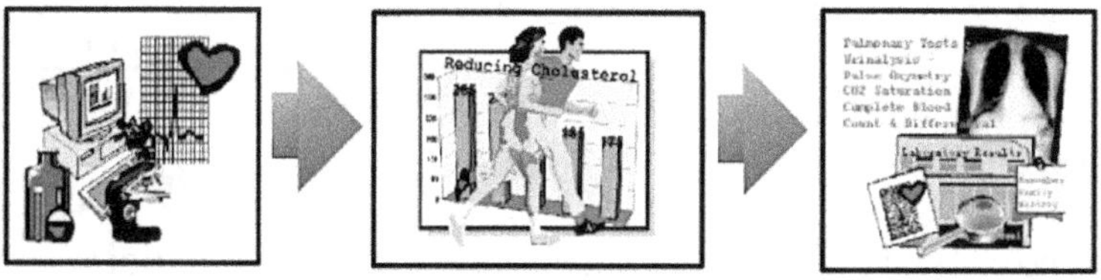

The Self-Referral Initiative states a clear hypothesis in scientific terms. The three additions to Modern Medicine are: Patient practice of the TM Technique; Aggressive patient education and refinement of daily routine and diet via Maharishi AyurVeda; and treatment as needed with Self-Referral Manual Therapy. We can determine with relatively simple patient monitoring (1) health status (2) Healthcare Expenditures over a study period of time.

The Self-Referral Medicine Group

The *Self-Referral Medicine Group* is an organization formed to plan and execute health professional training. This body is founded by Dr. Michael Borger and is soliciting healthcare professionals of all kinds to get involved studying Self-Referral Medicine. Current work is planning the knowledge base that will be taught to health professionals to integrate the principles of Self-Referral Medicine with their medical practice.

The next task will be to offer training programs to teach Self-Referral Medicine. This training will be structured in modular fashion and should be in the range of one to three days for each of the three modules. Instruction will be both in lecture format and hands-on instruction. Emphasis will be to quickly get health professionals to understanding and implement the practical aspects of Self-Referral Medicine.

The Self-Referral Medicine Group's aim is to teach and make available the three simple additions to Modern Medicine needed to improve medical practice. The plan is to quickly teach the principles and make services instantly available to the patients. Carrying out this streamlined program will reform Modern Medicine as quickly as possible, benefitting healthcare providers and patients alike.

The Self-Referral Research Group

The critical part of validating the Self-Referral Medicine Initiative is quantifying results from the start of services forward. The purpose of the *Self-Referral Research Group* is to plan and execute high quality medical research to study the effects of Self-Referral Medicine. The theory driving this movement is that implementing the three additions to Modern Medicine will (1) improve patient health and (2) reduce Healthcare Expenditures.

These are very clear and well-defined measures of improvement that are easily quantifiable.

The Self-Referral Research Group will plan and carry out the necessary data gathering and evaluation. Results will be treated according to high quality scientific research principles. Study outcomes will be published in well-established scientific journals. In this way, the Self-Referral Medicine Initiative will be objectively studied to evaluate its effects on both patient health and Healthcare Expenditures.

We will not need a long process to test this theory. After a reasonable time, probably from six months to a year, we will see the concrete medical and financial outcomes. *Based on what we know from past research and experience, we should see improvement in patient health and reduction in Healthcare Expenses.*

Dr. Michael Borger is actively seeking medical and research personnel to participate in designing and carrying out this research to validate the effects of the planned 3 additions to Modern Medicine. Please contact him if you have interest in this project. Pilot projects are being designed as this book goes to publication.

Everyone involved in pilot studies will meet and proactively plan (1) training of healthcare providers (2) Implementation of services (3) what specific parameters we will use to measure success of the project (4) Specific mechanics of data collection and (5) final analysis to determine results.

All these goals are realistic, well-defined, and attainable. Will we have to work to help this happen? Yes, it will require work to bring these initiatives into play as part of the medical system. Are they worth it? The savings in both costs and human suffering make it certain to pay high dividends.

The Dean Ornish Story

The Disease Approach of Modern Medicine is well known and needs little explanation. The Health Approach is a great idea, but does it work? Is there any proof the *Self-Referral/Maximum Health* ideas are an improvement over the Disease Approach of Modern Medicine? Perhaps no better example exists than the work of Dr. Dean Ornish. This physician is a graduate of Houston's Baylor College of Medicine and a Harvard Medical School fellow. He practices Internal Medicine in Sausalito, California. There he is president and director of the Preventative Medicine Research Institute.[1053]

Dr. Ornish has conducted clinical research on comprehensive lifestyle changes since 1977. He combined many of the health promotion methods discussed in *Self-Referral/Maximum Health.* Turning away from an exclusive Disease Approach, Dr. Ornish advocates a total lifestyle change to promote health – including diet, cultivation of a vital inner spiritual life, exercise, smoking cessation, stretching Yoga exercises, and mental stress reduction techniques.[1054] This is an ambitious program by anyone's estimation. Does it improve health or is it just wishful thinking?

In his landmark publication "Intensive Lifestyle Changes for Reversal of Coronary Heart Disease" he and his co-researchers provide strong evidence that his program works. Ornish studied patients with coronary artery disease over a five-year period. *Patients taught the Ornish program showed a reversal of hardening of the coronary arteries*. That is, the blockages reversed and opened to allow more blood flow to reach the heart. This resulted in a sharp reduction in further heart damage in the Ornish program study group. By contrast, the control group patients continued to deteriorate over the five-year period and had markedly worsening health.[1055]

Dr. Dean Ornish has done a great service to physicians and patients alike. He has shown that a complete and comprehensive lifestyle change is a better way to treat heart disease than to simply prescribe medication and hope for the best. While every patient may not be amenable to the kind of comprehensive approach that Ornish offers, those that are willing can reap huge improvements in their health.

The work of Dr. Dean Ornish and his colleagues is extremely important. This research shows what is possible by improving the total lifestyle instead of just treating the disease. I suggest that *this approach may be made even more comprehensive and effective*.

Let's Go Beyond the Ornish Program

This book clearly makes the case that TM is by far the most effective stress reduction technique. Research also shows that TM practice can reduce angina pectoris and improve coronary function. It only makes sense that the TM technique could be taught right along with all the other aspects of the Ornish program. Improvements are likely to be even more pronounced.

Is there current specific proof that Transcendental Meditation is important in treating cardiovascular disease? A recent study made this quite clear. Enlargement of the left side of the heart is a common problem caused by chronic high blood pressure. Stress is known to be a major factor that drives both high blood pressure and heart enlargement.

African Americans are known to have high rates of cardiovascular disease and heart enlargement. In 2019 a group of African American adults with high blood pressure were randomly assigned to either learn TM or receive standard health education. All were tested for cardiac enlargement. After six months had passed, all patients were retested and compared to the previous tests. The TM patients had significantly lower cardiac enlargement than those who did not learn TM.[1056] *This is strong evidence that specifically adding Transcendental Meditation to multiphase health promotion programs is critical.*

Is there evidence that Maharishi AyurVeda improves blockage of arteries? Carotid artery blockage from chronic buildup of plaques is a well-known high-risk factor for stroke and sudden death. These are the large arteries in the neck. A recent study used TM, a heart-healthy Maharishi AyurVeda diet, exercise, and herbal food supplements to treat patients with known blocked carotid artery disease. The patients initially had imaging of the carotid arteries to measure the disease plaques. Then the patients were treated for nine months with the Maharishi AyurVeda routine.

At the study's end the carotid arteries were rechecked. *The patients had reduced the blockages in the carotid arteries.* These changes were statistically significant – and the conclusion was that Maharishi AyurVeda measures were effective in reversing carotid artery plaques.[1057] *This is exactly the effect documented by the Dr. Dean Ornish program – except in the carotid arteries of the neck instead of the heart's coronary arteries.* This body of medical research thus proves that major cardiovascular disease can be improved by the three additions to Modern Medicine proposed by the Self-Referral Medicine Initiative.

Comparing the Disease Approach of *just take your medicine* to the Health Approach of tackling the real-life issues of lifestyle management, the contrast is quite evident. Intervention with aggressive lifestyle work, serious stress reduction, and major diet and exercise work make a powerful impact. We see patients not just improving <u>but actually defeating disease and returning to good health</u>. This is the basis of *Self-Referral/Maximum Health* – and this is why we must take the measures needed to move our population toward Maximum Health.

Solving the Healthcare Crisis: Self-Referral Medicine

We have found the best combination of several key disciplines that will allow us to achieve Maximum Health. We have examined current medical care and identified specific additions to support it. Now we can work together to create a far more effective medical system. To achieve this, we need a clear vision of where we are going - and a clear plan to bring that vision into reality.

Self-Referral
Maximum Health

Principles of Self-Referral Medicine

REMEMBER: ***Self-Referral Medicine is the new medical paradigm. Here are principles that health professionals and patients see in the context of Self-Referral/Maximum Health.***

- **Self-Referral Medicine** uses all of Modern Medicine to evaluate, diagnose, and treat health problems.
- **Self-Referral Medicine** recognizes Self-Referral as the fundamental principle of body operations.
- **Self-Referral Medicine** recognizes that normal Self-Referral creates health – and abnormal Self-Referral creates disease.
- **Self-Referral Medicine** sees all interruptions in Self-Referral as points of intervention to work with patients to restore their Self-Referral.
- **Self-Referral Medicine** encourages patients to learn TM to reduce stress and promote health.
- **Self-Referral Medicine** uses Maharishi AyurVeda to identify health imbalances and restore Self-Referral.
- **Self-Referral Medicine** uses Self-Referral Manual Therapy to diagnose and treat musculoskeletal problems and restore Self-Referral.
- **Self-Referral Medicine** encourages patients to practice their religion, pray, and live in accordance with positive religious precepts.

I use the term *Self-Referral Medicine* to lay the foundation for creating this improved medical system. Everyone understands the term "medicine" as it applies to the science and professions of healing. Whether we are an MD, a DO, Chiropractor, or any other health professional offering services in the medical field, *all of us are working in the field of medicine.*

We discussed the idea of changing paradigms. Paradigm shifts occur when new ideas or perceptions make their way into the culture at large. Once this happens, people from many fields often notice and begin to use the emerging paradigm to better understand and expand their own fields.

Self-Referral Medicine describes the emerging paradigm of medical care that we have been discussing throughout this book. Self-Referral Medicine is not a replacement or a substitute for Modern Medicine. Rather, we are adding to Modern Medicine the intent to practice with a clear aim to promote Self-Referral. This is a focused effort to create *Maximum Health* by restoring *Self-Referral.* We thus understand that Self-Referral Medicine clearly defines the emerging new paradigm, codifies it as something everyone can agree with and support, and will be a positive force to improve medical practice everywhere.

The goal of Self-Referral Medicine is to find the strengths and weaknesses in any patient's health, identify and treat all disease that is found, and help the patient improve their health through one-on-one coaching. Working through time, the patient will make lifestyle changes that will steadily improve their health. *The goal of Self-Referral Medicine is to optimize the health of all patients – moving them toward Maximum Health.*

If you are a healthcare professional – whether medical or administrative – you will want to visit the *Maximum Health Institute* Website at https://www.maximumhealthinstitute.com. You will find information about the Self-Referral Medicine Group, the Self-Referral Research Group, pilot projects, training program information, and many helps to learn about Self-Referral Medicine. You can also connect with Dr. Michael Borger's ongoing writings at

Substack. This is the ideal place to get involved with the Self-Referral Medicine Initiative.

If you are a patient or just want to learn more about Self-Referral Medicine, you can investigate the *Maximum Health Expert* Website at https://www.maximumhealthexpert.com

You can learn a lot about improving your health. There are many resources and links there as well as an invitation to connect with Dr. Michael Borger's more serious writing at Substack. Many report that this Website is of great help in the pursuit of Maximum Health.

In addition to the websites, Dr. Michael Borger's best online writing can be found at Substack:

www.Substack.com/@DrMichaelBorger

Dr. Michael Borger has a lively online presence on X (Twitter) at:

https://www.Twitter.com/@DrMichaelBorger

Dr. Michael Borger also can be found at:

https://www.Facebook.com/Dr.Michael.Borger

https://www.Instagram.com/Mike.borger1

Dr. Michael Borger is creating a community of healthcare professionals, educators, medical school faculty, and anyone interested in Self-Referral Medicine. The purpose of this community will be to learn the principles of Self-Referral Medicine and apply it to medical practice. I hope you take the initiative and get involved. This is the time in history that we can really make a difference for the better. Let's do it!

What Doctors Can Do

Self-Referral Medicine is an addition to Modern Medicine and not a replacement for Modern Medicine; it is a voluntary path taken by people who agree with the ideas. In this sense it is like the Quality Movement or the concept of the Medical Home. Self-Referral Medicine is theoretical, but practical application of it can change medicine for the better.

Today's practice of medicine is not the monolith portrayed by print and electronic media. Some doctors strictly follow majority opinions, but there are always doctors who think for themselves and are willing to try something new. A growing number of innovative doctors are expanding their medical practice beyond what they learned in medical school. These courageous professionals go outside the deep ruts of habit to find something new to help their patients achieve better health.

Doctors should connect with the Self-Referral Medicine Group to take the most effective path to participating in Self-Referral Medicine. The Self-Referral Medicine Group will be offering training modules to teach the three additions to medical practice. These include Transcendental Meditation (TM), Maharishi AyurVeda, and Self-Referral Manipulative Therapy. This will be the most effective way to learn and integrate this new set of knowledge and skills with your current medical practice.

The Self-Referral Medicine Group will offer a training module on the TM program. Doctors with an interest in TM can learn TM themselves and recommend TM to their patients. Many books about TM are available for study - for doctors and patients alike. Doctors thus can help patients reduce stress and improve their health simply by recommending TM.

If doctors have an interest in effective health promotion and disease prevention, the Self-Referral Medicine Group will be offering a training module in Maharishi AyurVeda. Doctors can learn pulse diagnosis, physical diagnosis, determination of Ayurvedic body type, and Ayurvedic therapies. Maharishi AyurVeda teaches specific recommendations to optimize each patient's daily routine, diet, and exercise to optimize their health.

The Self-Referral Medicine Group will offer a training module in Self-Referral Manual Therapy - a gentle, non-violent, easy-does-it system of Manipulative Therapy. Any health professional can learn and use this simple and gentle system of manual therapy. SRMT restores Self-Referral caused by abnormal function of the musculoskeletal system. And, most importantly, their patients will benefit from a new and effective dimension of medical care.

Finally, the Self-Referral Medicine Group will offer a training module teaching how to effectively integrate this new knowledge and skill set with modern medical practice. That will include how to carry out the new services in a timely way to avoid disrupting busy schedules. Specific help with billing and related services also will clarify Self-Referral Medicine operations.

Dare to be Different.

For *Self-Referral/Maximum Health* to become a reality, doctors are going to have to take risks. This is nothing new in human history. All innovators, from Galileo to Copernicus to Newton to Einstein took risks. Many of history's greatest innovators, including those in medicine – like Pasteur and Lister - were initially ridiculed for what critics called their "radical ideas."

In life, as in baseball, we must occasionally step up to the plate and give our best swing. This act requires risk, and it requires courage. Advocates of opposing viewpoints will disagree with some or all of what I have written. There are camps opposing TM, Maharishi AyurVeda, and Manipulative Therapy. All these people advocate their positions and work diligently to triumph over their rivals. The same is true for overzealous defenders of Modern Medicine, who strive to defend it from change of any kind.

Doctors interested in *Self-Referral/Maximum Health* should do whatever they can to make tomorrow's medicine a reality. We cannot reasonably expect all doctors to change immediately. Even so, Doctors should not allow what they cannot do prevent them from doing what they can do to improve medical practice. Find a way to participate and begin – for the sake of improving medical practice.

Change for many people is difficult at best. The change that *Self-Referral/Maximum Health* advocates will be difficult for some to accept. Nevertheless, I am convinced there are enough doctors and other health professionals with sufficient courage to implement these ideas. The change may not be noticeable at first, but if we start now, it will eventually come. R. Buckminster Fuller once said:

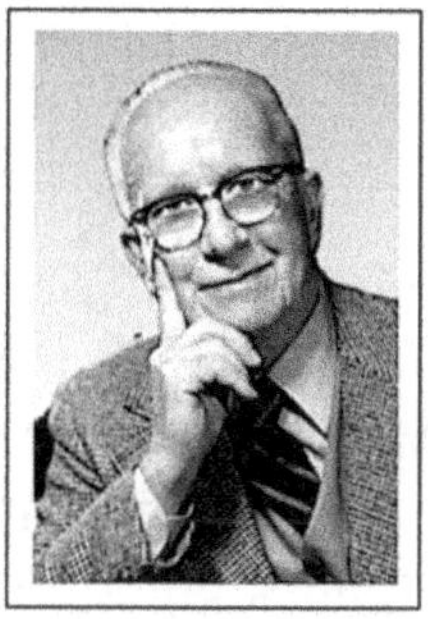

"Think of the Queen Elizabeth. The whole ship goes by and then comes the rudder. And there's a tiny thing on the edge of the rudder called a trim tab. Just moving that little trim tab builds a low pressure that pulls the rudder around. It takes almost no effort at all.

The individual can be a trim tab. Society thinks it's going right by you, that it's left you altogether. But if you're doing dynamic things mentally, the fact is that you can just put your foot out like that and the whole ship of state is going to turn around. To be a real trim tab, you've got to start with yourself, and soon you'll feel that low pressure, and suddenly things begin to work in a beautiful way. Of course, they happen only when you're dealing with really great integrity."[1058]

Health professionals with courage and vision can act as medical care's trim tab. While a small number of doctors cannot turn the ship of medicine all at once, they can slowly affect change through dynamic positive activity. That activity must begin by working with themselves. They must get the additional knowledge they need to create tomorrow's medicine. Then they must use this knowledge to improve the quality of life for all their patients. Finally, these courageous pioneers must educate their colleagues about these important additions to medical practice.

What Patients Can Do

Patients also can act as trim tabs to turn the ship of medicine toward *Self-Referral/Maximum Health*. People often think their choices are limited to what medicine presently offers. Doctors are listening to patients, now more than ever. This is because doctors are beginning to understand they must improve their communication skills. If patients express an interest in Transcendental Meditation, Maharishi AyurVeda, or Manipulative Therapy - doctors will be more likely to investigate these subjects.

Patients can start by reading about these subjects. There is a large bibliography listed in this book. The listings include available books about Manipulative Therapy, Maharishi AyurVeda, TM, and Self-Referral Medicine. It is good to become informed in these subjects anyway, but the more patients know the more they can share with doctors, nurses, and other health professionals.

Patients can become active in spreading the ideas of *Self-Referral/Maximum Health* in their communities. They can see that the local public library has copies of this book. Many people form study groups to read *Self-Referral/Maximum Health* and study its ideas. Such groups meet in schools, libraries, hospitals, clinics, or people's homes.

Finally, patients can help much by simply standing firm in their convictions and supporting their doctors when they offer new services. Attacks from political radicals, religious extremists, and overly conservative medical societies may come. When the going gets tough, nothing helps more than patients speaking freely about how these new ideas and therapies have helped them. Dark lies can never withstand the light of truth.

What Other Health Professionals Can Do

Non-physician health professionals can act as trim tabs to help realize *Self-Referral/Maximum Health.* Many health professionals such as Nurses and Dietitians routinely offer patient education and various levels of healthcare. Identifying and discouraging bad habits brings health improvements in patients. Good advice on diet, exercise, and other lifestyle changes can promote health and prevent future disease. These professionals can easily learn and apply the principles of Self-Referral Medicine to their work. The Self-Referral Group teaching modules will be of great assistance to them. Once learned, they can integrate this knowledge and skill set in their fields.

All healthcare personnel will benefit from learning Transcendental Meditation. *TM is the one stress reduction technique that has been validated by extensive scientific research.* Every health professional knows the daily grinding stress of medical practice. Learn TM and turn your life around for the better. Something to remember: Mindfulness or any other stress reduction technique are not equivalent to TM – and will not improve health or reduce

Healthcare Expenditures. Those techniques also will not give the desired relief from stress that TM practitioners experience. Learn TM and then recommend it specifically to others.

Nurse Practitioners, Physician Assistants, Nurses, Dietitians, Physical Therapists, Chiropractors, Kinesiologists, and other health professionals can learn the principles and skills of Self-Referral Medicine and use these ideas and skills as their professions allow. Those licensed to provide Physical Therapy can apply Self-Referral Manual Therapy to their work. Restoring Self-Referral through Physical Therapy is an excellent way for manipulating professionals to deliver tomorrow's medicine today.

Tomorrow's Self-Referral Medicine will not come about through force of will or political maneuvering. The vision of *Self-Referral/Maximum Health* will only come about through respectful cooperation between physicians, patients, and all health professionals.

All healthcare professionals can help realize the vision of *Self-Referral/Maximum Health* by supporting doctors and patients who accept and work with these ideas. Opposition to new ideas usually disappears once the ideas are better understood, and most importantly, the ideas are proven to work. Educating other people about these ideas will build acceptance.

Finally, all healthcare professionals can advocate the vision of tomorrow's medicine contained in *Self-Referral/Maximum Health.* Those who work in hospitals and contribute to committee work can recommend this book. When people read this book and learn the ideas found in *Self-Referral/Maximum Health*, they are likely to join in creating the medicine of tomorrow. They can advocate incorporation of Transcendental Meditation (TM), Maharishi AyurVeda, and Self-Referral Manual Therapy into hospitals, clinics, and medical practices. The more members of the health care team that get involved the faster change will come.

Self-Referral/Maximum Health: The Goal of Medicine

We have been on an amazing journey together, you and me. We have traced the idea of *Self-Referral/Maximum Health* from an unknown quantity to a new way to practice medicine. What have we learned together? I hope that we now see the human body as a potentially perfect, limitless idea of health. I hope we see the possibility of improving our health through a healthier lifestyle with Transcendental Meditation, Maharishi AyurVeda, and Self-Referral Manual Therapy.

My hope is that I have shown you many different pieces of what I see as the same puzzle – presenting a more complete and more coherent picture of medical practice. If you look at the research across the last century in stress, TM, Manipulative Therapy, Maharishi AyurVeda, and Modern Medicine, there are many bits of knowledge that obviously fit together in new and exciting ways. It is my desire that this new synthesis of thought, ideas, knowledge, and skills becomes useful to many people. I believe patients, doctors, and all health professionals need to hear this story to create a better medical system based on *Self-Referral/Maximum Health.*

Finally, I want to remind everybody why doctors and other health professionals go into medicine. We undergo the long, tough college courses, get a university degree, and then enter medical school as beginners all over again. We find ourselves studying an even tougher and more complex subject: medicine. Finally, we work grueling hours in hospitals, clinics, and doctor's offices to finish our training to . . . work long and grueling hours providing patient care. *Why do we do it?*

I cannot speak for others, but I know why I do it. I love people, and I especially love helping sick and injured people regain their health. The long hours and hard work are all worth it when I see a child's face light up because they feel better, or a middle-aged person gets their diabetes under control, or an elderly person without hope finds out they can improve their health with a little work and discipline. I really love people and that is why I love my work.

And what is that work? Wrap it up in all the technical jargon you want, but I call it being a *facilitator of healing*. A facilitator is someone who makes something easier and hence more likely to happen. *I believe true healing comes from God, and all of us in the medical professions are helpers, or facilitators of healing.*

Do I mean healing in the revival tent sense of the word? No, although I do believe that miraculous healing does occur. *The goal of medical care is healing because of well-trained, loving, and supportive professionals working together.* Their job is to aid sick and injured human beings by finding what ails them and creating a medical plan that works. That diagnosis and therapeutic plan needs to be based on fact, not fiction; it must be based on scientific truth, not wishes or guesses.

Everything that is in this book is based squarely on fact. Why did I write it? I wrote this book for the same reason I go to work every day, and sometimes in the middle of the night: to help sick and injured people regain their health.

I challenge you, the reader, to consider these ideas the way I have. Many of these ideas are new; many of them are literally ancient. I believe all of them are useful.

Promoting health and preventing disease is the heartfelt desire of every patient, doctor, and health professional. *Self-Referral/Maximum Health* is the quest to find ways to help the body govern itself. Let us join together and find *Self-Referral/Maximum Health:* ***the goal of medicine*.**

Acknowledgements

I first acknowledge the role of Jesus Christ in my life. To me, Jesus is the Master Physician who dedicated his ministry to healing people on all levels. With his healing miracles, he restored blindness, deafness, paralysis, deformities - and even reversed death itself, bringing the dead back to life. Through his death and resurrection, he took healing to the next level: spiritually healing everyone and giving salvation through faith.

This focus on healing illustrates how central love and true forgiveness is to life. You cannot love someone and be indifferent to their suffering. There is one God with many people, many cultures, in many times learning from God and talking about God. We all find ourselves somewhere in the world's rich context of religious experience and traditions.

As a Christian, I believe that Jesus has a unique place in history as everyone's Lord and Savior. His teaching to love God above all else and for us to have unconditional love for each other is central to a successful life. Applying these values to my life and the practice of medicine is my major goal. I felt the presence of Jesus throughout the writing of this book. I could not have done this work without him.

I also must acknowledge Maharishi Mahesh Yogi for his genius, generosity, and infinite capacity for love. Many who are fortunate enough to have learned from this timeless master and sage have only a small inkling of the comprehensive nature of his knowledge. Everyone has their own view of Maharishi. Along with every other insight about him that I have gained, *I see him as the unacknowledged genius of our age.*

Maharishi had the vision and courage to leave India in 1958 to teach the knowledge of his master, Guru Dev, until Maharishi passed on in 2008. I have focused on his work pertaining to medicine, but Maharishi also applied his genius to many other fields. All his efforts worked toward the same end: to apply the real meaning of Vedic knowledge to all fields of human endeavor. His efforts gave great assistance to people working in fields as diverse as philosophy, architecture, medicine, politics, education, and world peace. Jai Guru Dev.

Many people in my life contributed to thinking that went into this book. My wife Bonnie and daughters Mary and Maggie helped me by being there and supporting me. My wife Bonnie was my rudder, keeping me on course, and not accepting anything without a good wrangle to sift the facts. Her ideas created many passages of this book. Greater love hath no wife and kids than to tolerate a budding author.

I thank my parents, Donald L. Borger and Dorothy M. Borger, for teaching me of God and good values and that any worthwhile project is worth seeing to completion. This book is testimony to that principle.

Special thanks go to my grandfather, Alfred R. Hinton, for a conversation we had during college days at Stow, Ohio. Encouraging words and love mean so much. Without his influence, my life's path would have been much different.

Very special thanks go to my uncles: Robert L. Hinton, DO and Donald R. Hinton, DO. These men have always been and always will be my personal heroes and mentors in medicine, business, and life. Without them, I would not be the professional that I am.

Academic acknowledgments include James R. Gillham, Ph.D. for great friendship and training in university level statistical research; John Ramey, M.S.W. for training in caring and social work; Bernard TeePoorten, DO, FAAO and J. Gordon Zink, DO, FAAO for training in Osteopathic Principles and Practice; Donald Surridge, DO, FAAO and Allen Becker, DO, FAAO for showing me what Manipulative Therapy can become.

Neil Boston is an artist, educator, musician, and a peerless deep thinker. He also has been one of my best friends in life. His support, encouragement, and urging me to move from thinking to doing helped me enormously. More than one of our discussions found their way into print here, in one form or another. I thank him for his friendship, support, and forbearance.

Special thanks go to author Richard Bach. His encouragement and open heart to an unknown writer stand as testimony to his belief in the potential of others. He helped this writer become an author. The book *Jonathan Livingston Seagull* had a wonderfully positive influence on me, as have his many books before and since. Truly, *Self-Referral/Maximum Health* illustrates something Jonathan Livingston Seagull taught his fellow gulls in that wonderful story:

> "Your whole body, from wingtip to wingtip," Jonathan would say, "is nothing more than your thought itself in a form you can see. Break the chains of your thought, and you break the chains of your body."

The chains of your thought are stress, and the chains of your body are disease. Now we know what to do and how to do it. We no longer have a need to stand there, scratching our heads, just wishing we had ways to understand Self-Referral and move toward Maximum Health. ***Go forth and suffer no more!***

Robert Keith Wallace, Ph.D. influenced me greatly. When I appeared unannounced on his doorstep in 1979, he was kind enough to listen to a young doctor searching for the basis of real healing. He also offered great encouragement from then until now. He continues to be a wonderful, helpful friend and resource in the work we share. Dr. Wallace is, to me, the best example I know of someone who has accomplished great things and yet remains humble, kind, and accessible to anyone. This is a great example that we all should emulate.

I want to acknowledge the great dedication and Herculean efforts of Dr. David Orme-Johnson for his ongoing research. He has consistently produced many powerful research projects validating TM through the years. He has also been a fearless defender of truth and a critical organizer of people and resources to the same end. Many findings in his research career were critical in making the case for *Self-Referral/Maximum Health* through this book.

I must thank Dr. Christopher Clark, formerly the Medical Director at The Raj Maharishi AyurVeda Medical Center at Fairfield, Iowa. Dr. Clark made it possible for me to reclaim my health at a critical time in my life. He also is a wonderful source of knowledge and the co-author with Dr. Hari Sharma of *Contemporary Ayurveda - Medicine and Research in Maharishi AyurVeda*. If Dr. Clark and a handful of other Western doctors had not stepped forward to embrace Maharishi

AyurVeda in the 1980s, this precious knowledge would not be available today.

I must thank Dr. Mark Toomey, a peerless expert in Maharishi AyurVeda. I have benefitted from his evaluation and treatment in more recent years at The Raj Maharishi AyurVeda Medical Center at Fairfield, Iowa. Dr. Toomey has the finest combination of love, care, concern, empathy, and wisdom with his patients – placing me at the top of that list. I am a healthier and better man thanks to Dr. Toomy's intervention.

I thank Dr. Robert E. Herron and his book *New Knowledge for New Results – A Comprehensive Strategy for Reducing Skyrocketing Medical Costs.* Dr. Herron has done a masterful job analyzing the economics of medical care and how we can make big improvements in both quality medical care and reducing the cost of medical care. Whenever I looked for answers in the economics of medical care, Dr. Herron's book was my go-to resource.

I thank Alvin Toffler for his brilliant insight, tireless research, and laser-like mind that gave him the ability to show us the truth. Reading his bestseller *Future Shock* in 1970 was foundational to putting me on the thinking and writing road. His keen mind and encyclopedic knowledge were a critical key to tying together stress, disease, and the causal factor of modern life. He was the truly original alarm bell ringer on what I call the Adaptation Crisis.

At about the time I read *Future Shock*, I became acquainted with the interviews, articles, and books of R. Buckminster Fuller. He was the overarching influence in my thinking on the themes that make up this book. His teaching on integrity, serving others, and comprehensive literacy guided me throughout my writing – and have been a great influence on my life as a physician and as a writer. Thank you, Bucky Fuller, for reaching out to me.

Dr. Andrew Taylor Still gave me through his writing the comprehensive knowledge and practical application of same that has made me an excellent Osteopathic physician for 42 years. My whole family originated in Kirksville – and I was born in Kirksville in 1951. This gave me a big edge when I read his books. For me, reading Still is like getting a heart-warming letter from home. Without Still and his wisdom, this knowledge would have been lost to the ages. I agree with Still, who wrote:

"The God that I worship demonstrates all His works."

No matter how hard we try, we can never remember everyone who helped us along the way. If you read this and you are only between the lines, I apologize. For all these people I have named, and so many more people that I have failed to mention but also helped me along, I express my heartfelt thanks.

Dr. Michael Borger

Nappanee, Indiana

November 24, 2023

Bibliography

Bach, Richard. ***Jonathan Livingston Seagull.*** The Macmillan Company. New York, 1970.

Barnett, Lincoln. ***The Universe and Dr. Einstein.*** William Morrow and Company. New York, 1948.

Bates, Marston. ***Man in Nature.*** Prentice-Hall, Inc. Eaglewood Cliffs, New Jersey, 1964.

Benson, Herbert. ***The Relaxation Response.*** Avon Books. New York, 1976.

Bhishagratna, Kaviraj Kunjalal (Translator and Commentator). ***Sushruta Samhita.*** Volume I. *Uttara-Tantra.* Volume II. *Nidana-Sthan; Sariri-Sthana; Chikitsta-Thana; Kalpa-Sthana.* Volume III. Uttara-Tantra. Chowkhamba Sanskrit Series Office. Varanasi, India, 1981.

Bloomfield, Harold H.; Cain, Michael Peter; Jaffe, Dennis T. TM: ***Discovering Inner Energy and Overcoming Stress.*** Delacorte Press. New York, 1975.

Bourdillon, J. F. ***Spinal Manipulation.*** William Heinemann Medical Books Limited. London, 1973.

Branigan, K. ***The Atlas of Archaeology***. St. Martin's Press. New York, 1982.

Bremmer, J. Douglas. ***Does Stress Damage the Brain*?** W. W. Norton & Company. New York, 2002.

Brena, Steven F. ***Yoga and Medicine.*** Penguin Books, Inc. New York, 1972.

Brosse, Therese. ***Etude Instrumentale des Techniques du Yoga.*** Paris, 1963.

Campbell, Joseph. ***The Hero With a Thousand Faces.*** Bollington Series XVII. Princeton University Press. Princeton, 1973.

Campbell, Joseph; with Moyers, Bill. ***The Power of Myth.*** Doubleday. New York, 1988.

Cannon, W. B. ***The Wisdom of the Body.*** Norton. New York, 1932.

Capra, Fritjof. ***The Tao of Physics.*** Shamballa Publications, Inc. Boston, 1976.

Conn, Howard F. (Editor). ***Current Therapy.*** W. B. Saunders Company. Philadelphia, 1983.

Clark, Christopher; Sharma, Hari; ***Contemporary Ayurveda. Medicine and Research in Maharishi AyurVeda.*** Churchill Livingstone. Division of Harcourt Brace & Company. Philadelphia, 1998.

Clark, Ronald G: ***Manter and Gantz's Clinical Neuroanatomy*** *and Neurophysiology*. Fifth Edition. F. A. Davis Company. Philadelphia, 1978.

Rakel, Robert E. and Bope, Edward T. (Editors). ***Conn's Current Therapy 2007.*** Saunders Elsevier. Philadelphia, 2007.

Covey, Stephen. ***The 7 Habits of Highly Effective People.*** Simon and Shuster. New York, 1989.

Darwin, Bernard (Editor.) ***The Oxford Dictionary of Quotations.*** Oxford Press. New York, 1980.

Dennett, D. C. "Consciousness" in Gregory, Richard L. ***The Oxford Companion to The Mind.*** Oxford University Press. New York, 1987.

Dintenfass, Julius. ***Chiropractic - A Modern Way to Health.*** Pyramid Books. New York, 1970.

Dossey, Larry. ***Healing Words.*** HarperCollins Publishers. San Francisco, 1993.

Einstein, Albert; Infeld, Leopold. ***The Evolution of Physics.*** New York, Simon and Schuster, 1938.

Einstein, Albert; Lawson, Robert W. (Translation.) ***Relativity. The Special and the General Theory.*** Crown Publishers, Inc. New York, 1961.

Einstein, Albert. ***Relativity: The Special and the General Theory.*** Crown Publishers. New York, 1952. Originally published as formal journal publications in 1916.

Eliot, Robert S.; Breo, Dennis L. Is ***It Worth Dying For? A Self-Assessment Program to Make Stress Work For You, Not Against You.*** Bantam Books, Inc. New York, 1984.

Elzenberg, Norman. ***General Anatomy: Principles and Applications.*** McGraw-Hill Medical; 2nd edition. New York, 2007

Evans-Wentz, W. Y. ***Tibetan Yoga and Secret Doctrines.*** Oxford University Press. London, 1935.

Fleming, A. (Editor). ***Penicillin: Its Practical Application.*** The Blakiston Company. Philadelphia, 1946.

Forem, Jack. ***Transcendental Meditation.*** E. P. Dutton & Company, Inc. New York, 1973.

Fowler, N. O. ***Cardiac Diagnosis and Treatment.*** Third Edition. Harper & Rowe. Hagerstown, 1980.

Frawley, David. ***Ayurvedic Healing. A Comprehensive Guide.*** Passage Press. Salt Lake City, 1989.

Fuller, R. Buckminster. ***I Seem to Be a Verb.*** Bantam Books. New York, 1970.

Fuller, R. Buckminster: ***Inventions. The Patented Works of R. Buckminster Fuller.*** St Martin's Press. New York, 1983.

Fuller, R. Buckminster: ***Operating Manual for Spaceship Earth.*** E. P. Dutton. New York, 1963.

Ganong, W. F. ***Review of Medical Physiology.*** Sixth Edition. Lange Medical Publications. Los Altos, 1973

Gatterman, Meridel I. ***Foundations of Chiropractic – Subluxations.*** Mosby Yearbook. St. Louis, 1995.

Gevintz, Norman. ***The D.O.'s - Osteopathic Medicine in America.*** The Johns Hopkins University Press. Baltimore, 1982.

Gray, Henry; Goss, Charles Mayo (Editor). ***Anatomy of the Human Body.*** Lea & Feiber. Philadelphia, 1975. Pp. 527-560.

Greenman, Philip E. ***Principles of Manual Medicine.*** Williams & Wilkins. Baltimore, 1989.

Grene, Marjorie G. ***A Portrait of Aristotle.*** University of Chicago Press. Chicago, 1979

Grun, Bernard; Stein, Werner. ***The Timetables of History.*** Simon and Schuster, Inc. New York, 1979.

Guyton, Arthur C. ***Textbook of Medical Physiology.*** Fourth Edition. W. B. Saunders Company. Philadelphia, 1971

Harvey, A. McGehee (Editor); Johns, Richard J. (Editor); McKusick, Victor A. (Editor); Owens, Albert H. (Editor); Ross, Richard S. (Editor.) ***The Principles and Practice of Medicine.*** Twenty-second Edition. Appleton & Lange, Publishers. Norwalk, Connecticut, 1988.

Herron, Robert E. ***New Knowledge for New Results – A Comprehensive Strategy for Reducing Skyrocketing Medical Costs.*** 1st World Publishing. Fairfield, Iowa, 2008.

Horowitz, M. J. ***Stress Response Syndromes***. Aronson. New York, 1976.

Huang-ti. ***Huang-ti Nei-Ching Su-wen*** **(Basic Questions from The Classic Book of Internal Medicine).** Commercial Press. Shanghai, China, 1955.

Hubel, David H. "The Brain". *The Brain.* A Scientific American Book. W. H. Freeman and Company. New York, 1979.

Judovich, B.; Bates, W. ***Pain Syndromes.*** Fourth Edition. F.A. Davis Company. Philadelphia, 1953.

Julian, D. G. (Editor); Matthews, M. B. ***Angina Pectoris***. Churchill Livingstone. Edinburgh, 1977.

Kaku, Michio. ***Hyperspace.*** Oxford University Press. New York, 1994.

Kroll, Una. ***The Healing Potential of Transcendental Meditation.*** John Knox Press. Atlanta, 1974

Kuhn, Thomas. ***The Structure of Scientific Revolutions.*** Second Edition. University of Chicago Press. Chicago, 1970.

Lamb, Beatrice Pitney. ***India: A World in Transition.*** Praeger Publishers. New York, 1971.

Lao-Tzu; Mitchell, Stephen (Translation and Commentary). ***Tao Te Ching.*** Harper and Row, Publishers, Inc. New York, 1988.

Magoun, Harold Ives. ***Osteopathy in the Cranial Field.*** Third Edition. The Journal Printing Company. Kirksville, Missouri, 1976.

Maharishi Mahesh Yogi. ***The Bhagavad Gita: Chapters 1 - 6. A New Translation and Commentary.*** MIU Press. Fairfield, Iowa, 1979.

Maharishi Mahesh Yogi. ***Dawn of the Age of Enlightenment. Volume One 1957-1964: Thirty Years Around the World.*** Maharishi Vedic University Press. The Netherlands, 1986.

Maharishi Mahesh Yogi. ***Meditations of Maharishi Mahesh Yogi.*** Bantam Books. New York, 1968.

Maharishi Mahesh Yogi. ***Science of Being and Art of Living.*** MIU Press. Fairfield, Iowa, 1979.

Maimonides. ***The Preservation of Youth and Other Essays.*** Philosophical Library. New York, 1958.

Mascaro, Juan (Translation). ***The Bhagavad Gita.*** Penguin Books. Baltimore, 1971.

McWilliams, Peter. ***The TM Book - How to Enjoy the Rest of Your Life.*** Warner Books. New York, 1975.

Moyers, Bill. ***Healing and the Mind.*** Doubleday Publishing. New York, 1993.

Musashi, Miyamoto; Harris, Victor (Translation and Commentary): ***A Book of Five Rings.*** The Overlook Press. Woodstock, New York, 1974.

Northup, George W.: ***Osteopathic Medicine: An American Reformation.*** American Osteopathic Association. Chicago, Illinois, 1966.

Norton, Peter. Disk Explorer. ***Manual for The Norton Utilities.*** Version 6.1. Symantec Corporation. Cupertino, California, 1991.

Noss, John B. ***Man's Religions.*** The MacMillon Company, Inc. New York, 1949.

Oates, Jr., Robert M. ***Celebrating the Dawn.*** G. P. Putnam's Sons. New York, 1976.

Orme-Johnson, David W. (Editor); Farrow, John T. (Editor.) ***Scientific Research on the Transcendental Meditation Program: Collected Papers.*** **Volume I.** Maharishi European University Press. Livingston Manor, 1977.

Ornish, Dean. ***Dr. Dean Ornish's Program for Reversing Heart Disease.*** Ballentine Books. New York, 1990.

Paul, John. R. ***Yale Studies in the History of Science and Medicine.*** New Haven, Connecticut, 1971.

Patanjali, Maharishi; Pravananda, Swami (Translation and Commentary); Isherwood, Christopher (Translation and Commentary.) ***How To Know God: The Yoga Aphorisms of Patanjali.*** New American Library. New York, 1969.

Purves, Dale. ***Body and Brain.*** Harvard University Press. Cambridge, Massachusetts, 1988.

Rakel, Robert E. and Bope, Edward T. (Editors). ***Conn's Current Therapy 2007.*** Saunders Elsevier. Philadelphia, 2007.

Reith, Edward J.; Ross, Michael H. ***Atlas of Descriptive Histology.*** Second Edition. Harper & Row, Publishers. New York, 1970.

Restak, Richard. ***The Brain.*** Bantam Books. New York, 1984.

Robbins, Stanley L.: ***Pathologic Basis of Disease.*** W. B. Saunders Company. Philadelphia, 1974.

Romer, Alfred Sherwood. ***The Vertebrate Body. Shorter Version.*** Fourth Edition. W. B. Saunders Company. Philadelphia, 1971.

Rose, Kenneth Jon. ***The Body in Time.*** John Wiley & Sons, Inc. New York, 1988.

Rosen, Hugo. ***A Clinician's Guide to Affective Disorders.*** Second Edition. Mnemosyne Publishing Company. Miami, 1981.

Rosenthal, Norman E. Transcendence – ***Healing and Transformation Through Transcendental Meditation.*** The Penguin Group - Jeremy P. Tarcher/Penguin. New York, 2011.

Roth, Robert. ***Maharishi Mahesh Yogi's TM: Transcendental Meditation.*** Donald I. Fine, Inc. New York, 1987.

Sagan, Carl. ***Broca's Brain.*** Random House. New York, 1979.

Schmidt, Robert F. (Editor). ***Fundamentals of Neurophysiology.*** Springer Verlag. New York, 1978.

Schrödinger, Edwin. ***Science and Humanism.*** Cambridge University Press. Cambridge, England, 1951.

Schwarzenegger, Arnold; Bobbins, Bill. ***The New Encyclopedia of Modern Bodybuilding***. Fireside Books Simon & Shuster. New York, 1998.

Selye, Hans. ***The Stress of Life.*** Revised Edition. McGraw-Hill Book Company. New York, 1976.

Selye, Hans. ***Stress Without Distress.*** Lippincott. Philadelphia, 1974.

Sharma, Hari. ***Freedom from Disease.*** Veda Publishing Toronto, 1993.

Sharma, Ram Karan; Dash, Vaidya Bhagwan. (Translation and Commentary.) Agnivesa's ***Caraka Samhita.*** Based on Cakrapani Datta's Ayurveda Dipika. Volume I. Sutra Sthana. Volume II. Nidanasthana; Vimanasthana; Sarira Sthana; Indriyasthan. Chowkhamba Sanskrit Series Office. Varanasi, India, 1976.

Shearer, Alistair; Russell, Peter (Translation and Commentary). ***The Upanishads.*** Harper Colophon Books. Harper & Row, Publishers. New York, 1978.

Smolan, Rick; Moffitt, Phillip; Naythons, Matthew. ***The Power to Heal.*** **Ancient Arts & Modern Medicine.** Prentice Hall Press. New York, 1990.

Snell, Richard S. ***Clinical Embryology for Medical Students***. Little, Brown and Company. Boston, 1972.

Still, Andrew Taylor. ***Autobiography of A. T. Still.*** Published by the Author. Kirksville, Missouri, 1897.

Still, Andrew T.: ***Philosophical and Mechanical Principles of Osteopathy.*** Hudson-Kimberly Publishing Company. Kansas City, 1902.

Still, A. T. ***Philosophy of Osteopathy.*** Published by A. T. Still. Kirksville, Missouri, 1899.

Sun Tzu; Cleary, Thomas (Translation and Commentary): ***The Art of War.*** Shamballa Publications, Inc. Boston, 1988.

Sutherland, Adah Strand. ***With Thinking Fingers****: The Story Of William Garner Sutherland, D.O., D.Sc. (Hon.)*. The Cranial Academy. Kansas City, Missouri, 1962.

Sutherland, William G. ***The Cranial Bowl****: A Treatise Relating To Cranial Articular Mobility, Cranial Articular Lesions, and Cranial Technic*. Free Press Company. Mankato, Minnesota, 1939.

Thoreau, Henry David. ***Walden.*** Bramhall House. New York, 1951.

Thorne, Kip S. ***Black Holes & Time Warps.*** Einstein's Outrageous Legacy. W. W. Norton & Company. New York, 1994.

Thorpe, Robert G. ***Clinical Review Series. Osteopathic Medicine.*** Publishing Sciences Group, Inc. Acton, Massachusetts, 1975.

Toffler, Alvin. ***Future Shock.*** Random House. New York, 1970.

Treadway, Scott; Treadway, Linda. ***Ayurveda & Immortality.*** Celestial Arts. Berkeley, 1986.

Versalius, Andreas. ***On the Fabric of the Human Body.*** Milan, Italy, 1543.

Wallace, Robert Keith. ***The Maharishi Technology of the Unified Field: The Neurophysiology of Enlightenment.*** MIU Neuroscience Press. Maharishi International University, Fairfield, Iowa, 1986.

Wallace, Robert Keith. ***The Physiology of Consciousness.*** MIU Press. Fairfield, Iowa, 1993.

Wallace, Robert Keith; Marcus, Jay B.; Clark, Christopher S. ***The Coherence Effect.*** Armin Lear Press. Estes Park, Colorado, 2020.

Wenger, M. A.; Jones, F. N.; Jones, M. H. ***Physiological Psychology.*** Henry Holt and Company. New York, 1956.

White, Abraham; Handler, Philip; Smith, Emil l. ***Principles Of Biochemistry.*** Fifth Edition. McGraw-Hill Book Company. New York, 1973. P. 2 and P. 252.

Wiener, Norbert. ***Cybernetics.*** Freymann. Paris and New York, 1948.

Wintrobe, Maxwell M.; Thorn, George W.; Adams, Raymond D.; Braunwald, Eugene; Isselbach, Kurt J.; Petersdorf, Robert G. ***Harrison's Principles of Internal Medicine.*** Seventh Edition. McGraw-Hill Book Company. New York, 1974.

Woram, John. ***The PC Configuration Handbook.*** Bantam Books. New York, 1990.

Zukov, Gary. ***The Dancing Wu Li Masters.*** William Morrow & Company. New York, 1979.

Index
Alphabetical by Name or Topic

A

B

C

D

G

H

I

J

K

L

M

N

O

P

Q

R

S

T

U

V

W

X

Y

Z

Appendix A

The Comprehensive Theory of Health and Disease

What became the book *Self-Referral/Maximum Health* began as a scientific theory based on ideas illustrated through mathematics. In 1976 I was still in medical school and doing my best to learn what I now understand as *Self-Referral* – the human body's ability to create and sustain health. I reasoned that the human body was able to sustain perfect health, but that something was causing things to go wrong and create disease instead of health.

As I learned all the physiology that lies behind body operations, it became obvious to me that stress was the culprit disrupting health. This is how I learned how stress disrupts Self-Referral. Osteopathic knowledge taught me the rest. Putting this into an equation, stress translates into abnormal Self-Referral as follows:

<u>The Sum Total of the Stress of Life</u>

We assume the following:

Total Mental Stress + Total Physical Stress = Stress of Life

$$\frac{\text{Stress of Life}}{\text{Abnormal Brain Function}} \times \frac{\text{Abnormal Brain Function}}{\text{Somatic Dysfunction}} \times \frac{\text{Somatic Dysfunction}}{\text{Segmental Disruption}} \times \frac{\text{Segmental Disruption}}{\text{Self-Referral Disruption}} \times \frac{\text{Self-Referral Disruption}}{\text{Abnormal Self-Referral}}$$

<u>Key Assumptions for Equation to Work:</u>

Each term is in a causal relationship with the inverse term. That is: Stress of Life CAUSES Abnormal Brain Function. That is true for each fraction depicted. The fractions are set to cross multiply. The equivalences of the terms translate across the equation from left to right through cancellation. Each of the terms must be weighted using a similar scale, say "rated 1 = None, 10 = Maximum," etc. This equation will prove that the Stress of Life causes Abnormal Self-Referral = Disease.

Comprehensive Theory of Health and Disease: Integrating All Relevant Factors as an Equation:

With the previous equation and assumptions, it is possible to integrate more precise terminology and more complete factors. The Osteopathic concepts of Somatic Dysfunction and Segmental Disruption are critical to the equation.

Abnormal Brain Function as a response to the Stress of Life creates chaotic nerve impulses that cause tight muscles around the spinal cord, the cranium, and nerves throughout the body. Because the nervous system is organized by spinal segments, chaotic nerve impulses follow the segmental spinal pathways – although they may be distributed by the Cranial Nerves as well. Chaotic nerve operation creates Segmental Disruption. This in turn disrupts feedback from body to brain and brain to body – disrupting Self-Referral throughout the whole body. This process creates Disease instead of Health.

Summary Equation of Stress as the Basis of Disease

$$\frac{\text{Stress of Life}}{\text{Abnormal Brain Function}} \times \frac{\text{Abnormal Brain Function}}{\text{Somatic Dysfunction}} \times \frac{\text{Somatic Dysfunction}}{\text{Segmental Disruption}} \times \frac{\text{Segmental Disruption}}{\text{Abnormal Self-Referral}} \times \frac{\text{Abnormal Self-Referral}}{\text{Creates Disease}}$$

Abnormal Self-Referral Translates into Disease

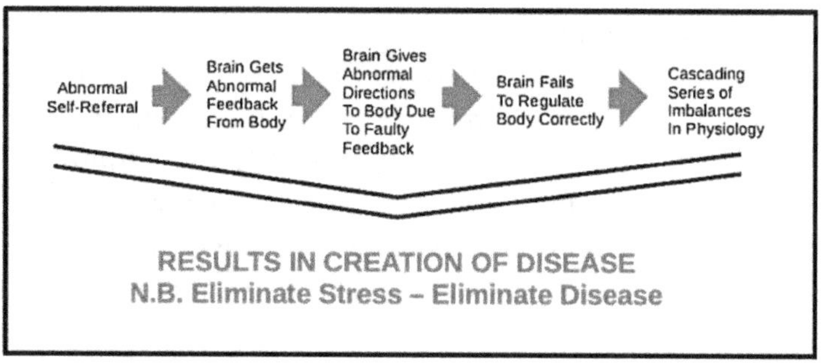

Q.E.D.

About the Author

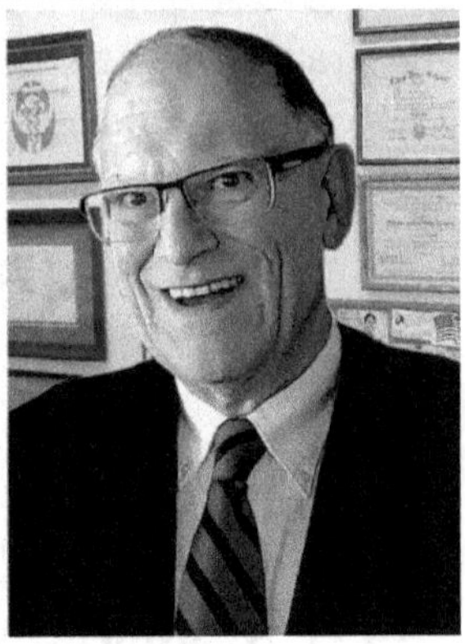

Dr. Michael Borger was born in Kirksville, Missouri – the birthplace of Osteopathic Medicine. His family moved to Cleveland, Ohio when he was two years old, and he grew up in the Cleveland-Akron area of Ohio. A keen interest was music. He studied Hammond organ, sang in a Capella choir, and often played organ in church. He led many jazz and rock bands in the Akron area during his junior and senior high school and college years.

Dr Borger attended the University of Akron, receiving a Bachelor of Arts degree in Sociology with a Certificate in Social Work while taking all the science courses needed to be accepted at Medical School. While studying at university, Dr. Borger had broad experience providing one-on-one counseling at a Methadone Clinic treating heroin addicts. During this period, he also extensively studied empirical research methods and helped design non-recursive multiple regression research projects.

Dr. Borger was accepted at Des Moines University College of Osteopathic Medicine and Surgery, completing his degree work and graduating in 1977. He received the Doctor of Osteopathy degree and was awarded a Special Certificate of Achievement in Osteopathic Manipulative Therapy. He then completed hospital training at South Bend, Indiana and entered Family Practice at Nappanee, Indiana. He was Board Certified in Family Practice and Osteopathic Manipulative Therapy by the American College of Osteopathic Family Physicians.

He practiced medicine at Northwood Family Medicine from 1978 to 2019. Dr. Borger was one of the original members of the Board of Advisors for the Still National Osteopathic Museum at Kirksville, Missouri 1979-1980. Dr. Borger served as City Medical Director, Nappanee Emergency Medical Services from 1980 to 1985. He was recipient of the Physician of the Year Award from the Indiana Association of Emergency Medical Technicians in 1981.

Dr. Borger's practice consisted of Family Practice all ages, Industrial Medicine and Emergency Room, Osteopathic Manipulative Therapy, and Health Promotion. During his years in practice, Dr. Borger served as Clinical Assistant Professor of Family Practice at multiple Colleges of Osteopathic Medicine. During his long career he taught clinical skills to scores of senior medical students from Kirksville College of Osteopathic Medicine, Kansas City College of Osteopathic Medicine, Des Moines College of Osteopathic Medicine, and Pikeville College of Osteopathic Medicine.

Dr. Michael Borger retired from active practice in 2019 and now serves as an author, teacher, and lecturer in great demand.

Dr. Michael Borger married his wife Bonnie in 1978. They have enjoyed 46 years of marriage so far and cherish every day together. They raised two daughters, Mary and Maggie, who are married, and each have two grandchildren with their wonderful husbands. The Borgers have a passion for working out, good music, exotic cooking, and do their best on foot to keep up with their Australian Cattle Dogs: Adelaide and Brisbane. Dr. Borger continues to play piano at church and works on music projects using piano, organ, synthesizer, computers, and Native American flute.

Dr. Michael Borger now is traveling widely to lecture and teach the principles of Self-Referral Medicine. He is open for contact to arrange lectures and teaching events. He looks forward to working with future Self-Referral research projects, leading the Self-Referral Medicine Group, and writing future books and instruction manuals.

Contact Information:

Dr. Michael Borger

353 North Hartman Street

Nappanee, Indiana 46550

Email: Dr.Michael.Borger@gmail.com

End Notes Section

I am determined that anyone who wants to can go to the sources that I collated through the years. I am certain that you will come to the same conclusions, as delineated throughout the book and especially in Appendix A: The Comprehensive Theory of Health and Disease. Good hunting! – Dr. Michael Borger

---

End Notes Introduction:

[1] Architect-Inventor-Polymath-Philosopher R. Buckminster Fuller. Fuller argued for comprehensive literacy: a completely thorough, broad-based knowledge of any subject – and all related subjects – to understand anything.

[2] Kipling, Rudyard; in the poem "The Ballad of East and West"; quoted in *The Oxford Dictionary of Quotations*. Third Edition. Oxford University Press. New York, 1980. P. 297.

[3] Michael H. I. Borger, D.O. practiced medicine in Nappanee, Indiana at Northwood Physicians, Inc. 1978 to 2014 and at Northwood Family Medicine and MedStat of KMG Health Physicians – Lutheran Health Network 2014 to 2019. This has all been at the same address: 1001 North Main Street- Suite One – Nappanee, Indiana 46550. Dr. Borger also worked at North Webster Medical Clinic in North Webster, Indiana 2015 to 2019.

[4] Dr. Michael Borger served as City Medical Director, Nappanee Emergency Medical Services - position created and appointed by Mayor and approved by City Council, 1980-1985. Dr. Borger was instrumental in working with the State of Indiana and local EMS units establishing Advanced Life Support services for the city of Nappanee and for many other small towns across the state of Indiana during those years.

[5] While practicing medicine as a Board-Certified Family Practice Physician 1978-2019, Dr. Michael Borger served as Assistant Clinical Professor of General Practice, Kirksville College of Osteopathic Medicine at Kirksville, Missouri; Assistant Professor of Clinical Medicine, University of Health Sciences, College of Osteopathic Medicine at Kansas City, Missouri; Assistant Professor of Family Practice, Pikeville College School of Osteopathic Medicine at Pikeville, Kentucky; and Assistant Professor of Clinical Osteopathic Manipulative Medicine, Pikeville College School of Osteopathic Medicine.

[6] *Merriam-Webster Pocket Dictionary*. Pocket Books. New York, 1974.

[7] Interestingly enough, Dr. Michael Borger was born in Kirksville, Missouri.

[8] Northup, George W.: *Osteopathic Medicine: An American Reformation.* American Osteopathic Association. Chicago, Illinois, 1966. Pp. 1-18.

[9] D.O. – Doctor of Osteopathy - is one of only two academic degrees one can receive in the United States to obtain the license for the unlimited practice of medicine. The other degree, of course, is the more familiar MD or Medical Doctor. You will find more information about Osteopathic Medicine later in this book.

[10] Fuller, R. Buckminster: *Inventions. The Patented Works of R. Buckminster Fuller.* St Martin's Press. New York, 1983. Pp.vii-xxxii.

[11] Fuller, R. Buckminster: *Operating Manual for Spaceship Earth.* E. P. Dutton. New York, 1963. Pp. 12-14.

<u>End Notes Chapter 1:</u>

[12] Carl Schurz, from a Graduation Address - Faneuil Hall in Boston, Massachusetts on April 18, 1859.

[13] Paraphrased from Matthew 7:12. *King James Bible.* American Bible Society. The World Publishing Company. Cleveland, Ohio, 1958. New Testament P. 7

[14] Paraphrased from Matthew 7:12. *The Holy Bible.* Zondervan Publishing House. Grand Rapids, Michigan, 1995. P. 1449.

[15] My late uncles are Robert L. Hinton, D.O. and Donald R. Hinton, D.O. Both men were Osteopathic physicians who I looked up to all my life. They were General Practitioners and were great men and heroes to me - I love and admire them both greatly. Donald R. Hinton, D.O. practiced family medicine in Nappanee, Indiana from 1951 until 1991 and was my mentor in medicine; he passed on in 1996. Robert L. Hinton, D.O. practiced family medicine in the Seattle, Washington area from 1964 to 2012 and passed on in 2018. He played a vital role with my Grandad Alfred R. Hinton as one of my "Dads" when my father passed on when I turned seven.

[16] Smolan, Rick; Moffitt, Phillip; Naythons, Matthew. *The Power to Heal.* Ancient Arts & Modern Medicine. Prentice Hall Press. New York, 1990.

[17] Fuller, R. Buckminster; Farrell, Barry (Interviewer): "The Playboy Interview - R. Buckminster Fuller." *Playboy Magazine*. January, 1971. Pp. 59-70 and 194-204.

[18] Broder, Samuel. "Beating the AIDS Epidemic." *OMNI Magazine*. December, 1990. P. 8.

[19] Zukov, Gary. *The Dancing Wu Li Masters.* William Morrow & Company. New York, 1979.

[20] Schrödinger, Edwin. *Science and Humanism.* Cambridge University Press. Cambridge, England, 1951. Pp. 7-8.

[21] Einstein, Albert; Infeld, Leopold. *The Evolution of Physics*. New York, Simon and Schuster, 1938. P. 27.

[22] *Encarta Dictionary*. Microsoft Software. Bellevue, Washington, 2005. On CD-ROM.

[23] Kuhn, Thomas. "The Structure of Scientific Revolutions," from *The Structure of Scientific Revolutions*. Second Edition. University of Chicago Press. Chicago, 1970.

[24] Ibid.

[25] Murray, Thomas J. "The New Wizard of Corporate Culture." *Dun's Business Month*. July, 1986. Pp. 3-7.

[26] Covey, Stephen. *The 7 Habits of Highly Effective People*. Simon and Shuster. New York, 1989. P. 30.

[27] Ibid., P. 32.

[28] Miyamoto Musashi; Harris, Victor (Translation and Commentary): *A Book of Five Rings*. The Overlook Press. Woodstock, New York, 1974.

[29] The computer game *The Ancient Art of War* was designed by Dave and Barry Murry, developed by Evryware, and published by Brøderbund in 1984. The game used the principles of Sun Tzu as taught in *The Ancient Art of War*. This computer game is now generally recognized as one of the first real-time strategy games. The game was later extended by the authors to a second game called The Ancient Art of War at Sea, also published by Broderbund Software. Who says these ideas can't be fun?

[30] Sun Tzu; Cleary, Thomas (Translation and Commentary): *The Art of War*. Shamballa Publications, Inc. Boston, 1988. Pp. 1-38.

[31] Ibid.

End Notes Chapter 2:

[32] Domagk, G. "Ein Beitrag zur Chemotherapie der Bekteriellen Infektionen". *German Medical Research* 61:250, 1935.

[33] Fleming, A. (Editor). *Penicillin: Its Practical Application*. The Blakiston Company. Philadelphia, 1946.

[34] Cutler, Anne G. (Editor). *Stedman's Medical Dictionary*. The Williams & Wilkins Company. Baltimore, 1972. P. 929.

[35] Ibid.

[36] Ibid. P. 719.

[37] From Psalm 139:14. *The Holy Bible*. New International Version. Zondervan. Grand Rapids, Michigan, 1995.

[38] Lao-Tzu; Mitchell, Stephen (Translation and Commentary). *Tao Te Ching*. Harper and Row, Publishers, Inc. New York, 1988. Pp. vii-viii.

[39] Ibid.

[40] Fuller, R. Buckminster. *I Seem To Be a Verb*. Bantam Books. New York, 1970.

[41] Ibid.

[42] Original story by Dr. Michael Borger.

[43] Versalius, Andreas. *On the Fabric of the Human Body*. Milan, Italy, 1543.

[44] Today, of course, all these big textbooks are available on computer programs via online versions, and even apps for your smart phone. No matter how you access the information, the material is still immense!

[45] Lao-Tzu; Mitchell, Stephen. *Tao Te Ching*. Harper & Row, Publishers, Inc. New York, 1988. P. 14.

[46] Paraphrased from 1 Corinthians 12:12-20. *The Holy Bible*. New International Version. Zondervan. Grand Rapids, Michigan, 1995.

[47] Freymann, John Gordon. "The Odyssey and Outlook of Graduate Medical Education." *Journal of the American Osteopathic Association* 89(6):761-767, 1989.

[48] Hoffman, Mark S. (Editor). "Population Projections, by Region and for Selected Counties: 1990 to 2025." *The World Almanac and Book of Facts 1988*. Newspaper Enterprise Association, Inc. Pharos Books. New York, 1988. Pp. 738-739.

[49] Staff Writer. "Doctors See 3 Million Patients Every Day." *Private Practice* 20(4):3, 1988.

End Notes Chapter 3:

[50] Sun Tzu; Cleary, Thomas (Translation and Commentary). *The Art of War*. Shambala Publications, Inc. Boston, 1988. P. 1.

[51] Many of today's doctors carry a version of the *PDR* on a hand-held device and refer to it as they work with patients. I like this on my smart phone because it is totally portable - and looking things up fast is a snap!

[52] Medical Economics Company. *Physicians' Desk Reference*. Forty-fourth Edition. Medical Economics Company. Oradell, New Jersey, 1990.

[53] Lazarou J; Pomeranz B H; Corey P N. "Incidence of Adverse Drug Reactions in Hospitalized Patients: A Meta-Analysis of Prospective Studies." *Journal of the American Medical Association* 279(15):1200-1205, 1998.

[54] Shute, Nancy. "On Health. Prescribed Killers." *U.S. News & World Report*. April 27, 1998. Page 71.

[55] Ibid.

[56] Ibid.

[57] Ivey, Kevin J. "Mechanisms of Nonsteroidal Anti-Inflammatory Drug-Induced Gastric Damage." *The American Journal of Medicine* 84(2a):41-48, 1988.

[58] MacDonald, W.; Owen, J. W. "The Effect of Total Hip Replacement on Driving Reactions." *Journal of Bone and Joint Surgery British* 70(2):202-205, 1988.

[59] Lafavore, Michael. "The Good, the Bad, and the Just Plain Weird." *Men's Health*. February 1992. P. 52.

[60] Sun Tzu; Cleary, Thomas Op. Cit... P. 1.

[61] Ibid.

[62] Wintrobe, Maxwell M.; Thorn, George W.; Adams, Raymond D.; Braunwald, Eugene; Isselbach, Kurt J.; Petersdorf, Robert G. *Harrison's Principles of Internal Medicine*. Seventh Edition. McGraw-Hill Book Company. New York, 1974. P. 2.

[63] Sun Tzu; Cleary, Thomas. Op. Cit.. Pp. 1-5.

[64] Robbins, Stanley L.: *Pathologic Basis of Disease*. W. B. Saunders Company. Philadelphia, 1974. Pp. 314-355.

[65] Cannon, W. B. *The Wisdom of the Body*. Norton, New York, 1932.

[66] Ibid.

[67] *Stedman's Medical Dictionary*. Twenty-second Edition. The Williams & Wilkins Company. Baltimore, 1972. P. 583.

[68] Guyton, Arthur C. *Textbook of Medical Physiology*. Fourth Edition. W. B. Saunders Company. Philadelphia, 1971: P. 3.

[69] Ganong, W. F. *Review of Medical Physiology*. Sixth Edition. Lange Medical Publications. Los Altos, 1973: P. 16.

[70] Wiener, Norbert. *Cybernetics*. Freymann. Paris and New York, 1948.

[71] Ibid.

[72] Ibid.

[73] Ibid.

[74] Guyton, Arthur C. Op. Cit. P. 6.

[75] Ibid., P. 8.

[76] Ibid., P. 11.

[77] Ganong, W. F. Op. Cit. Pp. 146-172.

[78] Ibid.

[79] Ibid., P. 18.

[80] Ibid.

[81] Restak, Richard. *The Brain*. Bantam Books. New York, 1984: Pp. 1-5.

[82] Lao-Tzu; Mitchell, Stephen (Translation and Commentary). *Tao te Ching*. Harper & Row Publishers, Inc. New York, 1988. P. 37.

[83] Ganong, W. F. Op. Cit. Pp. 83-99.

[84] Ibid.

End Notes Chapter 4:

[85] Paulsen, Barbara; Ma, Lora Elise. "Work and Play: A Nation Out of Balance." *Hippocrates Magazine*. October 1994. Pp. 30-32.

[86] Ibid.

[87] Ibid.

[88] Selye, Hans. *The Stress of Life*. Revised Edition. McGraw-Hill Book Company. New York, 1976. P. xi.

[89] Ibid., Pp. xvi-xvii.

[90] Ibid., Pp. 97-127.

[91] Ibid.

[92] Toffler, Alvin. *Future Shock*. Random House. New York, 1970. Pp. 323-365.

[93] Ibid., P. 328-329.

[94] Ibid.

[95] Holmes, Thomas H.; Rahe, Richard H. "The Social Readjustment Rating Scale." *Journal of Psychosomatic Medicine* 11:213-218, 1967.

[96] Holmes and Rahe, Op. Cit..

[97] Toffler, Op. Cit.., P. 329-330.

[98] Holmes and Rahe, Op. Cit..

[99] Selye, Op. Cit.., P. 74.

[100] Ibid.

[101] Ibid., P. xii.

[102] Lao-Tzu; Mitchell, Stephen. *Tao Te Ching*. Harper & Row, Publishers, Inc. New York, 1988. P. 14.

[103] Fox, Caroline S.; Evans, Jane C.; Larson, Martin G.; Levy, Daniel. "Temporal Trends in Coronary Heart Disease Mortality and Sudden Cardiac Death from 1955 to 1999." *Circulation* 110:522-526, 2004.

[104] *Maimonides. The Preservation of Youth and Other Essays*. Philosophical Library. New York, 1958. Pp. 35-50.

[105] Julian, D. G. (Editor); Matthews, M. B. "Historical Background". *Angina Pectoris*. Churchill Livingstone. Edinburgh, 1977.

[106] Ibid.

[107] Fowler, N. O. *Cardiac Diagnosis and Treatment*. Third Edition. Harper & Rowe. Hagerstown, 1980.

[108] Julian, D. G., Op. Cit.

[109] Ibid.

[110] Kowal, S. J. "Emotions of Angina Pectoris: An Historical Review." *American Journal of Cardiology* 5:421, 1960.

[111] Eliot, Robert S.; Buell, James C. "The Role of the CNS in Cardiovascular Disorders." *Hospital Practice*. 18(5):189-199, 1983.

[112] Sinatra, Stephen T. "Stress: A Cardiologist's Point of View." *Postgraduate Medicine* 76(1):231-234, 1984.

[113] Wintrobe, Maxwell M.; Thorn, George W.; Adams, Raymond D.; et al. (Editors). *Harrison's Principles of Internal Medicine*. Seventh Edition. McGraw-Hill Book Company. New York, 1974. Pp. 24-30.

[114] Robbins, Stanley L. *Pathologic Basis of Disease*. W. B. Saunders Company. Philadelphia, 1974. P. 639.

[115] Ibid., Pp. 648-655.

[116] Ibid., Pp. 646-649.

[117] Ibid.

[118] Reith, Edward J.; Ross, Michael H. *Atlas of Descriptive Histology*. Second Edition. Harper & Row, Publishers. New York, 1970. Pp. 70-78.

[119] Arnett, E. N.; Roberts, W. C. "Acute Myocardial Infarction With Normal Coronary Arteries." *Circulation* 53:395-400, 1976.

[120] Linsay, Jr., J.; Dwyer, S.; Punja, U. "Angiographic Demonstration of Coronary Occlusion During Spontaneous Acute Myocardial Infarction and Subsequent Angiographically Normal Coronary Arteries." *American Journal of Cardiology* 51:1227-1228, 1983.

[121] Betriu, A.; Pare, J. C.; Sanz, G. A.; et al. "Myocardial Infarction with Normal Coronary Arteries: A Prospective Clinical Angiographic Study." *American Journal of Cardiology* 48:28-32, 1981.

[122] Ganong, William F. *Review of Medical Physiology*. Lange Medical Publications. Los Altos, 1973. Pp. 146-154.

[123] Ibid.

[124] Julian, D. G., Op. Cit.

[125] Ibid.

[126] Conn, Howard F. (Editor). *Current Therapy*. W. B. Saunders Company. Philadelphia, 1983. Pp. 149-154.

[127] Ganong, William F. Op. Cit., Pp. 146-154.

[128] Ibid.

[129] Psaty, Bruce M; Koepsell, Thomas D; LoGerfo, James P; Wagner, Edward H; Inui, Thomas S. "Beta-Blockers and Primary Prevention of Coronary Heart Disease in Patients with High Blood Pressure." *Journal of the American Medical Association* 261(14):2087-2094, 1989.

[130] Lund, Lars H; Benson, Lina; Dahlstrom, Ulf; Edner, Magnus; Freiberg, Leif. "Association Between Use of Beta-Blockers and Outcomes in Patients with Heart Failure and Preserved Ejection Fraction." *Journal of the American Medical Association* 312(19):2008-2018, 2014.

[131] Conn, Howard F. (Editor)., Op. Cit.

[132] Ganong, William F. Op. Cit., Pp. 146-154.

[133] Crevey, Barry J. "Mechanism of Action of the Calcium Channel Blockers." *Cardiovascular Reviews & Reports* 4(11): 1429-1442, 1983

[134] Winniford, Michael D; Hillis, L. David. "Calcium Antagonists for the Treatment of Various Anginal Syndromes." *Cardiovascular Reviews & Reports* 4(12):1543-1549, 1983.

[135] Conn, Howard F. (Editor), Op. Cit.

[136] Zawada, Jr., Edward; Stinson, James; Ramirez, German. "Hypertension Screening and Treatment with Angiotensin Inhibitors Saralasin and Captopril." *Postgraduate Medicine* 68(4):12-18, 1980.

[137] The Fifth Report of the National Committee on Detection, Evaluation, and Treatment of High Blood Pressure (JNC V). *Archives of Internal Medicine* 153:154-183, 1993.

[138] Konstam, Marvin A; et al. Effects of the Angiotensin Converting Enzyme Inhibitor Enalapril on the Long-Term Progression of Left Ventricular Dysfunction in Patients with Heart Failure." *Circulation* 86:431-438, 1992

[139] Huff, Barbara B. (Editor). *Physicians' Desk Reference*. Medical Economics Company Inc. Oradell, New Jersey, 1992. Pp. 1564-1567.

[140] Houston, Mark C. "New Insights and New Approaches for the Treatment of Essential Hypertension: Selection of Therapy Based On Coronary Heart Disease Risk Factor Analysis, Hemodynamic Profiles, Quality of Life, and Subsets of Hypertension." *American Heart Journal* 117:911-949, 1989

[141] Schmieder, R. E.; Bahr, M; Langewitz, W; et al. "Efficacy of Four Antihypertensive Drugs (Clonidine, Enalapril, Nitrendipine, Oxrenolol) on Stress Blood Pressure" *American Journal of Cardiology* 63:1333-1338, 1989

[142] Ernst, Diana (Editor); Lee, Anissa (Editor). *MPR – Monthly Prescribing Reference*. Haymarket Media. New York, December 2008. Pp. 3-23.

[143] Fox, Keith A. A.' Steg, Phillippe Gabriel; Eagle, Kim A.; et al. "Decline of Death and Heart Failure in Acute Coronary Syndrome." *Journal of the American Medical Association* 297(17): 1892-1900, 2007.

[144] Staff Writer. "Spasm's Role in Heart Disease Spotlighted by Drug Successes." *Medical World News*. December 10, 1979. Pp 433-44.

[145] Selye, Hans. *The Stress of Life*. Revised Edition. McGraw- Hill Book Company. New York, 1976. P.74.

[146] Peterson, E. A.; et al. "Loud Noise as a Cause of Sustained Hypertension." *Science News* 119:198, 1979.

[147] Angus, Robert. "Sounds. Raising a Ruckus About Noise: It Threatens Your Hearing and Your Health." *OMNI Magazine*. February 1994. P. 18.

[148] Staff Writer. "Newsfront: Do Neural Factors Cause Atherosclerosis?" *Modern Medicine*. May 30-June 15, 1978. P. 34.

[149] Kaplan, J. R.; Manuch, S. B.; Clarkson, T. B.; et al. "Social Stress and Atherosclerosis in Normocholesterolemic Monkeys." *Science* 220:733-735, 1983.

[150] Eliot, Robert S.; Buell, James C. Op. Cit.

[151] The Multiple Risk Factor Intervention Trial Research Group. "Mortality Rates After 10.5 Years for Participants in the Multiple Risk Factor Intervention Trial. Findings Related to A Priori Hypotheses of the Trial." *Journal of the American Medical Association* 263(13):1795-1801, 1990.

[152] Multiple Risk Factor Intervention Trial Research Group. "Multiple Risk Factor Intervention Trial: Risk Factor Changes and Mortality Results." *Journal of the American Medical Association* 248(12):1465-1477, 1982.

[153] Weber, Michael A.; Brewer, Deborah S.; Megaffin, Bernard B. "Beta-Adrenoceptor Blocking Agents in the Treatment of Essential Hypertension." *Cardiovascular Reviews & Reports* 1(7):523-535, 1980.

[154] Kannel, William B.; Thom, Thomas J. "Implications of the Recent Decline in Cardiovascular Mortality." *Cardiovascular Medicine*. September 1979. Pp. 983-997.

[155] Thaulow, E.; Dale, J. "Effects of Timolol on Platelets in Coronary Sinus Blood and on Myocardial Ischemia During Pacing-Induced Angina." *Acta Medica Scandinavia* 216:193-198, 1984.

[156] Kannel, William B.; Thom, Thomas J. Op. Cit.

[157] Garraway, W. Michael; Whisnant, Jack P.; Drury, Ivo. "The Continuing Decline in the Incidence of Stroke." *Mayo Clinic Proceedings* 58:520-523, 1983.

[158] Conn, Howard F. (Editor). *Current Therapy*. W. B. Saunders Company. Philadelphia, 1983. Pp. 149-154.

[159] Miller, D.; et al. "Is Variant Angina the Coronary Manifestation of a Generalized Vasospastic Disorder?" *New England Journal of Medicine* 304:763, 1981.

[160] Johansson, B. W. "Editorial: Migraine and the Heart." *Acta Medica Scandinavia* 213:241-243, 1983.

[161] Bulkey, B. H.; Klacsmann, P. G.; Hutchins, G. M. "Angina Pectoris, Myocardial Infarction, and Sudden Cardiac Death with Normal Coronary Arteries: A Clinicopathological Study of 9 Patients with Progressive Systemic Sclerosis." *American Heart Journal* 95:563-569, 1978.

[162] Coffman, J. D.; Cohen, R. A. "Vasospasm - Ubiquitous?" *New England Journal of Medicine* 304:780-782, 1981.

[163] Guyton, Arthur C. *Textbook of Medical Physiology*. Fourth Edition. W. B. Saunders Company. Philadelphia, 1971. Pp. 481-493.

[164] Ibid. Pp. 494-516.

[165] Kendall, M. J. "Beta-Blockade and Respiratory Function." *Cardiovascular Reviews & Reports* 2(6):572-576, 1981.

[166] Hallett, Jeffrey S.; Jacobs, Robert L. "Asthma - A Predisposing Factor for Recurrent Acute Bronchitis." Presented at the 39th Meeting of the American Academy of Allergy and Immunology. March 1983.

[167] Huff, Barbara B. (Editor). *Physicians' Desk Reference*. Medical Economics Company Inc. Oradell, New Jersey, 1994. Pp. 1026-1029.

[168] Huff, Barbara B. (Editor). Op. Cit., Pp. 583-585.

[169] Conn, Howard F. (Editor). *Current Therapy*. W. B. Saunders Company. Philadelphia, 1983. Pp. 574-580.

[170] Borysenko, M.; Cupp, P. "Stress, Behavior, and Immunity: Animal Models and Mediating Mechanisms." *General Hospital Psychiatry* 4(1):59-67, 1982.

[171] Conn, Howard F. Op. Cit., Pp. 738-751.

[172] Ibid.

[173] Bardhan, K. D.; Blum, A.; Gillespie, G.; Larkworthy, W.; et al. "Long Term Treatment with Cimetidine in Duodenal Ulceration." *Lancet* 309(8017):900-901, 1977.

[174] Scharschmidt, B. "Cimetidine." *Western Journal of Medicine* 131:417-425, 1979.

[175] Ibid.

[176] Ernst, Diana (Editor); Lee, Anissa (Editor). *MPR – Monthly Prescribing Reference*. Haymarket Media. New York, December 2008. Pp. 190-197.

[177] Ibid.

[178] Taylor, I.; Darby, C.: Hammond, P.: Basu, P. "Is There a Myoelectrical Abnormality in the Irritable Colon Syndrome?" *Gut* 19:391-395, 1978.

[179] Zoler, Mitchel L. "Irritable Bowel Linked to Physiological Causes." *Medical World News* 29(7):16, 1988.

[180] Ibid.

[181] Whorwell, P. J.: Clouter, C.; Smith, C. L. "Esophogeal Motility in the Irritable Bowel Syndrome." *British Medical Journal* 282(6270):1101-1102, 1981.

[182] Benjamin, Stanley. "Is Reflux an Acid or Motility Disorder?" International Symposium. Jefferson Medical College. Philadelphia, 1990.

[183] Chokhavatia, S.; Anuras, S. "Neuromuscular Disease of the Gastrointestinal Tract." *American Journal of Medical Science* 1(3):201-214, 1991.

[184] Borysenko, M.; Cupp, P. "Stress, Behavior, and Immunity: Animal Models and Mediating Mechanisms." *General Hospital Psychiatry* 4(1):59-67, 1982.

[185] Williams, J. M.; Peterson, R. G.; Shea, P. A.; et al. "Sympathetic Innervation of Murine Thymus and Spleen: Evidence for a Functional Link Between the Nervous and Immune Systems." *Brain Research Bulletin* 6(1):83-94, 1981.

[186] Locke, S. E. "Stress, Adaptation, and Immunity: Studies in Humans." *General Hospital Psychiatry* 4(1):49-58, 1982.

[187] Schleifer, S. J.; et al. "Suppression of Lymphocyte Stimulation Following Bereavement." *Journal of the American Medical Association* 250:374-377, 1983.

[188] Linn, B. S.; Jensen, J. "Age and Immune Response to a Surgical Stress." *Archives of Surgery* 118:405-409, 1983.

[189] Eskola, J.; et al. "Effect of Sport Stress on Lymphocyte Transformation and Antibody Formation." *Clinical Experimental Immunology* 32:339-345, 1978.

[190] Palmblad, Jan; Petrini, Bjorn; Wasserman, Jerzy; Akerstedt, Torbjorn. "Lymphocyte and Granulocyte Reactions During Sleep Deprivation." *Psychosomatic Medicine* 41(4):273-278, 1979.

[191] Girard, D. E.; Arthur, R. J., Reuler, J. B. "Psychosocial Events and Subsequent Illness - A Review." *Western Journal of Medicine* 142(3):358-363, 1985.

[192] Garraway, W. Michael; Whisnant, Jack P.; Drury, Ivo. "The Continuing Decline in the Incidence of Stroke." *Mayo Clinic Proceedings* 58:520-523, 1983.

[193] Dexter, Donn D.; Whisant, Jack P.; Connolly, Daniel C.; O'Fallon, W. Michael. "The Association of Stroke and Coronary Heart Disease: A Population Study." *Mayo Clinic Proceedings* 62:1077-1083, 1987.

[194] Eliot, Robert S.; Buell, James C. Op. Cit..

[195] Basser, L. S.: The Relation of Migraine and Epilepsy. *Brain* 92:285-300, 1969.

[196] Jay, G. W. Epilepsy, Migraine, and EEG Abnormalities on Children: A Review and Hypothesis. *Headache* 22:110-114, 1982.

[197] Bacharach, J. Michael; Olin, Jeffrey W. "Raynaud's Phenomenon." *Heart Disease and Stroke* 3(5): 255-259, 1994.

[198] Schwartz, Marc L.; Rotmensch, Heschi H.; Vlasses, Peter H. "New Uses for Calcium Blockers: Asthma, Migraine, Raynaud's, and More." *Modern Medicine*. February 1984. Pp. 109-124.

[199] Stollerman, Gene H. (Editor). "Capsule and Comment - Coronary Artery Disease and Stroke." *Hospital Practice*. April 1984. Pp. 25-26.

[200] Staff Writer. "Clinical Horizons - MI Study Shows Neurogenic Alteration Preceding Vascular Modifications." *Primary Cardiology*. November 1980. P. 129.

---

[201] Branigan, K. *The Atlas of Archaeology*. St. Martin's Press. New York, 1982. P. 12.

[202] The previously quoted excerpt from the *Tao te Ching* - with my own first line added to make a point. Apologies to Lao-Tzu - although I honestly believe he would like it!

End Notes Chapter 5:

[203] Lao-Tzu; Mitchell, Stephen (Translation and Commentary). *Tao te Ching*. Harper & Row, Publishers. New York, 1988. P. 7.

[204] Selye, Hans. *The Stress of Life*. Revised Edition. McGraw-Hill Book Company. New York, 1976. P. xi.

[205] Sun Tzu, Cleary, Thomas (Translation and Commentary.) *The Art of War.* Shamballa Publications, Inc. Boston, 1988. Quoted by Thomas Cleary in the Introduction. P.3.

[206] Toffler, Alvin; *Future Shock*. Random House. New York, 1970. Pp.305-324.

[207] Selye, Hans; Op. Cit., Pp. 405-456.

[208] Weber, Michael A.; Brewer, Deborah S.; Megaffin, Bernard B. "Beta-Adrenoceptor Blocking Agents in the Treatment of Essential Hypertension." *Cardiovascular Reviews & Reports* 1(7):523-535, 1980.

[209] ACTH is an abbreviation for Adreno-Cortico-Tropic Hormone. This is a powerful stress hormone that helps prepare the human body for fight or flight.

[210] Borysenko, M.; Cupp, P. "Stress, Behavior, and Immunity: Animal Models and Mediating Mechanisms." *General Hospital Psychiatry* 4(1):59-67, 1982.

[211] Weber, Michael A.; Brewer, Deborah S.; Megaffin, Bernard B. "Beta-Adrenoceptor Blocking Agents in the Treatment of Essential Hypertension." *Cardiovascular Reviews & Reports* 1(7):523-535, 1980.

[212] Multiple Risk Factor Intervention Trial Research Group. "Multiple Risk Factor Intervention Trial: Risk Factor Changes and Mortality Results." *Journal of the American Medical Association* 248(12):1465-1477, 1982.

[213] Buell, J. C.; Eliot, R. C. "The Role of Emotional Stress in the Development of Heart Disease." *Journal of the American Medical Association* 242(4):365-368, 1979.

[214] Robbins, Stanley L. *Pathologic Basis of Disease*. W. B. Saunders Company. Philadelphia, 1974. Pp. 338-345.

[215] Coffman, J. D.; Cohen, R. A. "Vasospasm - Ubiquitous?" *New England Journal of Medicine* 304:780-782, 1981.

[216] Hamilton, D. R. "Immunosuppressive Effects of Predator-Induced Stress in Mice with Acquired Immunity to Hymenolepsis nana." *Journal of Psychosomatic Research* 18(3):143-153, 1974.

[217] Ibid.

[218] Guyton, Arthur C. *Textbook of Medical Physiology*. W. B. Saunders Company. Philadelphia, 1971. Pp. 108-124.

[219] Crary, B.; Vorysenko, M.; Sutherland, D. C.; et al. "Decrease in Mitogen Responsiveness of Mononuclear Cells from Peripheral Blood After Epinephrine Administration in Humans." *Journal of Immunology* 130(2):694-697, 1983.

[220] Locke, S. E. "Stress, Adaptation, and Immunity: Studies in Humans." *General Hospital Psychiatry* 4(1):49-58, 1982.

[221] Page, Charlotte. "Scared to Death by Assault, Lesion Suggests." *Hospital Tribune*. April 1980. P. 17.

[222] Eliot, R. S.; Todd, G. L.; Pieper, G. M.; Clayton, F. C. "Pathophysiology of Catecholamine-Mediated Myocardial Damage." *Journal of the South Carolina Medical Association* 75(11):513-518, 1975

[223] Thoreau, Henry David. *Walden*. Bramhall House. New York, 1951. P. 22.

[224] Freeman, L. J.; Nixon, P. J.; Sallabank, P.; et al. "Psychological Stress and Silent Myocardial Ischemia." *American Heart Journal* 114:477-482, 1987.

[225] Ibid.

[226] Deanfield, J. E., et al. "Ordinary Stress and Myocardial Ischemia." *Lancet* 2(8410):1001-1004, 1985.

[227] Deedwania, P. C.; Carbajal, E. V. "Silent Ischemia During Daily Life Is an Independent Predictor of Mortality in Stable Angina." *Circulation* 81:748-756, 1990.

[228] Deanfield, J. E., et al. "Ordinary Stress and Myocardial Ischemia." *Lancet* 2(8410):1001-1004, 1985.

[229] Ibid.

[230] Selye, Hans. "The Evolution of the Stress Concept." *American Journal of Cardiology* 26(3):289-299 1970.

[231] Sun Tzu; Cleary, Thomas Op. Cit.. P.3.

[232] Eliot, Robert S.; Breo, Dennis L. *Is It Worth Dying For? A Self-Assessment Program to Make Stress Work For You, Not Against You*. Bantam Books, Inc. New York, 1984.

[233] Breo, Dennis L. "Is It Worth Dying For?" *American Medical News*. May 15, 1981. Pp. 25-26.

[234] Ibid.

[235] Ibid.

[236] Ibid.

[237] Ibid.

[238] Lao-Tzu; Mitchell, Stephen Op. Cit., P. 33.

[239] Selye, Hans. "Stress and Cardiovascular Disease." *Cardiovascular Medicine* February 1979. Pp. 183-202.

[240] Selye, Hans. *Stress Without Distress.* Lippincott. Philadelphia, 1974. Pp. 35-83.

[241] Friedman, M.; St. George, S.; Byers, S. O.; Rosenman, R. H. "Excretion of Catecholamines, 17-Ketosteroids, 17-Hydroxycorticoids, and 5-Hydroxyindole in Men Exhibiting a Particular Behavior Pattern (A) Associated with High Incidence of Clinical Coronary Artery Disease." *Journal of Clinical Investigation* 39:758-764, 1960.

[242] Selye, Hans. "Stress and Cardiovascular Disease." *Cardiovascular Medicine.* February 1979. Pp. 183-202.

[243] Case, Robert; et al. "Type A Behavior and Survival After Acute Myocardial Infarction". *New England Journal of Medicine* 312:737-741, 1985.

[244] Friedman, Howard S.; Booth-Kewley, Stephanie. "Personality, Type A Behavior, and Coronary Heart Disease: The Role of Emotional Expression." *Journal of Personality and Social Psychology* 53(4):783-792, 1987.

[245] Breo, Dennis L. "Is It Worth Dying For?" *American Medical News.* May 15, 1981. Pp. 25-26.

[246] Eliot, Robert S. "Relationship of Emotional Stress to the Heart." *Heart Disease and Stroke* 2:243-246, 1993.

[247] Breo, Dennis L. "Is It Worth Dying For?" *American Medical News.* May 15, 1981. Pp. 25-26.

[248] Ibid.

[249] Eliot, Robert S. "Sudden Death on Monday." *Emergency Medicine.* February 28, 1982. Pp 25-36.

End Notes Chapter 6:

[250] Lao-Tzu; Mitchell, Stephen (Translation and Commentary.) *Tao te Ching.* A New English Version. Harper & Rowe, Publishers, Inc. New York, 1988. P. 41

[251] Zuckerman, Mortimer B. "The Victims of TV Violence." *U. S. News & World Report.* August 2, 1993. P. 64.

[252] Silver, Marc; Smons, John. "News You Can Use. The Rating Game." *U.S. News & World Report.* November 21, 1994. Pp. 91-93.

[253] Dvorak, John C. "Blow Their Heads Off." *PC Magazine*. November 8, 1994. P. 93.

[254] Perenson, Melissa J. "Warning: Parental Discretion Advised." *PC Magazine*. April 12, 1994. P. 30.

[255] Silver, Marc; Smons, John. "News You Can Use. The Rating Game." *U.S. News & World Report*. November 21, 1994. Pp. 91-93.

[256] Eliot, Robert S. "Relationship of Emotional Stress to the Heart." *Heart Disease and Stroke* 2:243-246, 1993.

[257] Morrow, Lance. "A Long Hallucination of War." *TIME Magazine*. December 10, 1990. Pp. 40-43.

[258] Moreno, Vaughn. "Men Desensitized by TV Falsehoods." *The Elkhart Truth*. February 17, 1991. P. A7.

[259] Witkin, Gordon; Greighton, Lina L.; Guttman, Monika. "More Murder Mysteries." *U.S. News & World Report*. April 11, 1994. Pp. 28-34.

[260] Ibid.

[261] Neria, Yuval. "Understanding the Mental Health Effects of Indirect Exposure to Mass Trauma Through the Media." *Journal of the American Medical Association* 306(11):1374-1375, 2011.

[262] Cooke, Patrick. "TV or Not TV." *Hippocrates Magazine*. January 1992. Pp. 39-49.

[263] Ibid.

[264] Author Michael Crichton was quoted in *TV Guide*. January 1995.

[265] Elmer-DeWitt, Elmer; Purvis, Andrew. "Why Junior Won't Sit Still." *TIME Magazine*. November 26, 1990. P. 59.

[266] Stein, Harry. "Our Times. Are Talk Shows Hazardous to your Mental Health?" *TV Guide*. March 12, 1994. P. 47.

[267] Wright, John W. (Editor). *The New York Times 2009 Almanac*. "Computers." The Penguin Group. New York, 2009. P. 805.

[268] Ibid.

[269] Levin, Carol. "Survey Reveals Psyche of Wired Society." *PC Magazine*. August 1994. P. 30.

[270] Wright, John W. (Editor). *The New York Times 2009 Almanac*. "Computers." The Penguin Group. New York, 2009. P. 805.

[271] Dvorak, John C. "The Impending CD-ROM Fiasco." *PC Magazine*. September 27, 1994. P. 93.

[272] Patton, Carole. "Dialog Box." *Windows Magazine*. October 1994. P. 69.

[273] Venditto, Gus. "Intel Lowers Prices, Increases Speeds." *PC Magazine*. March 31, 1994. P. 30.

[274] Flynn, Mary Kathleen. "On Technology. New Software, Old Computer." *U.S. News & World Report*. August 15, 1994. P. 62.

[275] Dvorak, John C. "Mouse Shoulder: A New Ailment." *PC Magazine*. December 6, 1994. P. 93.

[276] Allen, Dennis. "Managing Infoglut." *BYTE Magazine*. June 1992. P. 16.

[277] IBM Corporation. Advertisement for OS/2 Warp. *TIME Magazine*. December 27, 1994. P. 4.

[278] Madsen, Dan; McFadden, Gates. "Exclusive Interview: Gates McFadden - The Doctor is In." *Star Trek - The Official Fan Club Magazine*. June/July 1990. Pp. 2-5.

[279] Elmer-DeWitt, Philip. "Mystery - and Maybe Danger - in the Air." *TIME Magazine*. December 24, 1990. Pp. 67-68.

[280] Saffo, Paul. "Commentary. A Conspiracy of Silence." *BYTE Magazine*. July 1993. P. 278.

[281] Meena, Jitendra Kumar; Verma, Anjana; Kohli, Charu; Ingle, Gopal Krishna. "Mobile Phone Use and Possible Cancer Risk: Current Perspectives in India." *Indian Journal of Occupational and Environmental Medicine* 20(1):5-9, 2016.

[282] Machrone, Bill. "The Technology Rift." *PC Magazine*. September 27, 1994. Pp. 87-88.

[283] Zuckerman, Mortimer B. "America's Silent Revolution." *U. S. News & World Report*. July 18, 1994. P. 90.

[284] Staff Writer. "Business Workers' Lament: Too Much Overtime." *U. S. News & World Report*. October 10, 1994. P. 12.

[285] Killan, Michael. "Worked Over." *The South Bend Tribune*. March 2, 1992. P. B1-2.

[286] Creighton, Linda L. "Kids Taking Care of Kids." *U.S. News & World Report*. December 20, 1993. Pp. 26-33.

[287] Sugg, Nancy Kathleen; Inui, Thomas. "Primary Care Physicians' Response to Domestic Violence. Opening Pandora's Box." *Journal of the American Medical Association* 267(23):3157-3160, 1992.

[288] Prud'Homme, Alex; Szxzesny, Joe; Woodbury, Richard. "A Nation on the Move." *TIME Magazine*. April 29, 1991. Pp. 30-31.

[289] Lyznicki, James M.; Doege, Theodore C.; Davis, Ronald M. Williams, Michael A. "Council Report. Sleepiness, Driving, and Motor Vehicle Crashes." *Journal of the American Medical Association* 279(23):1908-1913, 1998.

[290] Holmes, Bob. "Silent Epidemic. Americans, Asleep at the Wheel." *U.S. News & World Report*. January 18, 1993. Pp. 68-69.

[291] Grandner, Michael A.; Pack, Allan I. "Sleep Disorders, Public Health, and Public Safety." *Journal of the American Medical Association* 306(23):2616-2617, 2011

[292] Ibid.

[293] Ibid.

[294] Binkley, S. "A Timekeeping Enzyme in the Pineal Gland." *Scientific American*. April 1979. Pp. 45-52.

[295] Brody, Jane E. "From Fertility to Mood, Sunlight Found to Affect Human Biology." *The New York Times*. June 26, 1981. Pp. C1-C4.

[296] Thompson, C.; et al. "Seasonal Affective Disorder and Season-Dependent Abnormalities of Melatonin Suppression by Light." *Lancet* 336:703, 1990.

[297] Rosenthal, Norman E. "Diagnosis and Treatment of Seasonal Affective Disorder." *Journal of the American Medical Association* 270(22):1717-2720, 1993.

[298] Wehr, T.A.; et al. "Contrasts Between Symptoms of Summer Depression and Winter Depression." *Journal of Affective Disorders* 23:173-183, 1991.

[299] Kasper, Siegfried; et al. "Epidemiological Findings of Seasonal Changes in Mood and Behavior: A Telephone Survey of Montgomery County, Maryland." *Archives of General Psychiatry* 46:823-833, 1989.

[300] Rosenthal, Normal E.; Carpenter, Constance J.; James, Steven P.; Parry, Barbara L.; Rogers, Susan L.; Wehr, Thomas A. "Seasonal Affective Disorder in Children and Adolescents." *American Journal of Psychiatry* 143:356-358, 1986.

[301] King, Christopher R.; Knutson, Kristen L.; Rathouz, Paul J.; Sidney, Steve; Liu, Kiang; Lauderdale, Diane S. "Short Sleep Duration and Incident Coronary Artery Calcification." *Journal of the American Medical Association* 300(24):2859-2866, 2008.

[302] Spiegel, K.; Leproult, R.; Van Cauter, E. "Impact of Seep Debt on Metabolic and Endocrine Function." *Lancet* 354(9188):1435-1439, 1999.

[303] Eliot, Robert S.; Kumar, Naresh; Morales-Ballejo, Hugo. "Emotions and Coronary Heart Disease." *Heart Disease and Stroke* 3:361-364, 1994.

[304] Schnall, Peter l.; Pieper, Carl; Schwartz, Joseph E; Karasek, Robert A.; Schlussel, Yvette; Devereaux, Richard B.; Ganau, Antonello; Alderman, Michael; Warren, Katherine; Pickering, Thomas G. "The Relationship Between 'Job Strain,' Workplace Diastolic Blood Pressure, and Left Ventricular Mass Index." *Journal of the American Medical Association* 263(14):1929-1935, 1990.

[305] Nordstrom, Cheryl K.; et al. "Work-Related Stress and Early Atherosclerosis." *Epidemiology* 12:180-185, 2001.

[306]Falliers, C. J. "Time Dependent Processes in Allergy and Asthma." *Annals of Allergy* 47:253-259, 1981.

[307] Toffler, Alvin. *Future Shock.* Random House. New York, 1970. P. 285.

End Notes Chapter 7:

[308] Gampel, M. B.; Slome, C.; Scotch, N.; Abramson, J. H. "Urbanization and Hypertension Among Zulu Adults." *Journal of Chronic Diseases* 15:67-70, 1962.

[309] Ganong, William F. *Review of Medical Physiology*. Lange Medical Publications. Los Altos, 1973. Pp. 146-154.

[310] Erman, Milton K.; Rush, A. John. "The Physiologic Disturbances of Depression." *The Female Patient* 8:19-30, 1983.

[311] Altshuler, Kenneth Z.; Hollister, Leo E. "Senile Dementia or Stress-Induced Depression?" *Patient Care*. November 30, 1981. Pp. 115-117.

[312] Erman, Milton K.; Rush, A. John. Op. Cit.

[313] Larkin, Marilynn. "Easing EMT Stress Can Prevent Depression." *Emergency Medical News*. April 1993. Pp. 1-2.

[314] Barefoot, J. C.; Schroll, M. "Symptoms of Depression, Acute Myocardial Infarction, and Total Mortality in a Community Sample." *Circulation* 93(11):1976-1980, 1996.

[315] Creagan, E. T. "Stress Among Medical Oncologists: The Phenomenon of Burnout and a Call to Action." *Mayo Clinic Proceedings* 68:614-615, 1993.

[316] Gillin, J.; Duncan, W.; Pettigrew, K. "Successful Separation of Depressed, Normal, and Insomniac Patients by EEG sleep data." *Archives of General Psychiatry* 136:85-90, 1979.

[317] Sachar, E.; Hellman, L.; Roffwarg, H.; et al. "Disrupted 24- Hour Patterns of Cortisol Secretions in Psychotic Depression." *Archives of General Psychiatry* 28:19-24, 1973.

[318] Borysenko, M.; Cupp, P. "Stress, Behavior, and Immunity: Animal Models and Mediating Mechanisms." *General Hospital Psychiatry* 4(1):59-67, 1982.

[319] Erman, Milton K.; Rush, A. John. Op. Cit.

[320] Conway, Melanie W.; Miller, Merry N. "Mood Disorders." Rakel, Robert E. and Bope, Edward T. (Editors). *Conn's Current Therapy* 2007. Saunders Elsevier. Philadelphia, 2007. Pp. 1300-1308.

[321] Ricelson, Elliott. "Tricyclic Antidepressants and Histamine H-1 Receptors." *Mayo Clinic Proceedings* 54:669-674, 1979.

[322] Scharschmidt, B. "Cimetidine." *Western Journal of Medicine* 131:417-425, 1979.

[323] Epstein, Charles M. "Histamine H-2 Antagonists and the Central Nervous System." *American Family Physician* 32(6):109-112, 1985.

[324] Rubin, Nancy. "Severe Asthma and Depression." *Archives of Family Medicine* 2:433-440, 1993.

[325] Beers, M. H; Passman, L.J. "Antihypertension Medications and Depression." *Drugs* 40(6):792-799; December, 1990.

[326] Thomas, Patricia. "ACE Inhibitor Takes Blues Away." *Medical World News*. January 1991. P. 51.

[327] Crowe, R. R.; Pauls, D. L.; Venkatesh, A.; et al. "Exercise and Anxiety Neurosis." *Archives of General Psychiatry* 36:652-653, 1979.

[328] Lipowski, Z. J. "Psychosomatic Medicine in the Seventies: An Overview." *American Journal of Psychiatry* 134:233-244, 1977.

[329] Ibid.

[330] Conway, Melanie W.; Miller, Merry N. Op. Cit..

[331] Schuckit, M. A. "Current Therapeutic Options in the Management of Typical Anxiety." *Journal of Clinical Psychiatry* 42:15-24, 1981.

[332] Gullette, Elizabeth C. D.; Blumenthal, James A.; Babyak, Michael; Jiang, Wei; Waugh, Robert A.; Frid, David J.; O'Conner, Christopher M.; Morris, James J.; Krantz, David S. "Effects of Mental Stress on Myocardial Ischemia During Daily Life." *Journal of the American Medical Association* 277(20):152-1560, 1997.

[333] Mittleman, Murray A. "Mental Stress During Daily Life Triggers Myocardial Ischemia." *Journal of the American Medical Association* 277(19):1558-1559, 1997.

[334] Jonas, Bruce S.; Franks, Peter; Ingram, Deborah D. "Are Symptoms of Anxiety and Depression Risk Factors for Hypertension? Longitudinal Evidence from the National Health and Nutrition Examination Survey I Epidemiologic Follow-Up Study." *Archives of Family Medicine* 6:43-49, 1997.

[335] Niles, David P. "War Trauma and Post-Traumatic Stress Disorder." *American Family Practice* 44(5):1663-1669, 1991.

[336] Borger, M. H. I. Personal recollection of interviews with Vietnam veterans suffering from Post-Traumatic Stress Syndrome. January 1988.

[337] Buck, O. D.; Walker, J. I. "Posttraumatic Stress Disorder in Viet Nam Veterans." *Southern Medical Journal* 75:704-706, 1982.

[338] Horowitz, M. J. *Stress Response Syndromes*. Aronson. New York, 1976.

[339] Goldfeld, Anne E.; Mollica, Richard F.; Pesavento, Barbara H.; Faraone, Stephen V. "The Physical and Psychological Sequelae of Torture - Symptomatology and Diagnosis." *Journal of the American Medical Association* 259(18):2725-2729, 1988.

[340] Walker, John I. "Posttraumatic Stress Disorder After a Car Accident." *Postgraduate Medicine* 69(2):82-86, 1981.

[341] Ibid.

[342] DeVita, Elizabeth. "Abused Children Being Diagnosed with PTSD." *Emergency Medicine News*. August 1993. Pp. 1-2.

[343] Altshuler, Kenneth Z.; Hollister, Leo E. "Senile Dementia or Stress-Induced Depression?" *Patient Care*. November 30, 1981. Pp. 115-117.

[344] Friedman, M.; St. George, S.; Byers, S. O.; Rosenman, R. H. "Excretion of Catecholamines, 17-Ketosteroids, 17-Hydroxycorticoids, and 5-Hydroxyindole in Men Exhibiting a Particular Behavior Pattern (A) Associated with High Incidence of Clinical Coronary Artery Disease." *Journal of Clinical Investigation* 39:758-764, 1960.

[345] Schmidt, Robert F. (Editor). *Fundamentals of Neurophysiology*. Springer Verlag. New York, 1978. P. 300.

[346] Ibid. P. 303.

[347] Ibid.

[348] Norton, Peter. *Disk Explorer. Manual for The Norton Utilities*. Version 6.1. Symantec Corporation. Cupertino, California, 1991. Pp. 1-36.

[349] Schmidt, Robert F. (Editor). Op.Cit. P. 303.

[350] Ibid.

[351] The term *Stress Syndrome* is simpler and is easier to remember. Do not confuse Stress Syndrome with the stress response. The stress response, properly triggered, is a natural feedback loop of the Self-Referral process and promotes Self-Referral. *Stress Syndrome* is caused by the negative effects of stress and destroys Self-Referral.

[352] Clark, Ronald G: *Manter and Gantz's Clinical Neuroanatomy and Neurophysiology*. Fifth Edition. F. A. Davis Company. Philadelphia, 1978. P. 3.

[353] Restak, Richard. *The Brain*. Bantam Books. New York, 1984. P. 2.

[354] Snell, Richard S. *Clinical Embryology for Medical Students.* Little, Brown and Company. Boston, 1972. P. 235.

[355] Ibid.

[356] Clark, Ronald G. (Editor.) Op. Cit.. Pp. 145-159.

[357] Ibid.

[358] Restak, Richard. *The Brain.* Bantam Books. New York, 1984. Pp. 168-187.

[359] Schmidt, R. F. (Editor). Op. Cit.. Pp. 300-305.

[360] Ibid.

[361] Ibid.

[362] Ibid.

[363] Ibid.

[364] Gelman, David. "Treating War's Psychic Wounds." *Newsweek Magazine.* August 29, 1988. Pp. 62-64.

[365] Penrose, Roger. *The Emperor's New Mind.* Oxford University Press. New York, 1989. Pp. 23-29.

[366] Ibid.

[367] Schmidt, R. F. (Editor). Op. Cit.. Pp. 300-305.

[368] Woram, John. *The PC Configuration Handbook.* Bantam Books. New York, 1990. Pp. 6-77.

[369] Ibid.

[370] Bremmer, J. Douglas. *Does Stress Damage the Brain?* W. W. Norton & Company. New York, 2002. Pp 43-50.

[371] Rakel, Robert E. (Editor.) *Textbook of Family Practice*. Third Edition. W. B. Saunders Company. Philadelphia, 1984. Pp. 1190-1196.

[372] Harvey, A. McGehee (Editor); Johns, Richard J. (Editor); McKusick, Victor A. (Editor); Owens, Albert H. (Editor); Ross, Richard S. (Editor.) *The Principles and Practice of Medicine.* Twenty-second Edition. Appleton & Lange, Publishers. Norwalk, Connecticut, 1988. Pp. 1070-1080.

[373] Gelman, David. Op. Cit..

[374] McCloskey, Laura Ann; Walker, Maria. "Posttraumatic Stress in Children Exposed to Family Violence and Single Event Trauma." *Journal of the American Academy of Child and Adolescent Psychiatry* 39:108-115, 2000.

[375] Kolb, Lawrence C. "A Neuropsychological Hypothesis Explaining Posttraumatic Stress Disorders." *American Journal of Psychiatry* 144:989-995, 1987.

[376] Yehuda, Rachel; et al. "Urinary Catecholamine Excretion and Severity of PTSD Symptoms in Vietnam Combat Veterans." *Journal of Nervous Mental Disease* 180:321-325, 1992.

[377] Yaffe, Kristine; Vittinghoff, Eric; Lindquist, Karla; Barnes, Deborah; Covinsky, Kenneth E.; Neylan, Thomas; Kluse, Molly; Marmar, Charles. "Posttraumatic Stress Disorder and Dementia. What Is the Origin of the Association?" *Journal of the American Medical Association* 202(22):2287-2292, 2010.

[378] Weber, Michael A.; Brewer, Deborah S.; Megaffin, Bernard B. "Beta-Adrenoceptor Blocking Agents in the Treatment of Essential Hypertension." *Cardiovascular Reviews & Reports* 1(7):523-535, 1980.

[379] Lao-Tzu; Mitchell, Stephen (Translation and Commentary). *Tao te Ching*. Harper & Row, Publishers. New York, 1988. P. 60.

End Notes Chapter 8:

[380] Lao-Tzu; Mitchell, Stephen (Translation and Commentary). *Tao te Ching*. Harper & Row Publishers, Inc. New York, 1988. P. 42.

[381] Wintrobe, Maxwell M.; Thorn, George W.; Adams, Raymond D; et al. (Editors). *Harrison's Principles of Internal Medicine*. Seventh Edition. McGraw-Hill Book Company. New York, 1974: Pp. 125- 130.

[382] Tononi, Giulio; Cirelli, Chiara. "Perchance to Prune." *Scientific American* 309(2):34-39, 2013.

[383] Guyton, Arthur. *Textbook of Medical Physiology*. W. B. Saunders Company. Philadelphia, 1971: Pp. 703-715.

[384] Ibid.

[385] Ibid.

[386] Ibid.

[387] Wintrobe, Maxwell M.; Thorn, George W.; Adams, Raymond D; et al. (Editors). *Harrison's Principles of Internal Medicine.* Seventh Edition. McGraw-Hill Book Company. New York, 1974: Pp. 125- 130.

[388] Ibid.

[389] Toufexis, Anastasia. “Drowsy America.” *TIME Magazine.* December 17, 1990. Pp. 78-85.

[390] Toffler, Alvin. *Future Shock.* Random House, Inc. New York, 1970. Pp. 323-337.

[391] Ibid.

[392] Friedman, Meyer; Ulmer, D. *Treating Type A Behavior - And Your Heart.* Alfred A. Knopf, Inc. New York, 1984.

[393] Toffler, Alvin. *Future Shock.* Op. Cit..

[394] Ibid.

[395] Ibid.

[396] Ibid. Pp. 343-365.

[397] Ibid.

[398] Ibid. Pp. 323-337.

[399] Friedman, Meyer; Ulmer, D. Op. Cit..

[400] Ibid.

[401] Ibid.

[402] Friedman, M.; Thoresen, C. E.; Gill, J. J.; et al. "Alteration of Type A Behavior and Reduction in Cardiac Recurrences in Post Myocardial Infarction Patients." *American Heart Journal* 108:237-248, 1984.

[403] Friedman, Meyer; Ulmer, D. Op. Cit.

[404] Ibid.

[405] Brady, J. P.; et al. "Behavioral Vs. Medical Therapy for Hypertension." *Letters. New England Journal of Medicine* 303:586, 1980.

[406] Shapiro, Alvin P. "Behavior Modification: Can It Control Hypertension?" *Journal of Cardiovascular Medicine* December 1980:1075-1079.

[407] Wadden, Thomas A.; de la Torre, Cristina S. "Relaxation Therapy as an Adjunct Treatment for Essential Hypertension." *Journal of Family Practice* 11(6):901-908, 1980.

[408] Brown, Barbara B. *Stress and the Art of Biofeedback.* Harper & Rowe. New York, 1977.

[409] Bruhn, P.; Oleson, J.; Melgaard, B. "Controlled Trial of EMG Biofeedback in Muscle Contraction Headache." *Annals of Neurology* 6:34-36, 1979.

[410] Ibid.

[411] Fuller, George D. *Biofeedback: Methods and Procedures in Clinical Practice.* Biofeedback Press. San Francisco, 1977.

[412] Ross, Jane. "From England: 79% `More Tolerant' of Tinnitus After 10 Biofeedback Sessions." *Medical Tribune*. April 8, 1981. P. 3.

[413] Kall, Anne. "Sleep/Wake Biofeedback." *OMNI Magazine*. October, 1981. P. 12.

[414] Staff Writer. "Relieving the Stress of Cancer." *Your Patient and Cancer*. January 1982. P.70

[415] Staff Writer. "Biofeedback Use in Sex Therapy, Psychotherapy Discussed at Meeting." *Behavioral Medicine* 8(5):3-4; May 1981.

[416] Young, Stuart H. "Asthmatics Give Biofeedback Mixed Reviews." Letter in Medical Previews Section. *Continuing Education.* April 1979. P.99.

[417] Staff Writer. "Youngsters Fight Hypertension Sans Drugs." *Medical World News.* June 11, 1979. P.74.

[418] David, Leonard. "Nausea in Space." *OMNI Magazine.* November 1981. P.39.

[419] Wolf, Steven L. "Electromyographic Biofeedback in Exercise Programs." *The Physician and Sportsmedicine* 8(11):61-69, 1980.

[420] Goldsmith, Marsha F. "Computerized Biofeedback Training Aids in Spinal Injury Rehabilitation." *Journal of the American Medical Association* 253(8):1097-1099, 1985.

[421] Gannon, Linda R.; et al. "Biofeedback and Muscle Contraction Headache." *Journal of Psychosomatic Research* 25:271-280, 1981.

[422] Young, Stuart H. "Asthmatics Give Biofeedback Mixed Reviews." Letter in Medical Previews Section. *Continuing Education.* April 1979. P. 99.

[423] Bernstein, D. A.; Borkovec, T. D. *Progressive Relaxation Training.* Research Press. Champaign, Illinois, 1973.

[424] Ibid.

[425] Ibid.

[426] Lammers, C. A.; et al. "The Effects of Progressive Muscle Relaxation on Stress and Diabetic Control." *Behavioral Research Therapy* 22:641-650, 1984.

[427] Burish, T. G.; Lyles, J. N. "Effectiveness of Relaxation Training in Reducing Adverse Reactions to Cancer Chemotherapy." *Journal of Behavioral Medicine* 4:65, 1981.

[428] Carney, Robert M. "Clinical Applications of Relaxation Training." *Hospital Practice.* July 1983. Pp. 83-94.

[429] Ibid.

[430] Ibid.

[431] Restak, Richard. *The Brain*. Bantam Books. New York, 1984. Pp. 192 and 337.

[432] Ibid.

[433] Whorwell, P. J.; Prior, A.; Faragher, E. B. "Controlled Trial of Hypnotherapy in the Treatment of Severe Refractory Irritable-Bowel Syndrome." *Lancet* 2(8414):1232-1234, 1984.

[434] Restak, Richard. *The Brain*. Bantam Books. New York, 1984. P. 192.

[435] Ibid.

[436] Barber, Joseph; Gitelson, Jean. "Cancer Pain: Psychological Management Using Hypnosis" *CA - A Cancer Journal for Clinicians* 30(3):130-135, 1980.

[437] Kattan, M.; Ben-Zvi, W.; Spohn, W. A.; et al. "Hypnosis as an Adjunctive Treatment for Bronchial Asthma." *American Review of Respiratory Diseases* 125(4):392, 1982.

[438] Restak, Richard. *The Brain*. Bantam Books. New York, 1984. P. 337.

[439] Staff Writer. "Off the Couch and Into the Tub." *TIME Magazine*. January 12, 1981. P. 45.

[440] Gorman, John. "Tanking." *OMNI Magazine*. October 1981. Pp. 61-64.

[441] Staff Writer. "Off the Couch and Into the Tub." *TIME Magazine*. January 12, 1981. P. 45.

[442] Ibid.

[443] Suedfeld, P. *Restricted Environmental Stimulation: Research and Clinical Application*. John Wiley & Sons. New York, 1980.

[444] Lilly, J. C. *The Deep Self*. Warner Books. New York, 1977.

[445] Staff Writer. "Raising Your Spirits. Isolation Tanks: Therapeutic Tools or Toys?" *Behavioral Medicine*. April 1981. Pp. 17- 23.

[446] Wallace, Robert Keith; Benson, Herbert. "The Physiology of Meditation." *Scientific American* 226(2):84-90, 1972.

[447] Akishige, Y. "A Historical Survey of the Psychological Studies in Zen." Kyushu Psychological Studies, V, *Bulletin of the Faculty of Literature of the Kyushu University* 11:1-56, 1968.

[448] Benson, Herbert. *The Relaxation Response*. William Morrow. New York, 1975.

[449] Williams, Mark; Penman, Danny. *Mindfulness. An Eight Week Plan for Finding Peace in a Frantic World.* Rodale, Inc. New York, 2011. Pp. 83-85.

[450] Goleman, Daniel. *The Varieties of the Meditative Experience.* E. P. Dutton & Company. New York, 1977.

[451] Goleman, Daniel. "Meditation Without Mystery." *Psychology Today.* March 1977. Pp. 55-88.

[452] Benson, Herbert; Wallace, Robert Keith. "Decreased Blood Pressure in Hypertensive Subjects Who Practiced Meditation." *Supplement II to Circulation 45 and 46*:516, 1972.

[453] Carrington, P.; Collings, G. H.; Benson, H.; et al. "The Use of Meditation-Relaxation Techniques for the Management of Stress in a Working Population." *Occupational Medicine* 22:221-231, 1980.

[454] Glueck, B. C.; Stroebel, C. F. "Biofeedback and Meditation in the Treatment of Psychiatric Illnesses." *Comprehensive Psychiatry* 16:303-321, 1975.

[455] Benson, Herbert; Wallace, Robert Keith. "Decreased Drug Abuse with Transcendental Meditation: A Study of 1,862 Subjects." in Zarafonetis, Chris J. (Editor.) *Drug Abuse: Proceedings of the International Conference. Lea and Febeiger. Philadelphia, 1972.* Also, in *The Congressional Record Serial Number 92-1.* Government Printing Office. Washington, D.C., 1971.

[456] Shafti, Mohammad; Lavely, Robert A.; Jaffe, Robert D. "Meditation and the Prevention of Alcohol Abuse." *American Journal of Psychiatry* 132:942-945, 1975.

[457] Miskiman, Donald E. "The Treatment of Insomnia by the Transcendental Meditation Program." *Scientific Research on the Transcendental Meditation Program: Collected Papers, Volume I.* Maharishi European Research University Press Publication Number G-1181. Livingston Manor, New York, 1977. Pp. 292-295.

[458] Honsberger, Ronald W.; Wilson, Archie F. "The Effect of Transcendental Meditation Upon Bronchial Asthma." *Clinical Research* 21(2):278, 1973.

[459] Zamarra, John W.; Besseghini, Italo; Wittenberg, Stephen. "The Effects of the Transcendental Meditation Program on the Exercise Performance of Patients with Angina Pectoris." *Scientific Research on the Transcendental Meditation Program: Collected Papers, Volume I.* Maharishi European Research University Press Publication Number G-1181. Livingston Manor, New York, 1977. Pp. 270-278.

[460] Benson, Herbert; et al. "Behavioral Induction of Arterial Hypertension and Its Reversal." *American Journal of Physiology* 217:30-34, 1969.

[461] Galland, Leo; Benson, Herbert; Carrington, Patricia; Shealy, C. Norman. "Easing Stress. How to Help Patients Learn to Relax." *Patient Care.* November 30, 1980. Pp. 138-170.

[462] Alderman, Mary; Altshuler, Kenneth Z.; Soloman, Harold S.; et al. "Stress Management: State of the Art." *Patient Care*. July 15, 1983. Pp. 88-163.

[463] Johnson, Nancy. "Patient Who Has Recurring Stress-Related Symptoms Rarely Gets Treatment He Needs." *Family Practice* News October 15, 1980. P. 1.

[464] Fisher, Carrie; Arrington, Carl Wayne. "A Spy in Her Own House." *TIME Magazine*. October 15, 1990. Pp. 72-74.

[465] Ibid.

[466] Huxley, Aldous. *Brave New World.* Perennial Library. New York, 1968. P. 94.

[467] Suedfeld, P. *Restricted Environmental Stimulation: Research and Clinical Application*. John Wiley & Sons. New York, 1980.

[468] Banquet, Jean-Paul. "Spectral Analysis of the E.E.G. in Meditation." *Electroencephalography and Clinical Neurophysiology* 35:143-151, 1973.

[469] Bruhn, P.; Oleson, J.; Melgaard, B. "Controlled Trial of EMG Biofeedback in Muscle Contraction Headache." *Annals of Neurology* 6:34-36, 1979.

[470] Allison, J. "Respiratory Changes During Transcendental Meditation." *Lancet* 1(7651):833-834, 1970.

[471] Ornish, Dean; Scherwitz, Larry W.; Doody, Rachelle S.; et al. "Effects of Stress Management Training and Dietary Changes in Treating Ischemic Heart Disease." *Journal of the American Medical Association* 249(1):55-59, 1983.

[472] McCauley, J. D.; Thelan, M. K.; Frank, R. G.; et al. "Hypnosis Compared to Relaxation in the Outpatient Management of Chronic Low Back Pain." *Archives of Physical Medicine Rehabilitation* 64:548-552, 1983.

[473] Johnson, Nancy. "Patient Who Has Recurring Stress-Related Symptoms Rarely Gets Treatment He Needs." *Family Practice News* October 15, 1980. P. 13.

[474] Glueck, Bernard C.; Stroebel, Charles F. "Biofeedback and Meditation in the Treatment of Psychiatric Illnesses." *Comprehensive Psychiatry* 16(4):303-321, 1975.

[475] Ibid.

[476] Glueck, Bernard C.; Stroebel, Charles F. Op. Cit.

[477] Ibid.

[478] Ibid.

[479] Ibid.

[480] Wallace, Robert Keith. "Physiological Effects of Transcendental Meditation." *Science* 167:1751-1754, 1970.

[481] Banquet, Jean-Paul. "Spectral Analysis of the E.E.G. in Meditation." *Electroencephalography and Clinical Neurophysiology* 35:143-151, 1973.

[482] Glueck, Bernard C.; Stroebel, Charles F. Op. Cit.

[483] Ibid.

[484] Ibid.

[485] Ibid.

[486] Ibid.

[487] Ibid.

[488] Ibid.

[489] Lao-Tzu; Mitchell, Stephen (Translation and Commentary). *Tao te Ching*. Harper & Row Publishers, Inc. New York, 1988. P. 42.

End Notes Chapter 9:

[490] Lao-Tzu; Mitchell, Stephen (Translation and Commentary.) *Tao te Ching*. Harper & Rowe Publishers, Inc. New York, 1988. P. 62.

[491] Eppley, Kenneth R.; Abrams, Jonathan Shear. "Differential Effects of Relaxation Techniques on Trait Anxiety: A Meta-Analysis." *Journal of Clinical Psychology* 45:957-974, 1989.

[492] Selye, Hans. *The Stress of Life*. Revised Edition. McGraw-Hill Book Company. New York, 1976.

[493] Forem, Jack. *Transcendental Meditation*. E. P. Dutton & Company, Inc. Introduction. New York, 1973.

[494] Orme-Johnson, David W. (Editor); Farrow, John T. (Editor.) *Scientific Research on the Transcendental Meditation Program: Collected Papers. Volume I.* Maharishi European University Press. Livingston Manor, 1977.

[495] Plato. *Republic, III.* Also: Hare, R. M. *Plato.* Oxford Press. New York, 1982.

[496] Aristotle. *De Anima*. Also: Grene, Marjorie G. *A Portrait of Aristotle.* University of Chicago Press. Chicago, 1979.

[497] Patanjali, Maharishi; Pravananda, Swami (Translation and Commentary); Isherwood, Christopher (Translation and Commentary.) *How To Know God: The Yoga Aphorisms of Patanjali.* New American Library. New York, 1969. Pp. 1-65.

[498] Huang-ti. Huang-ti Nei-Ching Su-wen (*Basic Questions from the Classic Book of Internal Medicine*). Commercial Press. Shanghai, China, 1955.

[499] Darwin, Bernard (Editor.) *The Oxford Dictionary of Quotations.* Oxford Press. New York, 1980. P. 251.

[500] Restak, Richard. *The Brain.* Bantam Books. New York, 1984. P. 343.

[501] Evans-Wentz, W. Y. *Tibetan Yoga and Secret Doctrines.* Oxford University Press. London, 1935.

[502] Lamb, Beatrice Pitney. *India: A World in Transition.* Praeger Publishers. New York, 1971.

[503] Evans-Wentz, W. Y. Op. Cit.

[504] Brosse, Therese. "Psychophysiological Study." *Main Currents in Modern Thought* 4:77-84, 1946.

[505] Bagchi, B. K.; Wenger, M. A. "Electrophysiological Correlates of Some Yogi Exercises." *Electroencephalography and Clinical Neurophysiology, Supplement* 7:132-149, 1957.

[506] Wenger, M. A.; Jones, F. N.; Jones, M. H. *Physiological Psychology*. Henry Holt and Company. New York, 1956.

[507] Das, N. N.; Gastaut, H. "Variation de L'activite Electrique du Cerveau, du Coeur et des Muscles Squelletiques au Cours de la Meditation et L'extase Yogique." *Electroencephalography and Clinical Neurophysiology Supplement* 6:211-219, 1957.

[508] Anand, B. K.; Chhina, G. S.; Singh, B. "Some Aspects of Electroencephalographic Studies on Yogis." *Electroencephalography and Clinical Neurophysiology* 13:452-456, 1961.

[509] Brosse, Therese. *Etude Instrumentale des Techniques du Yoga.* Paris, 1963.

[510] Henrotte, J. G. "Yoga et Biologie." *Atomes.* May 1965. P. 265.

[511] Akishige, Y.: A Historical Survey of the Psychological Studies in Zen. Kyusha Psychological Studies, V, *Bulletin of the Faculty of Literature of the Kyushu University* 11:1-56, 1968.

[512] Kasamatsu, A.; Hitai, T. "An Electroencephalographic Study of the Zen Meditation (Zazen)." *Folio Psychiatry Neurology Japonica* 20:315-336, 1966.

[513] Sugi, Y.; Akutsu, K. "Studies on Respiration and Energy-Metabolism During Sitting in Zazen." *Research Journal of Physical Education* 12:190-206, 1968.

[514] Vakil, R. "Remarkable Feat of Endurance of a Yogi Priest." *Lancet* 2:871, 1950.

[515] Wallace, Robert Keith. *The Maharishi Technology of the Unified Field: The Neurophysiology of Enlightenment.* MIU Neuroscience Press. Maharishi International University, Fairfield, Iowa, 1986. P. 56.

[516] Brena, Steven F. *Yoga and Medicine*. Penguin Books, Inc. New York, 1972.

[517] Sagan, Carl. *Broca's Brain*. Random House. New York, 1979.

[518] Wallace, Robert Keith. "Physiological Effects of Transcendental Meditation." *Science* 167:1751-1754, 1970.

[519] Ibid.

[520] Ibid.

[521] Orme-Johnson, David W. (Editor); Farrow, John T. (Editor.) *Scientific Research on the Transcendental Meditation Program: Collected Papers. Volume I.* Maharishi European University Press. Livingston Manor, 1977.

[522] Rosenthal, Norman E. *Transcendence – Healing and Transformation Through Transcendental Meditation*. The Penguin Group - Jeremy P. Tarcher/Penguin. New York, 2011. P, 258.

[523] Maharishi Foundation USA. The Transcendental Meditation Program Web Site. http://www.tm.org/meditation-techniques

[524] Roth, Robert. *Maharishi Mahesh Yogi's TM: Transcendental Meditation.* Donald I. Fine, Inc. New York, 1987. Pp. 1-2.

[525] McWilliams, Peter. *The TM Book - How to Enjoy the Rest of Your Life.* Warner Books. New York, 1975.

[526] Ibid.

[527] Ibid.

[528] Wallace, Robert Keith. "Physiological Effects of Transcendental Meditation." *Science* 167:1751-1754, 1970.

[529] Wallace, Robert Keith; Benson, Herbert; Wilson, Archie F. "A Wakeful Hypometabolic Physiologic State." *American Journal of Physiology* 221:795-799, 1971.

[530] Wallace, Robert Keith; Benson, Herbert; Wilson, Archie F. "Decreased Blood Lactate During Transcendental Meditation." *Abstract. Federation Proceedings* 30:376, 1971.

[531] Wallace, Robert Keith. "The Physiology of Meditation." *Scientific American* 226:84-90, 1972.

[532] Ibid.

[533] Dhanaraj, V. Hubert; Singh, Mohan. "Reduction in Metabolic Rate During the Practice of the Transcendental Meditation Technique." Ph.D. *Thesis, Department of Physical Education*, University of Alberta, Edmonton, Canada, 1973.

[534] Bakker, Robert. "Decreased Respiratory Rate During the Transcendental Meditation Technique: A Replication." *Scientific Research on the Transcendental Meditation Program. Collected Papers. Volume I.* Maharishi European Research University Press. Livingston Manor, New York, 1977.

[535] Farrow, John T. "Physiological Changes Associated with Transcendental Consciousness, the State of Least Excitation of Consciousness." *Scientific Research on the Transcendental Meditation Program. Collected Papers. Volume I.* Maharishi European Research University Press. Livingston Manor, New York, 1977.

[536] Benson, Herbert; Wallace, Robert Keith. "Decreased Blood Pressure in Hypertensive Subjects Who Practiced Meditation." *Circulation Supplement II to Volumes 45 and 46*:516, 1972.

[537] Simon, David B.; Oparil, Suzanne; Kimball, Chase P. "The Transcendental Meditation Program and Essential Hypertension." *Scientific Research on the Transcendental Meditation Program. Collected Papers. Volume I.* Maharishi European Research University Press. Livingston Manor, New York, 1977.

[538] Blackwell, Barry; Hanenson, Irwin B.; Bloomfield, Saul S.; Magenheim, Herbert G.; Nidich, Sanford I; Gartside, Peter. "Effects of Transcendental Meditation on Blood Pressure: A Controlled Pilot Experiment." *Psychosomatic Medicine* 37(1):86, 1975.

[539] Anderson J.W.; Liu, C; Kryscio, R. J. "Blood Pressure Response to Transcendental Meditation: A Meta-Analysis." *American Journal of Hypertension* 21(3):310-6, 2008.

[540] Brook RD, Appel LJ, Rubenfire M, Ogedegbe G, Bisognano JD, Elliott WJ, Fuchs F, Hughes JW, Lackland DT, Staffileno BA, Townsend RR, Rajagopalan S. "Beyond Medications and Diet: Alternative Approaches to Lowering Blood Pressure. A Scientific Statement from the American Heart Association." *Hypertension* 61(6):1360-1383, 2013

[541] Marwaha, Komal; Schneider, Robert. *Manual of Hypertension of the European Society of Hypertension. Second Edition.* CRC Press. London, 2018.

[542] Zamarra, John W.; Besseghini, Italo; Wittenberg, Stephen. "The Effects of Transcendental Meditation Program on the Exercise Performance of Patients with Angina Pectoris." *Scientific Research on the Transcendental Meditation Program. Collected Papers. Volume I.* Maharishi European Research University Press. Livingston Manor, New York, 1977.

[543] Ibid.

[544] Cooper M. J., et al. "Transcendental Meditation in the Management of Hypercholesterolemia." *Journal of Human Stress* 5(4):24–27, 1979.

[545] Castillo-Richmond A, Schneider RH, Alexander CN, Cook R, Myers H, Nidich S, Haney C, Rainforth M, Salerno J. "Effects of Stress Reduction on Carotid Atherosclerosis in Hypertensive African Americans." *Stroke* 31(3):568-573, 2000

[546] Schneider RH, Grim CE, Rainforth MV, Kotchen T, Nidich SI, Gaylord-King C, Salerno JW, Kotchen JM, Alexander CN. "Stress Reduction in the Secondary Prevention

of Cardiovascular Disease: Randomized, Controlled Trial of Transcendental Meditation and Health Education in Blacks." *Circulation: Cardiovascular Quality and Outcomes* 5(6):750-758, 2012

[547] Transcendental Meditation Health Professionals Web Site. http://www.tm.org/healthpro/research.php September 15, 2018.

[548] Bokhari, S.; Schneider, R.; Salerno, J., Rainforth, M; Gaylord-King, C.; Nidich, S. "Effects of Cardiac Rehabilitation With and Without Meditation on Myocardial Blood Flow Using Quantitative Positron Emission Tomography: A Pilot Study. *Journal of Nuclear Cardiology.* September 16, 2019:1-12 Published online ahead of print.

[549] Rosen, Hugo. *A Clinician's Guide to Affective Disorders.* Second Edition. Mnemosyne Publishing Company. Miami, 1981.

[550] Wallace, Robert Keith; Benson, Herbert; Wilson, Archie F. "Decreased Blood Lactate During Transcendental Meditation." *Abstract. Federation Proceedings* 30:376, 1971.

[551] Karacan, I.; Williams, R. "Insomnia: Old Wine in a New Bottle." *Psychiatric Quarterly* 45:274-288, 1971.

[552] Hinkle, J.; Lutker, E. "Insomnia: A New Approach." *Psychotherapy* 9:236-237, 1972.

[553] Miskiman, Donald E. "The Treatment of Insomnia by the Transcendental Meditation Program." *Scientific Research on the Transcendental Meditation Program. Collected Papers. Volume I.* Maharishi European Research University Press. Livingston Manor, New York, 1977.

[554] Miskiman, Donald E. "The Long-Term Effects of the Transcendental Meditation Program in the Treatment of Insomnia." *Scientific Research on the Transcendental Meditation Program. Collected Papers. Volume I.* Maharishi European Research University Press. Livingston Manor, New York, 1977.

[555] Rosen, Hugo. *A Clinician's Guide to Affective Disorders*. Second Edition. Mnemosyne Publishing Company. Miami, 1981.

[556] Ford, Daniel E.; Kamerwo, Douglas B. "Epidemiologic Study of Sleep Disturbance and Psychiatric Disorders. An Opportunity for Prevention?" *Journal of the American Medical Association* 262(11):1479-1484, 1989.

[557] Cattell, R.; Scheier, I. H. *IPAT Anxiety Scale. Institute for Personality and Ability Testing.* Champaign, Illinois, 1957.

[558] Rosen, Hugo. Op. Cit.

[559] Ross, Jean. "The Effects of the Transcendental Meditation Program on Anxiety, Neuroticism, and Psychoticism." *Scientific Research on the Transcendental Meditation Program. Collected Papers. Volume I.* Maharishi European Research University Press. Livingston Manor, New York, 1977.

[560] Bensen, Herbert; Wallace, Robert Keith. "Decreased Drug Abuse with Transcendental Meditation: A Study of 1,862 Subjects." I in Zarafonetis, Chris J. (Editor). *Drug Abuse: Proceedings of the International Conference.* Lea and Febeiger. Philadelphia, 1972. Pp. 369-376.

[561] Shafii, Mohammad; Lavely, Richard A.; Jaffe, Robert D. "Meditation and Marijuana." *American Journal of Psychiatry* 131:60-63, 1974.

[562] Shafii, Mohammad; Lavely, Richard A.; Jaffe, Robert D. "Meditation and the Prevention of Alcohol Abuse." *American Journal of Psychiatry* 132:942-945, 1975.

[563] Gryczynski, J., Schwartz, R. P., Fishman, M. J., Nordeck, C. D., Grant, J., Nidich, S., et al. (2018). "Integration of Transcendental Meditation® (TM) into Alcohol Use Disorder (AUD) Treatment." *Journal of Substance Abuse* 87:23-30 2018. Epub January 16, 2018.

[564] Banquet, Jean-Paul. "EEG and Meditation." *Electroencephalography and Clinical Neurophysiology* 33:454, 1972.

[565] Banquet, Jean-Paul. "Spectral Analysis of the EEG in Meditation." *Electroencephalography and Clinical Neurophysiology* 35:143-151, 1973.

[566] Banquet, Jean-Paul; Sailhan, Maurice. "EEG Analysis of Spontaneous and Induced States of Consciousness." *Revu d'Electroencephalographie et de Neurophysiologie Clinique* 4:445-453, 1974.

[567] Westcott, Mark. "Hemispheric Symmetry of the EEG During the Transcendental Meditation Technique." *Scientific Research on the Transcendental Meditation Program. Collected Papers. Volume I.* Maharishi European Research University Press. Livingston Manor, New York, 1977.

[568] IBID.

[569] Levine, Paul H.; Herbert, J. Russell; Haynes, Christopher T.; Strobel, Urs. "EEG Coherence During the Transcendental Meditation Technique." *Scientific Research on the Transcendental Meditation Program. Collected Papers. Volume I.* Maharishi European Research University Press. Livingston Manor, New York, 1977.

[570] IBID.

[571] Wallace, Robert Keith; Marcus, Jay B; Clark, Christopher S. *The Coherence Effect.* Armin Lear Press. Estes Park, Colorado, 2020. pp. vii-viii

[572] Nidich, S.; Mills., P.; Rainforth, M.; Heppner, P.; Schneider, R.; Salerno, J.; Gaylord-King, C.; Rutledge, T. "Non-Trauma-Focused Meditation Compared to Exposure Therapy in Veterans with Post-Traumatic Stress Disorder: A Randomized Controlled Trial." *The Lancet Psychiatry* 5(12):975-986. December 2018.

[573] Barnes, Vernon. Editorial. *The Lancet Psychiatry* 5(12):975-986. December 2018.

[574] Nidich, S.; Mills.; P., Rainforth, M.; Heppner, P.; Schneider, R.; Salerno, J.; Gaylord-King, C.; Rutledge, T. "Non-Trauma-Focused Meditation Compared to Exposure Therapy

in Veterans with Post-Traumatic Stress Disorder: A Randomized Controlled Trial." *The Lancet Psychiatry* 5(12):975-986. December 2018.

[574] Barnes, Vernon. Editorial. *The Lancet Psychiatry* 5(12):975-986. December 2018.

[575] Barnes, V. A.; Monto, A.; Williams, J. J.; Rigg, J. L. "Impact of Transcendental Meditation on Psychotropic Medication Use Among Active Duty Military Service Members with Anxiety and PTSD." *Military Medicine* 181(1):56-62, 2016.

[576] Rees, B.; Travis, F.; Shapiro, D.; and Chant, R. "Significant Reductions in Posttraumatic Stress Symptoms in Congolese Refugees after 10 Days Transcendental Meditation Practice." *Journal of Traumatic Stress* 27(1): 112-115, 2014.

[577] Yoshimura, Mitsunobu; Etsuko, Kurokawa; Noda, Takayuki; Hineno, Koji;, Tanaka, Yasuo; Kawai, Yuji; Dillbeck, Michael C. "Disaster Relief for the Japanese Earthquake-Tsunami of 2011: Stress Reduction Through the Transcendental Meditation Technique." *Psychological Reports:Mental & Physical Health* 117(1): 1-11, 2015.

[578] Nidich, S.; O'Connor, T.; Rutledge, T; Duncan, J; Compton, B.; Seng, A.; et al. "Reduced Trauma Symptoms and Perceived Stress in Male Prison Inmates Through the Transcendental Meditation Program: A Randomized Controlled Trial." *The Permanente Journal* 20(4):16-007, 2016.

[579] Nidich, S.; Seng, A.; Compton, B.; O'Connor, T.; Salerno, J. W.; Nidich, R. "Transcendental Meditation and Reduced Trauma Symptoms in Female Inmates: A Randomized Controlled Study." *The Permanente Journal* 21:16-008, 2017.

[580] Loiselle M, et al. "Effect of Transcendental Meditation on Physician Burnout, Depression, and Insomnia: A Randomized Controlled Study." *In preparation for publication*, 2020.

[581] Bonamer, J. R.; Aquino-Russell, C. "Self-Care Strategies for Professional Development: Transcendental Meditation Reduces Compassion Fatigue and Improves Resilience for Nurses." *Journal for Nurses in Professional Development* 35(2):93-97, 2019.

[582] Nidich, S.; Nidich, R. J.; Salerno, J; Hadfield, B; Elder, C. "Stress Reduction with the Transcendental Meditation Program in Caregivers: A Pilot Study." *International Archives of Nursing and Health Care Perspectives* 1(011):1-4, 2015.

[583] Valosek, Laurent; Nidich, Sanford; Wendt, Staci; Grant, Jamie; Nidich, Randi. "Effect of Meditation on Social-Emotional Learning in Middle School Students." *Education* 139(3): 111-119, 2019.

[584] Wendt, S.; Hipps, J.; Abrams, A.; et al. "Practicing Transcendental Meditation in High Schools: Relationship to Well-Being and Academic Achievement Among Students." *Contemporary School Psychology* 19: 312-319. July 22, 2015.

[585] Nidich, S.; Mjasiri, S.; Nidich, R.; Rainforth, M; Grant, J.; Valosek, L.; Chang, W.; Zigler, R. L. "Academic Achievement and Transcendental Meditation: a Study with At-Risk Urban Middle School Students." *Education* 131(3):556-564, 2011.

[586] Colbert, R. D.; Nidich, S. "Effect of the Transcendental Meditation Program on Graduation, College Acceptance and Dropout Rates for Students Attending an Urban Public High School." *Education* 133(4):495-501, 2013.

[587] Ibid.

[588] Travis, F. T.; Haaga, D.; Hagelin, J. S.; Tanner, M.; Nidich, S.I.; King, C.G.; Grosswald, S; Rainforth, M.; Schneider, R.H. "Effects of Transcendental Meditation Practice on Brain Functioning and Stress Reactivity in College Students." *International Journal of Psychophysiology* 71(2):170-6, 2009.

[589] Mahone, Michelle C.; Travis, Fred; Gevirtz, Richard; Hubbard, David. "fMRI during Transcendental Meditation practice." *Brain and Cognition* 123:30-33, 2018.

[590] Klimes-Dougan, Bonnie; Shen Chong, Li; Samikoglu, Ali; Thai, Michelle; Amatya, Palistha; Cullen, Kathryn R.; Lim, Kelvin O. "Transcendental Meditation and Hypothalamic-Pituitary-Adrenal Axis Functioning: A Pilot, Randomized Controlled Trial with Young Adults. Stress: *The International Journal on the Biology of Stress* 23(1):105-115, 2019

[591] Orme-Johnson, David W. "Autonomic Stability and Transcendental Meditation." *Psychosomatic Medicine* 35:341-349, 1973.

[592] Bloomfield, Harold H.; Cain, Michael Peter; Jaffe, Dennis T. *TM: Discovering Inner Energy and Overcoming Stress*. Delacorte Press. New York, 1975.

[593] Web site: "Global Good News: Good News from Around the World. "http://www.transcendental-meditation.globalgoodnews.com

[594] Ibid.

[595] Scientific Research on Maharishi's Transcendental Meditation and TM-Sidhi Programme Volumes 1-7. Maharishi European Research University Press. Netherlands, 1977-2018.

[596] TM Web Site. https://www.tm.org September 15, 2018.

[597] Ibid.

[598] Ibid.

End Notes Chapter 10:

[599] Lao-Tzu; Mitchell, Stephen (Translation and Commentary.) *Tao te Ching*. Harper & Rowe Publishers, Inc. New York, 1988. P. 76.

[600] An original story, so far as I know. Please correct me if I stole it from somewhere I forgot about!

[601] Ibid.

602 Maharishi Mahesh Yogi. *Dawn of the Age of Enlightenment. Volume One 1957-1964: Thirty Years Around the World.* Maharishi Vedic University Press. The Netherlands, 1986. Pp. 177-276.

603 Ibid.

604 Maharishi Mahesh Yogi. *Science of Being and Art of Living.* MIU Press. Fairfield, Iowa, 1979. Pp. 50-59.

605 Maharishi Mahesh Yogi. *The Bhagavad Gita: Chapters 1 - 6. A New Translation and Commentary.* MIU Press. Fairfield, Iowa, 1979.

606 Maharishi Mahesh Yogi. *Science of Being and Art of Living.* MIU Press. Fairfield, Iowa, 1979.

607 Maharishi Mahesh Yogi. *Meditations of Maharishi Mahesh Yogi.* Bantam Books. New York, 1968. Pp. 83-85.

608 Hubel, David H. *The Brain.* A Scientific American Book. W. H. Freeman and Company. New York, 1979. P. 3.

609 Einstein, Albert; Lawson, Robert W. (Translation.) *Relativity. The Special and the General Theory.* Crown Publishers, Inc. New York, 1961.

610 Einstein, Albert. Relativity: *The Special and the General Theory.* Crown Publishers. New York, 1952. Originally published as formal journal publications in 1916.

611 Barnett, Lincoln. *The Universe and Dr. Einstein.* William Morrow and Company. New York, 1948.

612 Maharishi Mahesh Yogi. *Meditations of Maharishi Mahesh Yogi.* Bantam Books. New York, 1968. Pp. 83-85.

613 Maharishi Mahesh Yogi. *Science of Being and Art of Living.* MIU Press. Fairfield, Iowa, 1979. Pp. 50-59.

614 Bloomfield, Harold H.; Cain, Michael Peter; Jaffe, Dennis T. *TM: Discovering Inner Energy and Overcoming Stress.* Delacorte Press. New York, 1975. Pp. 13-18.

615 Ibid.

616 Maharishi Mahesh Yogi. *Science of Being and Art of Living.* MIU Press. Fairfield, Iowa, 1979. P. 43.

617 Ibid. Pp. 43-59.

618 Ibid. P. 43.

619 Ibid. Pp. 119-143.

[620] Ibid. Pp. 188-209.

[621] Maharishi Patanjali; Swami Prabhavananda (Translation and Commentary); Isherwood, Christopher (Translation and Commentary). *How to Know God - The Yoga Aphorisms of Patanjali.* New American Library. New York, 1953. P. vii.

[622] Ibid. Pp. 14-20.

[623] Ibid.

[624] Ibid.

[625] Ibid.

[626] Ibid.

[627] Bloomfield, Harold H.; Cain, Michael Peter; Jaffe, Dennis T. Op. Cit. Pp. 23-26.

[628] Ibid. Pp. 13-20.

[629] Ibid.

[630] Ibid.

[631] Maharishi Mahesh Yogi. *Meditations of Maharishi Mahesh Yogi.* Bantam Books. New York, 1968. Pp. 77-78.

[632] Benson, Herbert. *The Relaxation Response.* Avon Books. New York, 1976.

[633] Benson, Herbert. Ibid. P. 83.

[634] Wallace, Robert Keith; Benson, Herbert; Wilson, Archie F. "A Wakeful Hypometabolic Physiologic State." *American Journal of Physiology* 221:795-799, 1971.

[635] Wallace, Robert Keith; Benson, Herbert; Wilson, Archie F. "Decreased Blood Lactate During Transcendental Meditation." *Abstract. Federation Proceedings* 30:376, 1971.

[636] Benson, Herbert; Wallace, Robert Keith. "Decreased Blood Pressure in Hypertensive Subjects Who Practiced Meditation." *Circulation Supplement II to Volumes 45 and 46*:516, 1972.

[637] Benson, Herbert; Wallace, Robert Keith. "Decreased Drug Abuse with Transcendental Meditation: A Study of 1,862 Subjects," in Zarafonetis, Chris J. (Editor.) *Drug Abuse: Proceedings of the International Conference.* Lea and Febeiger. Philadelphia, 1972. Pp. 369-376.

[638] Benson, Herbert. *The Relaxation Response.* Avon Books. New York, 1976.

[639] Ibid. Pp. 98-99.

[640] Ibid. Pp 76-140.

[641] Ibid. Pp. 161-163.

[642] Benson, H.; Rosner, B. A.; Marzetta, B. R.; Klemchuck, H. M. "Decreased Blood Pressure in Pharmacologically Treated Hypertensive Patients Who Regularly Elicited the Relaxation Response." *Lancet* I:289-291, 1974.

[643] Wallace, Robert Keith. "The Physiology of Meditation." *Scientific American* 226:84-90, 1972.

[644] Banquet, Jean-Paul. "EEG and Meditation." *Electroencephalography and Clinical Neurophysiology* 33:454, 1972.

[645] Benson, Herbert. *The Relaxation Response*. Avon Books. New York, 1976.

[646] Ibid.

[647] Ibid. Pp. 161-163.

[648] Orme-Johnson, David W. "Autonomic Stability and Transcendental Meditation." *Psychosomatic Medicine* 35:341-349, 1973.

[649] Glueck, Bernard C.; Stroebel, Charles F. "Biofeedback and Meditation in the Treatment of Psychiatric Illnesses." *Comprehensive Psychiatry* 16(4):303-321, 1975.

[650] White, Abraham; Handler, Philip; Smith, Emil l. *Principles of Biochemistry.* Fifth Edition. McGraw-Hill Book Company. New York, 1973. P. 2 and P. 252.

[651] Ibid.

[652] Bloomfield, Harold H.; Cain, Michael Peter; Jaffe, Dennis T. Op. Cit.. Pp. 10-33.

[653] Ibid. Pp. 18-19.

[654] Ibid.

[655] Ibid.

[656] Roberts, Bertram W.; Forester, Wilbur E. "Group Relaxation - Acute and Chronic Benefits on Essential Hypertension." *Cardiovascular Medicine.* May 1979. Pp. 575-580.

[657] Ibid.

[658] Williams, Mark; Penman, Danny. *Mindfulness – An Eight Week Plan for Finding Peace in a Frantic World.* Rodale, Inc. New York, 2011. Pp. x-xi.

[659] Dillbeck, M. C.; Orme-Johnson, D. W. “Physiological Differences Between Transcendental Meditation and Rest.” *American Psychologist* 42:879-881, 1987. See also: Alexander, C. N.; Rainforth, M. V.; Gelderloos, P. “Transcendental Meditation, Self-Actualization, and Psychological Health: A Conceptual Overview and Statistical Meta-Analysis.” *Journal of Social Behavior and Personality* 6(5):189-247, 1987.

[660] Orme-Johnson, D. W. and Barnes, V. A. "Effects of the Transcendental Meditation Technique on Trait Anxiety: A Meta-Analysis of Randomized Controlled Trials." *Journal of Alternative and Complementary Medicine* 20(5):330-41, 2013.

[661] Hofmann, S. G., Sawyer, A. T., Witt, A. A., and Oh, D. "The Effect of Mindfulness-Based Therapy on Anxiety and Depression: A Meta-Analytic Review." *Journal of Consulting and Clinical Psychology* 78(2):169-183, 2010.

[662] Sedlmeier, P., Eberth, J., Schwarz, M., Zimmermann, D., and Haarig, F. "The Psychological Effects of Meditation: A Meta-Analysis." *Psychological Bulletin* 138(6):1139-1171, 2012.

[663] Maharishi Foundation USA (MFUSA), Web Site http://www.tm.org/meditation-techniques

[664] Roth, Robert. *Maharishi Mahesh Yogi's TM: Transcendental Meditation.* Donald I. Fine, Inc. New York, 1987. Pp. 1-5.

[665] Kroll, Una. *The Healing Potential of Transcendental Meditation.* John Knox Press. Atlanta, 1974: Pp. 20-23.

[666] Oates, Jr., Robert M. *Celebrating the Dawn.* G. P. Putnam's Sons. New York, 1976. P. 102.

[667] Kroll, Una. Op. Cit.

[668] Oates, Jr., Robert M. Op. Cit. P. 108.

End Notes Chapter 11:

[669] Knechtges, David R. "Chinese Language." *The World Book Encyclopedia.* World Book, Inc. Chicago, 1988. Volume 3. Pp. 509-511.

[670] Ibid.

[671] Thorpe, Robert G. "Psychodynamics of Stress and Relationships with the Musculoskeletal System." *Clinical Review Series. Osteopathic Medicine.* Publishing Sciences Group, Inc. Acton, Massachusetts, 1975.

[672] Purves, Dale. *Body and Brain.* Harvard University Press. Cambridge, Massachusetts, 1988. Pp. 1-16; 169-175.

[673] Romer, Alfred Sherwood. "Who's Who Among the Vertebrates." *The Vertebrate Body. Shorter Version.* Fourth Edition. W. B. Saunders Company. Philadelphia, 1971. Pp. 30-76.

[674] Buzzell, Keith A. "The Cost of Human Posture and Locomotion." *The Physiological Basis of Osteopathic Medicine.* The Postgraduate Institute of Osteopathic Medicine and Surgery. New York, 1970. Pp. 63-72.

[675] Bates, Marston. "Human Evolution." *Man in Nature*. Prentice- Hall, Inc. Eaglewood Cliffs, New Jersey, 1964.

[676] Schmidt, Robert F. (Editor). *Fundamentals of Neurophysiology*. Springer-Verlag. New York, 1978. Pp. 129-211.

[677] Ibid.

[678] Schwarzenegger, Arnold; Bobbins, Bill. *The New Encyclopedia of Modern Bodybuilding*. Fireside Books Simon & Shuster. New York, 1998. Pp. 56-83.

[679] Schmidt, Robert F. (Editor). Op. Cit..

[680] Ibid.

[681] Eisenberg, Robert S. "Human Body." *The World Book Encyclopedia*. Chicago, 1987. Volume 9. P. 404.

[682] Selye, Hans. *The Stress of Life*. McGraw-Hill Book Company. New York, 1976. Pp. 369-461.

[683] Thorpe, Robert G. "Psychodynamics of Stress and Relationships with the Musculoskeletal System." *Clinical Review Series: Osteopathic Medicine*. Publishing Science Group, Inc. Acton, Massachusetts, 1975. Pp. 1-8.

[684] Selye, Hans. Op. Cit., P. 424.

[685] Guyton, Arthur C. *Textbook of Medical Physiology*. Fourth Edition. W. B. Saunders Company. Philadelphia, 1971. Pp. 546-590.

[686] Thorpe, Robert G. "Psychodynamics of Stress and Relationships with the Musculoskeletal System." *Clinical Review Series: Osteopathic Medicine*. Publishing Science Group, Inc. Acton, Massachusetts, 1975. Pp. 1-8.

[687] Selye, Hans. *The Stress of Life*. McGraw-Hill Book Company. New York, 1976. Pp. 369-461.

[688] Bhattacharya, A. “Costs of Occupational Musculoskeletal Disorders (MSDs) in the United States.” *International Journal of Industrial Ergonomics* 44(3):448-454, 2014.

[689] Nachemson, A. L. "Low Back Pain: Its Etiology and Treatment." *Clinical Medicine* 78:18, 1971.

[690] Pope, Thomas L.; Riddervold, Hans O. "Low-Back Pain: When to Get Spine Films." *Diagnosis*. June 1982. Pp. 71-87.

[691] Barton, J. E.; Haight, R. O.; Marsland, D. W.; et al. "Low Back Pain in the Primary Care Setting." *Journal of Family Practice* 3:363, 1976.

[692] Pope, Thomas L. Op. Cit.

[693] Shields, Christopher B.; Williams, Phillip E. "Low Back Pain." *American Family Practice* 33(3):173-182, 1986.

[694] Lucas, P. R. "Low Back Pain." *Surgical Clinics of North America* 63:515-528, 1983.

[695] *Provider Bulletin* # 93-11. Bureau of Workers' Compensation. Columbus, Ohio. April 1993.

[696] *United States Department of Labor. Bureau of Labor Statistics. Databases, Tables & Calculators by Subject.* CPI Inflation Calculator. http://www.bls.gov/data/inflation_calculator.htm and Arrepin. Current to Real Dollars Converter (using GDP deflator). http://stats.areppim.com/calc/calc_usdlrxdeflator.php

[697] Boachie-Adjei, Oheneba. "Evaluation of the Patient with Low Back Pain." *Postgraduate Medicine* 84(3):111-119, 1988.

[698] Ibid.

[699] Shields, Christopher B.; Williams, Phillip E. "Low Back Pain." *American Family Practice* 33(3):173-182, 1986.

[700] Kunkel, Robert S. "Headache and the Neck." *Pain Management* 2(2):119-123, 1990.

[701] Appenzeller, O. "Headache. Clinical and Pathologic Aspects." *Advanced Pain Research and Therapy* 3:345-48, 1979. In Proceedings of the Second World Congress on Pain. Raven Press. New York, 1979.

[702] Kunkel, Robert S., Op. Cit..

[703] Stellar, Stanley; Ahrens, Suzanne P.; Meibohm, Anne R.; Reines, Scott A. "Migraine Prevention with Timolol." *Journal of the American Medical Association* 252(18):2576-2580, 1984.

[704] The American Osteopathic Association and the American College of Osteopathic Family Physicians prefers the term Osteopathic Manipulative Treatment to Osteopathic Manipulative Therapy. This is to avoid confusion between Osteopathic Physician's techniques and other modalities such as Physical Therapy. I choose to use the term Manipulative Therapy as a term that includes Osteopathic Manipulative Treatment with all other modalities of manual medicine, including Physical and Occupational Therapy, Chiropractic, Massage Therapy, and other musculoskeletal treatment modalities.

[705] Gevintz, Norman. *The D.O.'s - Osteopathic Medicine in America.* The Johns Hopkins University Press. Baltimore, 1982. Pp. 94-98.

[706] At the American Medical Association Web site: https://wire.ama-assn.org/life-career/what-its-be-sports-medicine-shadowing-dr-vasudevan

[707] Greenman, Philip E. *Principles of Manual Medicine.* Williams & Wilkins. Baltimore, 1989. P. vii.

[708] Smolan, Rick; Moffitt, Phillip; Naythons, Matthews. *The Power to Heal.* Ancient Arts and Modern Medicine. Prentice Hall Press. New York, 1990. P.46.

[709] Grun, Bernard; Stein, Werner. *The Timetables of History.* Simon and Schuster, Inc. New York, 1979. Pp. 1-15.

[710] Ibid.

[711] Greenman, Phillip E., Op. Cit..

[712] Bourdillon, J. F. *Spinal Manipulation.* William Heinemann Medical Books Limited. London, 1973. P. 1.

[713] Evans, Mary. "Barber." *The World Book Encyclopedia.* World Book, Inc. Chicago, 1988. Volume 2. P. 106.

[714] Bourdillon, J. F., Op. Cit., Pp. 1-13.

[715] Greenman, Phillip E., Op. Cit.

[716] Ibid.

[717] Greenman, Phillip E., Op. Cit.

[718] Paget, Sir James. "Cases That Bone-Setters Cure." *British Medical Journal* 1:1-4, 1867.

[719] Bourdillon, J. F., Op. Cit.. Pp. 2-8.

[720] Bourdillon, J. F., Op. Cit.. Pp. 2-8.

[721] Still, Andrew Taylor. *Autobiography of A. T. Still.* Published by the Author. Kirksville, Missouri, 1897.

[722] Greenman, Phillip E., Op. Cit..

[723] "Commission on Osteopathic Accreditation Colleges of Osteopathic Medicine." September 10, 2014. American Osteopathic Association. Chicago, 2014. http://www.osteopathic.org/inside-aoa/accreditation/predoctoral%20accreditation/Documents/current-list-of-colleges-of-osteopathic-medicine.pdf

[724] DeRosier, Andrea; Lischka, Terri A.; Martinez, Bulmaro. "Appendix 1: Osteopathic Medical Education 2014." *Journal of the American Osteopathic Association* 114(4):299-303. April 2014. Osteopathic Medical Education Issue

[725] Caleel, G. T., D.O. "The Legacy and the Challenge." *Osteopathic Annals* 13(7):264-268, 1985.

[726] "Commission on Osteopathic Accreditation Colleges of Osteopathic Medicine." September 10, 2014. American Osteopathic Association. Chicago, 2014. http://www.osteopathic.org/inside-

aoa/accreditation/predoctoral%20accreditation/Documents/current-list-of-colleges-of-osteopathic-medicine.pdf

[727] American Osteopathic Association. "Osteopathic Medical Profession Report." *The D.O.* December 2007. Pp. 1-20.

[728] Gross, Cheryl; Bell, Elaine. "Appendix 3: AOA Specialty Board Certification." *Journal of the American Osteopathic Association* 114(4):313-316, 2014. Osteopathic Medical Education Issue

[729] Bourdillon, J. F., Op. Cit.. Pp. 1-13.

[730] Greenman, Phillip E., Op. Cit..

[731] Dintenfass, Julius. *Chiropractic - A Modern Way to Health.* Pyramid Books. New York, 1970. Pp. 36-37.

[732] Bourdillon, J. F., Op. Cit.. Pp. 1-13.

[733] Greenman, Phillip E., Op. Cit..

[734] Wardwell, Walter I. *Chiropractic – History and Evolution of a New Profession.* Mosby Yearbook. St. Louis, 1992. "Chapter 4. The Palmers and Their Fountainhead School." Pp. 51-84.

[735] Gatterman, Meridel I. Foundations of Chiropractic – Subluxations. Mosby Yearbook. St. Louis, 1995.

[736] Greenman, Phillip E. Op. Cit..

[737] Wardwell, Walter I. *Chiropractic – History and Evolution of a New Profession.* Mosby Year Book. St. Louis, 1992. "Chapter 14. The Future of Chiropractic." Pp. 275-287.

[738] Ibid.

End Notes Chapter 12:

[739] Substance Abuse and Mental Health Services Administration. "Opioids." https://www.samhsa.gov/atod/opioids. January 20, 2018.

[740] United States Committee on Finance. Newsroom/Chairman's Views. "Hatch Calls on Senate to Support Historic Opioid Legislation." July 12, 2016. https://www.finance.senate.gov/chairmans-news/hatch-calls-on-senate-to-support-historic-opioid-legislation January 20, 2018.

[741] Dowell, Deborah; Arias, Elizabeth; Kochanek, Kenneth; Anderson, Robert; Guy, Jr., Gery P.; Losby, Jan L.; Baldwin, Grant. "Research Letter. Contribution of Opioid-Involved Poisoning to the Change in Life Expectancy in the United States, 2000-2015." *Journal of the American Medical Association* 318(11):1065-1067, 2017.

[742] Democratic Staff of the Senate Committee on Finance. "Dying Waiting for Treatment: The Opioid Use Disorder Treatment Gap and the Need for Funding." October 10, 2016.

https://www.finance.senate.gov/media/doc/110116%20Opioid%20Treatment%20Gap%20Report%20Final.pdf. January 20, 2018.

743 Sullivan, Michele G. "Opioid Deaths and Suicides. Twin Tragedies that Need a Communitywide Response." *Family Practice News* 47(17):1 and 4. October 15, 2017.

744 CDC National Center for Health Statistics Reported in *American Medical News* 52(7):1, 2009.

745 Drug Overdose Death Rates | National Institute on Drug Abuse (NIDA). https://nida.nih.gov/research-topics/trends-statistics/overdose-death-rates

746 Bohnert, Amy S. B.; Valenstein, Marcia; Bair, Matthew J.; Ganoczy, Dara; McCarthy, John F.; Ilgen, Mark A.; Blow, Frederick C. "Association Between Opioid Prescribing Patterns and Opioid Overdose-Related Deaths." *Journal of the American Medical Association* 305(13), 2011.

747 Twillman, Robert K.; Kirch, Rebecca; Gilson, Aaron. "Efforts to Control Prescription Drug Abuse: Why Clinicians Should Be Concerned and Take Action as Essential Advocates for Rational Policy." *CA: A Journal for Clinicians* 64(6):369-376, 2014.

748 Staff Writer. "Insurers, PBMs Asked to Help Staunch Nation's Raging Opioid Epidemic." *Managed Care* 26(9):6, 2017.

749 Martin, Keith L. "Physicians – Not the Government – Should Lead Fight Against Opioid Abuse." *Medical Economics* 94(18):1, 2017.

750 Prinsen, Joseph K.; Hensel, Kendi L.; Snow, Richard J. "OMT Associated with Reduced Analgesic Prescribing and Fewer Missed Workdays in Patients with Low Back Pain: An Observational Study." *Journal of the American Osteopathic Association* 114(2):90-98, 2014.

751 Abbasi, Jennifer. "As Opioid Epidemic Rages, Complementary Health Approaches to Pain Gain Traction." *Journal of the American Medical Association* 316(22):2343-2344, 2016. Published Online December 13, 2016.
Doi:10.1001/jama.2016.15029
http://jamanetwork.com/journals/jama/fullarticle/2579926

752 Association of American Medical Colleges Web site. "Active Physicians in the Largest Specialties, 2015."
https://www.aamc.org/data/workforce/reports/458480/1-1-chart.html January 15, 2018.

753 Osteopathic Medical Profession Report: 2017. American Osteopathic Association. 142 East Ontario Street. Chicago, Illinois 60611-2864. American Osteopathic Association Masterfile Data, January 20, 2018.
http://www.osteopathic.org/inside-aoa/about/aoa-annual-statistics/Pages/default.aspx

754 Northup, George W. *Osteopathic Medicine: An American Reformation*. American Osteopathic Association. Chicago, 1966. Pp. 1-75.

755 Ibid.

[756] Ibid. Pp. 1-50.

[757] Ibid. Pp. 1-75.

[758] Ibid. Pp. 1-50.

[759] Ibid. Pp. 1-75.

[760] Shearer, Alistair; Russell, Peter (Translation and Commentary). *The Upanishads.* Harper Colophon Books. Harper & Row, Publishers. New York, 1978. P. 12.

[761] Still, A. T. *Philosophy of Osteopathy.* Published by A. T. Still. Kirksville, Missouri, 1899. P. 28.

[762] Lao-Tzu; Mitchell, Stephen (Translation and Commentary). *Tao te Ching.* Harper & Row, Publishers. New York, 1988. P. 64.

[763] Northup, George., Op. Cit., Pp. 1-75.

[764] Still, A. T., Op. Cit., P. 51.

[765] Northup, George., Op. Cit., P. 27.

[766] Still, A. T., Op. Cit., P. 197.

[767] Ibid. P. 41.

[768] Ibid.

[769] Still, A. T., Op. Cit., Pp. 165-166.

[770] Gray, Henry; Goss, Charles Mayo (Editor). *Anatomy of the Human Body.* Lea & Feiber. Philadelphia, 1975. Pp. 527-560.

[771] Still, A. T., Op. Cit., P. 153.

[772] Ibid. P. 76.

[773] Ibid.

[774] Ibid. Pp. 49-50.

[775] Ibid. P. 168.

[776] Sutherland, Adah Strand. *With Thinking Fingers: The Story of William Garner Sutherland, D.O., D.Sc.* (Hon.). The Cranial Academy. Kansas City, Missouri, 1962. P. 11. Dr. Still was affectionately called "The Old Doctor" in his later years by family, friends, faculty, students, and colleagues.

[777] Ibid. Pp. 12-13.

[778] Ibid. P. 25.

[779] Sutherland, William G. T*he Cranial Bowl: A Treatise Relating to Cranial Articular Mobility, Cranial Articular Lesions, and Cranial Technic.* Free Press Company. Mankato, Minnesota, 1939. Pp. 24-25.

[780] Ibid.

[781] Ibid. P. 28.

[782] Ibid. Pp. 22-26.

[783] Kappler, Robert. "Osteopathy in the Cranial Field. Its History, Scientific Basis, and Current Status." *The Osteopathic Physician.* February 1979. Pp. 13-18.

[784] Magoun, Harold Ives. *Osteopathy in the Cranial Field.* Third Edition. The Journal Printing Company. Kirksville, Missouri, 1976. Pp. 23-25.

[785] Ibid. Pp. 32-35.

[786] Merritt, John L.; McLean, Timothy J.; Erickson, Rolland P.; Offord, Kenneth P. "Measurement of Trunk Flexibility in Normal Subjects: Reproducibility of Three Clinical Methods." *Mayo Clinic Proceedings* 61:192-197, 1986.

[787] Fisk, J. W. "The Straight Leg Raising Test: Its Relevance to Possible Disc Pathology." *New Zealand Medical Journal* 81:557-560, 1975.

[788] Thornton, Shannon N. "The Fast but Thorough Musculoskeletal Exam." *Aches and Pains.* May 1982. Pp. 14-19.

[789] Dinnar, Uri; Beal, Myron C.; Goodridge, John P.; Johnston, William L.; Karni, Zvi; Mitchell, Frederic L. Jr.; Upledger, John E.; McConnell, David G. "Description of Fifty Diagnostic Tests Used with Osteopathic Manipulation." *Journal of the American Osteopathic Association* 81(5):314-321, 1982.

[790] Magoun, Harold I. Jr. "Before Manipulation: Thorough Screening." *Osteopathic Symposium* 2(6):6-7, 1974.

[791] Cathie, Angus G. "The Interpretation of Asymmetry of the Bony Landmarks of the Pelvis." *American Academy of Osteopathy 1974 Yearbook. Papers Selected from the Writings and Lectures of Angus G. Cathie, D.O.*, M.Sc. (Anatomy), F.A.A.O. (1902-1970).

[792] Johnston, W. L. "Passive Gross Motion Testing: Part I. Its Role in Physical Examination." *Journal of the American Osteopathic Association* 81(5)298-303, 1982.

[793] Adams, Thomas; Steinmetz, Michael A.; Heisey, S. Richard; Holmes, Kenneth R.; Greenman, Philip E. "Physiologic Basis for Skin Properties in Palpatory Physical Diagnosis." *Journal of the American Osteopathic Association* 81(6):366-377, 1982.

[794] Johnston, William L.; Hill, James L. "Spinal Segmental Dysfunction: Incidence in Cervicothoracic Region." *Journal of the American Osteopathic Association* 81(11):67-76, 1981.

[795] Zink, J. Gordon; Fetchik, William D.; Lawson, William B. "The Posterior Axillary Folds: A Gateway for Osteopathic Treatment of the Upper Extremities." *Osteopathic Annals* 9(3):114-117, 1981.

[796] Heilig, David. "Some Basic Considerations of Spinal Curves." *Osteopathic Annals* 6(7):43-53, 1978.

[797] Miller, Herbert C. "Head Pain." *Journal of the American Osteopathic Association* 72:75-83, 1972.

[798] Becker, Alan R. "Parameters of Resistance." *Journal of the American Osteopathic Association* 73:117-129, 1973.

[799] Beal, Myron C.; Goodridge, John P.; Johnston, William L. "Inter-Examiner Agreement of Patient Improvement." 1979 *American Osteopathic Association Research Conference.* March 15-17, Chicago, Illinois.

[800] Allen, Thomas W.; Kelso, Albert F. "Osteopathic Research and Respiratory Disease." *Journal of the American Osteopathic Association.* 81(1):350, 1981.

[801] De Bias, D. A.; Greene, S. H.; Helig, D.; Nicholas, A. S.; Harrer, W. V. "A Somatic Component of Experimental Myocardial Infarction." *Journal of the American Osteopathic Association* 85(10):752, 1985.

[802] Johnson, William L.; Hill, James L.; Elkiss, Mitchell L.; Marino, Ronald V. "Identification of Stable Somatic Findings in Hypertensive Subjects by Trained Examiners Using Palpatory Examination." *Journal of the American Osteopathic Association* 81(12):830-836, 1982.

[803] Rooney, Theodore W. "Musculoskeletal Manifestations Associated with Malignancy." *Osteopathic Annals* 11(10):437-442, 1983.

[804] Lerch, G. L.; Marino, R. V. "Diagnostic Techniques for Congenital Hip Disease: Reliability and Interexaminer Agreement." *Journal of the American Osteopathic Association* 85(8):528-531, 1985.

[805] Upledger, John E.; Vredevoogd, Jon D.; Retzlaff, Ernest; Raynesford, Alice K.; Howard, Thomas F. "Autistic Children: Preliminary Physiologic, Structural, and Craniosacral Evaluations." *Journal of the American Osteopathic Association* 79(2):123, 1979.

[806] Lane, Stanley L. "Diagnosing and Treating Temporomandibular Joint Dysfunction." *Patient Care.* November 15, 1980. Pp. 100-101.

[807] Magoun, Harold I. "Whiplash Injury: A Greater Lesion Complex." *Journal of the American Osteopathic Association* 63(6): 524-535, 1964.

[808] Nicholas, Nicholas S. "Traumatic Somatic Dysfunction of the Knee." *Journal of the American Osteopathic Association* 72:96-116, 1973.

[809] Lao-Tzu; Mitchell, Stephen (Translation and Commentary). *Tao te Ching*. Harper & Row, Publishers. New York, 1988. P. 39.

[810] Osteopathic Medicine Report: 2017. American Osteopathic Association. 142 East Ontario Street. Chicago, Illinois 60611-2864. American Osteopathic Association Masterfile Data, January 20, 2018.
http://www.osteopathic.org/inside-aoa/about/aoa-annual-statistics/Pages/default.aspx

[811] Association of American Medical Colleges Web site. "Active Physicians in the Largest Specialties, 2015." January 15, 2018.
https://www.aamc.org/data/workforce/reports/458480/1-1-chart.html.

[812] Osteopathic Medical Profession Report: 2023. American Osteopathic Association. 142 East Ontario Street. Chicago, Illinois 60611-2864. January, 2023.

[813] Michael H. I. Borger, D.O. Personal recollection of conversations with patients over forty years of medical practice.

[814] Osteopathic Medicine Report: 2017. American Osteopathic Association. 142 East Ontario Street. Chicago, Illinois 60611-2864. American Osteopathic Association Masterfile Data, January 20, 2018.
http://www.osteopathic.org/inside-aoa/about/aoa-annual-statistics/Pages/default.aspx

[815] Based on American Osteopathic Association statistics. Direct Mail Advertisement. Celebrating 100 Years of Osteopathic Medicine. Sandoz Pharmaceuticals Corporation. East Hanover, New Jersey. Mailed February 1992.

[816] Davis, Glenn E.; Hartwig, Walter Carl; Riemer, Richard B.; Char, Chandra; McTighe, Adam; Kremelberg, David. "Assessing Patient Experience of the Tenets of Osteopathic Medicine." *Journal of Osteopathic Medicine 123*(8): 371-378. May 16, 2023.

End Notes Chapter 13:

[817] "X-ray" and "Roentgen or Röentgen, Wilhelm Conrad." Articles. *The Concise Columbia Encyclopedia*. Columbia University Press. New York, 1989.

[818] Northup, George W. *Osteopathic Medicine: An American Reformation.* American Osteopathic Association. Chicago, 1966.

[819] Staff Writer. "Infirmary Improvements." *Journal of Osteopathy* 5(5):259, 1898.

[820] Littlejohn, D. "X-Radiance." *Journal of Osteopathy* 5(6):274- 276, 1898.

[821] Staff Writer. "Notes." *Journal of Osteopathy* 5(7):357, 1898.

[822] Smith, W. "Skiagraphy and the Circulation. First Delineation of the Arterial System with X-rays Achieved by the American School of Osteopathy." *Journal of Osteopathy* 5(8):364-378, 1899.

[823] Staff Writer. "Infirmary Items." *Journal of Osteopathy* 5(10):492, 1899.

[824] Still, Andrew T.: *Philosophical and Mechanical Principles of Osteopathy.* Hudson-Kimberly Publishing Company. Kansas City, 1902.

[825] Beilke, M.C. "Roentgenological Spinal Analysis and the Technic for Taking Standing X-ray Plates." *Journal of the American Osteopathic Association* 35:414-418, 1936.

[826] Hoskins, E.R. "The Development of Posture and its Importance: Short Leg." *Journal of the American Osteopathic Association* 33(11):125, 1934.

[827] Beilke, M.C. "Roentgenological Spinal Analysis and the Technic for Taking Standing X-ray Plates." *Journal of the American Osteopathic Association* 35:414-418, 1936.

[828] Rush, W.A.; Steiner, H.A. "A Study of Lower Extremity Length Inequality." *American Journal of Roentgenology, Radium Therapy, and Nuclear Medicine* 56(5):616-623, 1946.

[829] Judovich, B.; Bates, W. *Pain Syndromes.* Fourth Edition. F.A. Davis Company. Philadelphia, 1953.

[830] Denslow, J.S.; Chace, J.A.; Gutensohn, O.R.; Kumm, M.G. "Methods in Taking and Interpreting Weight-Bearing X-ray Films." *Journal of the American Osteopathic Association* 54(11):109-118,1955.

[831] Ibid.

[832] Denslow, J. S.; Beal, Myron C. (Editor). *1993 Yearbook of the American Academy of Osteopathy. Selected Papers of John Stedman Denslow, D.O.* P. v. The American Academy of Osteopathy. Indianapolis, 1993.

[833] Ibid.

[834] I am very proud that my late uncle, Donald R. Hinton, D.O., served as a laboratory assistant for Dr. I. M. Korr at Kirksville College of Osteopathic Medicine when he was a medical student there in the late 1940s. Dr. Hinton assisted Dr. Korr with sensor and wire lead placement on patients while performing the research that proved segmental somatic dysfunction – in other words the distribution of stress effects throughout the body via the spinal cord, cranial nerves, and segmental innervation. That is like being Thomas Edison's laboratory assistant when Edison discovered the light bulb filament that worked. Wow!

[835] Denslow, J.S.; Clough, G.H. "Reflex Activity in the Spinal Extensors." *Journal of Neurophysiology* 4:430-437, 1941.

[836] Denslow, J.S.; Hassett, C.C. "The Central Excitatory State Associated with Postural Abnormalities." *Journal of Neurophysiology* 5:393-402, 1942.

[837] Denslow, J. S. "An Analysis of the Variability of Spinal Reflex Thresholds." *Journal of Neurophysiology.* 7:207-215, 1944.

[838] Denslow, J. S. "Double Discharges in Human Motor Units." *Journal of Neurophysiology* 11: 50-54, 1948.

[839] Denslow, J. S.; Gutensohn, Olwen R. "Neuromuscular Reflexes in Response to Gravity. *Journal of Applied Physiology* 23(2):243-247, 1967.

[840] Denslow, J. S. "An Analysis of the Variability of Spinal Reflex Thresholds." *Journal of Neurophysiology* 7:207-215, 1944.

[841] Peterson, Barbara. "Editor's Forward." *The Collected Papers of Irvin M. Korr. American Academy of Osteopathy*. Colorado Springs, Colorado, 1979. Pp. 5-6.

[842] Denslow, J. S.; Korr, I. M.; Krems, A. D. "Quantitative Studies of Chronic Facilitation in Human Motoneuron Pools." *The American Journal of Physiology* 150(2):43-49, 1947.

[843] Korr, I. M. "The Neural Basis of the Osteopathic Lesion." *Journal of the American Osteopathic Association* 47:191-198, 1947.

[844] Extracted from Korr, Irvin M. "Preface." *The Collected Papers of Irvin M. Korr. American Academy of Osteopathy*. Colorado Springs, Colorado, 1979. Pp. 7-8.

[845] Korr, Irvin M.; Thomas, Price E. "The Automatic Recording of Electrical Skin Resistance Patterns on the Human Trunk." *EEG Clinical Neurophysiology* 3:361-368, 1951.

[846] Thomas, Price E.; Korr, Irvin M. "Relationship Between Sweat Gland Activity and Electrical Resistance of the Skin. *Journal of Applied Physiology* 10(3):505-510, 1957.

[847] Korr, Irvin M.; Goldstein, Martin J. "Dermatomal Autonomic Activity in Relation to Segmental Motor Reflex Threshold." *Federation Proceedings* 7:67, 1948.

[848] Korr, Irvin M. "Skin Resistance Patterns Associated with Visceral Disease." *Federation Proceedings* 8:87, 1949.

[849] Sherwood, Lauralee. *Human Physiology: From Cells to Systems.* CENGAGE Learning. New York, 2016.

[850] Ibid.

[851] Watson, P. E.; Watson, I. D., Batt, R. D. "Total Body Water Volumes for Adult Males and Females Estimated from Simple Anthropometric Measurements." *American Journal of Clinical Nutrition*. 33(1):27-29, 1980.

[852] Elzenberg, Norman. *General Anatomy: Principles and Applications.* McGraw-Hill Medical; 2nd edition. New York, 2007. P. 70

[853] Still, A. T. *Philosophy of Osteopathy*. Published by Andrew Taylor Still. Kirksville, Missouri, 1899. P. 41.

[854] Paul, John. R. A History of Poliomyelitis. Pp. 16-18. Yale *Studies in the History of Science and Medicine*. New Haven, Connecticut, 1971.

[855] Aylward, R. B. "Eradicating Polio: Today's Challenges and Tomorrow's Legacy." *Annals of Tropical Medicine and Parasitology* 100(5-6):401-413, 2006.

[856] Hamborsky, J. and Kroger, A. Editors. "Poliomyelitis." *Epidemiology and Prevention of Vaccine-Preventable Diseases.* 13th Edition. Communication and Education Branch, National Center for Immunization and Respiratory Diseases, Centers for Disease Control and Prevention. Washington, D.C, 2015.

[857] Korr, Irvin M. "The Trophic Functions of Nerves and Their Mechanisms." *Journal of the American Osteopathic Association* 72(2):163-171, 1972 reprinted in The Collected Papers of Irvin M. Korr. American Academy of Osteopathy. Colorado Springs, 1979.

[858] Ibid.

[859] Korr, I. M. "The Spinal Cord as Organizer of Disease Processes: IV. Axonal Transport and Neurotrophic Function in Relation to Somatic Dysfunction." *Journal of the American Osteopathic Association* 80(7):451-459, 1981.

[860] Korr, Irvin M. "Neurochemical and Neurotrophic Consequences of Nerve Deformation: Clinical Implications in Relation to Spinal Manipulation." *Journal of the American Osteopathic Association* 75:409-414, 1975.

[861] Greenman, Philip E. "Roentgen Findings in the Craniosacral Mechanism." *Journal of the American Osteopathic Association* 70:24-35, 1970.

[862] Retzlaff, Ernest W.; Mitchell, Fred L. Jr.; Upledger, John E.; Vredevoogd, Jon; Walsh, Jane. "Neurovascular Mechanisms in Cranial Sutures." *Journal of the American Osteopathic Association* 80(3):918, 1980.

[863] Retzlaff, E. W.; Mitchell, Fred L.; Upledger, John E.; Vredvevoogd, Jon; Walsh, Jane A. "Age Related Changes in Human Cranial Sutures." *American Osteopathic Association Research Conference*. Chicago, Illinois. March 15-17, 1979.

[864] Upledger, John E. "Mechano-Electric Patterns During Craniosacral Osteopathic Diagnosis and Treatment." *Journal of the American Osteopathic Association* 78:782-791, 1979.

[865] Still, A. T. *Philosophy of Osteopathy*. Published by Andrew Taylor Still. Kirksville, Missouri, 1899. P. 41.

[866] Robbins, Stanley L. *Pathologic Basis of Disease*. W. B. Saunders Company. Philadelphia, 1974. P. 13.

[867] Ghanbari, Hossein A.; Miller, Barney E.; Haigler, Henry J.; Arato, Mihaly; Bissette, Garth; Davies, Dick F.; Nemeroff, Charles B. et al. "Biochemical Assay of Alzheimer's Disease - Associated Protein(s) in Human Brain Tissue." *Journal of the American Medical Association* 263(21):2907-2910, 1990.

[868] Staff Writer. “Alzheimer's Clue: It May Not Begin in the Brain.” *TIME Magazine*. October 1, 1989. P. 86.

[869] Maharishi Mahesh Yogi. Heard from a video tape of Maharishi speaking at Maharishi University of Management. Fairfield, Iowa, 1981.

[870] Korr, Irvin M. “The Spinal Cord as Organizer of Disease Processes: III. Hyperactivity of Sympathetic Innervation as a Common Factor in Disease.” *Journal of the American Osteopathic Association* 79(4):232-137, 1979.

[871] Korr, Irvin M. “Sustained Sympathicotonia as a Factor in Disease.” from *The Neurobiologic Mechanisms in Manipulative Therapy*. Plenum Publishing Corporation. New York, 1978. pp. 229-268.

[872] Truhlar, Robert E. *Doctor A. T. Still in the Living*. Robert E. Truhlar, D.O. Cleveland, 1950. P. 27.

[873] Lao-Tzu; Mitchell, Stephen (Translation and Commentary). *Tao Te Ching.* Harper and Row, Publishers, Inc. New York, 1988. P. 35.

End Notes Chapter 14:

[874] Maharishi Mahesh Yogi. *Meditations of Maharishi Mahesh Yogi.* Bantam Books. New York, 1968. Pp. 1-23.

[875] Dennett, D. C. “Consciousness” in Gregory, Richard L. *The Oxford Companion to The Mind.* Oxford University Press. New York, 1987. Pp. 159-164.

[876] Wallace, Robert Keith. *The Physiology of Consciousness*. MIU Press. Fairfield, Iowa, 1993. Pp. 17-30.

[877] This classic story about Sir Isaac Newton’s discovery of gravity is thought by some scholars to be apocryphal.

[878] Einstein, Albert. *Relativity. The Special and the General Theory.* Crown Publisher. New York, 1961. Pp. 59-100; Pp. 105-113; and Pp. 115-160.

[879] “Thomas Young.” *The Concise Columbia Encyclopedia.* Columbia University Press. New York, 1989.

[880] Zukav, Gary. *The Dancing Wu Li Masters*. An Overview of the New Physics. William Morrow and Company, Inc. New York, 1979. Pp. 79-88.

[881] Ibid.

[882] Ibid. Pp. 88-89.

[883] Walker, Evan H. “The Nature of Consciousness.” *Mathematical Biosciences* 7:175-176, 1970.

[884] Einstein, Albert; Infeld, Leopold. *The Evolution of Physics.* Simon and Schuster. New York, 1938. P. 152.

[885] From Brewster, *Memoirs of Newton* [1855], *Volume II,* Chapter 27. According to Bartlett, John. *Bartlett's Familiar Quotations.* Little, Brown and Company, Inc. New York, 1980.

[886] Capra, Fritjof. *The Tao of Physics*. Shamballa Publications, Inc. Boston, 1976.

[887] Zukav, Gary. *The Dancing Wu Li Masters*. An Overview of the New Physics. William Morrow and Company, Inc. New York, 1979.

[888] Moyers, Bill. *Healing and the Mind.* Doubleday Publishing. New York, 1993.

[889] Thorne, Kip S. *Black Holes & Time Warps*. Einstein's Outrageous Legacy. W. W. Norton & Company. New York, 1994.

[890] Kaku, Michio. *Hyperspace*. Oxford University Press. New York, 1994.

[891] Wallace, R. Keith. *The Maharishi Technology of the Unified Field: The Neurophysiology of Enlightenment.* MIU Neuroscience Press. Fairfield, Iowa, 1986.

[892] Wallace, R. Keith. *The Physiology of Consciousness.* Maharishi International University Press. Fairfield, Iowa, 1993.

[893] Allman, William. "Alternative Realities." *U.S. News & World Report*. May 9, 1994. Pp. 59-62.

[894] Observed by Dr. Michael H. I. Borger. Glassed-In Tibet display at the Field Museum of Natural History in Chicago, Illinois. Summer, 1994.

[895] Wallace, Robert Keith. T*he Maharishi Technology of the Unified Field: The Neurophysiology of Enlightenment.* MIU Neuroscience Press. Fairfield, Iowa, 1986. Pp. 5-23.

[896] Ibid.

[897] Ibid. P. 1.

[898] Ibid.

[899] Sharma, Hari. *Freedom from Disease.* Veda Publishing. Toronto, 1993. Pp. 207-208.

[900] Frawley, David. *Ayurvedic Healing. A Comprehensive Guide.* Passage Press. Salt Lake City, 1989.

[901] Treadway, Scott; Treadway, Linda. *Ayurveda & Immortality*. Celestial Arts. Berkeley, 1986.

[902] Sharma, Ram Karan; Dash, Vaidya Bhagwan. (Translation and Commentary.) *Agnivesa's Caraka Samhita*. Based on Cakrapani Datta's Ayurveda Dipika. Volume I.

Sutra Sthana. Volume II. Nidanasthana; Vimanasthana; Sarira Sthana; Indriyasthan. Chowkhamba Sanskrit Series Office. Varanasi, India, 1976.

903 Bhishagratna, Kaviraj Kunjalal (Translator and Commentator). *Sushruta Samhita.* Volume I. Uttara-Tantra. Volume II. Nidana-Sthan; Sariri-Sthana; Chikitsta-Thana; Kalpa-Sthana. Volume III. Uttara-Tantra. Chowkhamba Sanskrit Series Office. Varanasi, India, 1981.

904 Frawley, David. Op. Cit.

905 Wallace, Robert Keith. Op. Cit., Pp. 10-11.

906 Sharma, Hari. Op. Cit., Pp. 140-143.

907 Wallace, Robert Keith. *The Physiology of Consciousness*. MIU Press. Fairfield, Iowa, 1993. Pp. 64-70.

908 Maharishi AyurVeda is the name of the specific revision of Ayurveda that resulted from Maharishi Mahesh Yogi working with the Vaidyas as described. Other forms of Ayurveda exist, both in India and in the West. When I write Ayurveda, I intend this as a shortened reference to Maharishi Ayurveda.

909 Averbach, Richard; Rothenberg, Stuart. "A Concise Introduction to Maharishi Ayurveda." *Maharishi Ayurveda Medical Association* 1(1):2-3, 1993.

910 Wallace, Robert Keith. *The Physiology of Consciousness*. MIU Press. Fairfield, Iowa, 1993. Pp. 69-92.

911 Ibid.

912 Ibid. Pp. 93-134.

913 Sharma, Hari. Op. Cit., Pp.1-6.

914 Sharma, Hari. Op. Cit., Pp. 15-72.

915 Sharma, Hari. Op. Cit., Pp. 1-72.

916 Sharma, Hari. Op. Cit., P. 7.

917 Sharma, Hari. Op. Cit., Pp. 6-10.

918 Ibid.

919 Ibid.

920 Niwa, Y. "Effect of Maharishi 4 and Maharishi 5 On Inflammatory Mediators - With Special Reference to Their Free Radical Scavenging Effect." *Indian Journal of Clinical Practice* 1(8):23-27, 1998.

[921] Panganamala, R. V.; Sharma, H. M. "Antioxidant and Antiplatelet Properties of Maharishi Amrit Kalash (M-4) in Hypercholesterolemic Rabbits." Paper presented at the International Atherosclerosis Society, 9th International Symposium on Atherosclerosis. Rosemont, Illinois. October 6-22, 1991.

[922] Sharma, H. M.; Feng, Y.; Panganamala, R. V. "Maharishi Amrit Kalash (MAK) Prevents Human Platelet Aggregation." *Clinia & Terapia Cardiovascolare* 8(3):227-230, 1989.

[923] Dileepan, K. N.; Patel, V.; Sharma, H. M.; Stechschulte, D. J. "Priming of Spleenic Lymphocytes After Ingestion of an Ayurvedic Herbal Food Supplement: Evidence for an Immunomodulatory Effect." *Biochemical Archives* 6:267-274, 1990.

[924] Glaser, J. L.; Robinson, D. K.; Wallace, R. K. "Effect of Maharishi Amrit Kalash on Allergies, described in Maharishi Ayurveda: An Introduction to Recent Research." *Modern Science and Vedic Science* 2(1):89-108, 1988.

[925] Patel, V. K.; Wang, J.; Shen, R. N.; Sharma, H. M. "Reduction of Metastases of Lewis Lung Carcinoma by an Ayurvedic Food Supplement in Mice." *Nutrition Research* 12:51-61, 1990.

[926] Sharma, H. M.; Dwivedi, C.; Satter, B. C.; Gudehithlu, K. P.; Abou-issa, H.; Malarkey, W.; Tejawani, G. A. "Antineoplastic Properties of Maharishi-4 Against DMBA-Induced Mammary Tumors in Rats." *Pharmacology, Biochemistry and Behavior* 35:767-773, 1990.

[927] Iles, Robert L.; Kumar, Naresh; Morales-Ballejo, Hugo. "Emotions and Coronary Heart Disease." *Heart Disease and Stroke.* November/December 1994. Pp. 361-364.

[928] Dracup, Kathleen; Baker, David W.; Dunbar, Sandra B.; Dacey, Robert A.; et al. "Management of Heart Failure. II. Counseling, Education, and Lifestyle Modifications. *Journal of the American Medical Association* 272(18):1442-1446, 1994.

[929] Staff Writer. "Tough Intervention Alters Course of Advanced CAD." *Medical World News* 30(24):8-9, 1989.

[930] Cooper, Edward S. "Prevention: The Key to Progress." *Heart Disease and Stroke.* 2(4):278-282, 1993.

[931] Sun Tzu; Cleary, Thomas. *The Art of War*. Shamballah Publications, Inc. Boston, 1988. Pp. 1-5.

[932] Pollner, Fran. "International Experts Urge MDs to Hit CAD Risk Factors Harder." *Medical World News*. January 1991. P. 11.

[933]Reinberg, A.; Smolensky, M. H. *Biological Rhythms and Medicine.* Springer-Verlag. New York, 1983.

[934] Johnstone, Michael T.; Mittleman, Murray; Tofler, Geoffrey; Muller, James E. "The Pathophysiology of the Onset of Morning Cardivascular Events." *American Journal of Hypertension* 9(4) Part 3: 23S-28S, 1996.

[935] Fantidis, Panayotis; et al. "Morning Cortisol Production in Coronary Heart Disease Patients." *European Journal of Clinical Investigation* 32:304-308, 2002.

[936] Beard, C. Mary; Fuster, Valentin; Elveback, Lila R. "Daily and Seasonal Variation in Sudden Cardiac Death, Rochester, Minnesota, 1950-1975." *Mayo Clinic Proceedings* 57:704-706, 1982.

[937] Marler, J. R.; Price, T. R.; Clark, G. L.; et al. "Morning Increase in Onset of Ischemic Stroke." *Stroke* 20:473-476, 1989.

[938] Lamberg, Lynne. "Time of Day Medication Dose is Taken May Boost Its Efficacy, Cut Toxicity." *Journal of the American Medical Association* 275(15) 1143-1144, 1996.

[939] White, William. "A Chronotherapeutic Approach to the Management of Hypertension." *American Journal of Hypertension* 9(4) Part 3: 29S-33S, 1996.

[940] Troisi, Rebecca J.; Cowie, Catherine C.; Harris, Maureen I. "Diurnal Variation in Fasting Plasma Glucose. Implications for Dignosis of Diabetes in Patients Examined in the Afternoon." *Journal of the American Medical Association* 284(24):3157-3162, 2000.

[941] Smolensky, Michael. "Chronobiology and Chronotherapeutics. Applications to Cardiovascular Medicine." *American Journal of Hypertension* 9(4) Part 3:11S-21S, 1996.

[942] Kaplan, Norman M. "The Ups and Downs of Air Travel." *Cardiology Guide*. December 1988. Pp. 7-9.

[943] Rose, Kenneth Jon. *The Body in Time*. John Wiley & Sons, Inc. New York, 1988.

[944] Whitney, Hunter. "Medicine. The Biological Roller Coaster: Chronobiologists Study the Body's Natural Rhythms." *OMNI Magazine.* February 1994. P. 26.

[945] Ibid.

[946] Ibid.

[947] Kasper, Siegfried; et al. "Epidemiological Findings of Seasonal Changes in Mood and Behavior: A Telephone Survey of Montgomery County, Maryland." *Archives of General Psychiatry* 46:823-833, 1989.

[948] Thompson, C.; et al. "Seasonal Affective Disorder and Season-Dependent Abnormalities of Melatonin Suppression by Light." *Lancet* 336(8717):703-706, 1990.

[949] Wehr, T.A.; et al. "Contrasts Between Symptoms of Summer Depression and Winter Depression." *Journal of Affective Disorders* 23(4):173-183, 1991.

[950] Rosenthal, Normal E. "Diagnosis and Treatment of Seasonal Affective Disorder." *Journal of the American Medicial Association* 270(22):2717-2720, 1993.

[951] Thomas, Patricia. "Elderly Chosen for Light Therapy." *Medical World News*. October 1989, Pp. 25-26

[952] Al-Tamer, Yassar Y.; Al-Hayali, Jasim M. T.; Al-Ramadhan, A. H. "Seasonality of Hypertension." *The Journal of Clinical Hypertension* 10(2):125-129.

[953] Beard, C. Mary; Fuster, Valentin; Elveback, Lila R. "Daily and Seasonal Variation in Sudden Cardiac Death, Rochester, Minnesota, 1950-1975." *Mayo Clinic Proceedings* 57:704-706, 1982.

[954]Orlock, Carol. "Exploring Our Inner Clocks." *Arthritis Today*. September-October 1994. Pp. 34-37.

[955] Culleton, Bruce F., Walsh, Michael; Klarenback, Scott W.; Mortis, Garth; et al. "Effect of Frequent Nocturnal Hemodialysis vs. Conventional Hemodialysis on Left Ventricular Mass and Quality of Life. A Randomized Trial." *Journal of the American Medical Association* 298(11):1291-1299, 2007.

[956] Holmes, Bob. "Molecular Ticktock." *U.S. News & World Report.* January 18, 1993. Pp. 67-68.

[957] Ibid.

End Notes Chapter 15:

[958] Gleick, James. "Chaos." *Science Illustrated.* June 1988. Pp. 12-19.

[959] Smith, Blake W. H. "Chaotic Family Dynamics." *Archives of Family Medicine* 3:231-238, 1994.

[960] Allman, William F. "Science & Society. The Mathematics of human Life." *U.S. News & World Report.* June 14, 1993. Pp. 84-85.

[961] Collier, Peter; Del Calzo, Nick. *Medal of Honor. Portraits of Valor Beyond the Call of Duty.* Artisan: A Division of Workman Publishing Company, Inc. New York, 2003. "Over Japan, 1945: Aboard The City of Los Angeles." Pp. 70-71.

[962] Gregory, Richard L. (Editor). *The Oxford Companion to the Mind.* Oxford University Press. New York, 1987. Pp. 403-405.

[963] Campbell, Joseph. *The Hero with a Thousand Faces.* Bollington Series XVII. Princeton University Press. Princeton, 1973.

[964] Campbell, Joseph; with Moyers, Bill. *The Power of Myth.* Doubleday. New York, 1988. P. 5.

[965] Guyton, Arthur C. *Textbook of Medical Physiology.* Fourth Edition. W. B. Saunders Company. Philadelphia, 1971. Pp. 380-382.

[966] Rose, Kenneth Jon. *The Body in Time.* John Wiley & Sons, Inc. New York, 1988. P. 4.

[967] Ibid. P. 138.

[968] Ibid. P. 28.

[969] Ibid. P. 143.

[970] Ibid. P. 117.

[971] Ibid. P. 89.

[972] Ibid. P. 122.

[973] Korr, I. M.; Wilkinson, P. N.; Chornock, F. W. "Axonal Delivery of Neuroplasmic Components to Muscle Cells." *Science* 155:342-345, 1967.

[974] Rose, Kenneth Jon. Op. Cit.. P. 103.

[975] Pert CB, Snyder SH (March 1973). "Opiate receptor: Demonstration in Nervous Tissue". *Science* 179(4077):1011–4, 1973.

[976] Pert, C. B.; Ruff, M. R.; Weber, R. J.; Herkenham, M. "Neuropeptides and Their Receptors: A Psychosomatic Network." *Journal of Immunology* 135(2Suppl):820s-826s, 1985.

[977] Ibid.

[978] Pert, Candace B. "The Wisdom of the Receptors: Neuropeptides, the Emotions, and Body-Mind." in Ornstein, Robert (Editor); Swencionis, Charles (Editor). *The Healing Brain. A Scientific Reader.* The Guilford Press. New York, 1990. Pp. 147-158.

[979] Ibid.

[980] The Student.
https://www.drtonynader.com/about/the-student/

[981] Dr. Nader and Transcendental Meditation.
https://www.drtonynader.com/about/transcendental-meditation/

[982] Ibid.

[983] Ibid.

[984] Nader, Dr. Tony. *Human Physiology: Expression of Veda and the Vedic Literature.* Maharishi Vedic University. Station 24, 6063 NP Vlodrop, The Netherlands. Reprinted by Maharishi Institute of Management. Maharishi Nagar, India, 1994.

[985] The Scientist.
https://www.drtonynader.com/about/the-scientist/

[986] Ibid.

[987] Dr. Nader and Transcendental Meditation.
https://www.drtonynader.com/about/transcendental-meditation/

[988] Nader, Dr. Tony. Op. Cit..

[989] Nader, Dr. Tony. Op. Cit..

[990] The Leader.
https://www.drtonynader.com/about/the-leader/

[991] Ibid.

[992] G. & C. Merriam Company. *Webster's New Collegiate Dictionary*. Springfield, Massachusetts, 1974. P. 241.

[993] Venes, Donald (Editor). *Taber's Cyclopedic Medical Dictionary.* 21st Edition. F. A. Davis Company. Philadelphia, 2009. P. 511.

[994] Gallup. In depth: topics A to ZL religion 2016.
http://www.gallup.com/poll/1690/religion.aspx. January, 2018.

[995] VanderWeele, Tyler J.; Balboni, Tracy A.; Koh, Howard K. "Viewpoint: Health and Spirituality." *Journal of the American Medical Association* 318(6):519-520, 2017.

[996] Pastor Terry Tyler writing in the Unison Confession of the Order of Worship, First Presbyterian Church. Nappanee, Indiana. March 21, 1999.

[997] Dossey, Larry. *Healing Words*. HarperCollins Publishers. San Francisco, 1993.

[998] Ibid.

[999] Ibid. Pp. 179-181.

[1000] Byrd, Randolph C. "Positive Therapeutic Effects of Intercessory Prayer in a Coronary Care Unit Population." *Southern Medical Journal* 81(7):826-829, 1988.

[1001] Ibid.

[1002] Ibid.

[1003] Ibid.

[1004] Riley, Barth B.; Perna, Robert; Tate, Denise G.; Forchheimer, Marty; Anderson, Cheryl; Luera, Gail. "Types of Spiritual Well-Being Among Persons with Chronic Illness: Their Relation to Various Forms of Quality of Life." *Archives of Physical Medicine Rehabilition* 79:258-264, 1998.

[1005] Koenig, Harold G.; Hays, Judith C.; Larson, David B.; George, Linda K.; Cohen, Harvey J.; McCullough, Michael E.; Meador, Keith G.; Blaer, Dan G. "Does Religious Attendance Prolong Survival? A Six-Year Follow-Up Study of 3,968 Older Adults." *Journal of Gerontology* 54A(7):M370-M376, 1999.

[1006] Mascaro, Juan (Translation). *The Bhagavad Gita* 2:40. Penguin Books. Baltimore, 1971.

End Notes Chapter 16:

[1007] By way of full disclosure, my faith background is Christian. I grew up attending Methodist and later Presbyterian churches. Later my wife and I attended a General Conference Mennonite Church. These days we attend an Evangelical Presbyterian Church. All of these churches are middle of the road Protestant denominations with few theological differences. If you want my personal faith statement, I refer you to the Acknowledgements at the back of this book.

[1008] I emphasize the need to be global minded regarding religion. Engaging patients in arguments about faith, religion, theology, or anything else that is a personal matter is unprofessional and inadvisable. Pointing people toward God and prayer is enough to get them the help they need. They will receive your reminder within the context of the faith they already know, and that accomplishes all that is needed in the arena of patient care.

[1009] I credit my wife, Bonnie M. Borger, with the "Baby Steps" approach. I was in very poor physical health in the late 1980s. When I was struggling to return to health, she encouraged me the way I have encouraged the patients ever since. As I went through all of that, I learned as a patient from her all the practical aspects of patient coaching that made it into this book.

[1010] Heaton, Caryl J. "An Introduction to the Patient-Centered Medical Home." *Osteopathic Family Physician* 6(1):8-13, 2014.

[1011] Singh, Hardeep; Graber, Mark. "Reducing Diagnostic Error Through Medical Home-Based Primary Care Reform." Journal of the American Medical Association 304(4):463-464, 2010.

[1012] Scuderi, Christopher B.; Kenyatta, Y. Lee; Bilello, Lori A.; Webb, Fern J.; Shah, Nipa R. "Team-Based Care – the 'Who' of the Patient-Centered Medical Home." *Osteopathic Family Physician* 3:22-27, 2014.

[1013] Carroll, John. "Lessons Learned in Building the Patient-Centered Medical Home." *Managed Care* 19(8):12-22, 2010.

[1014] Sarfaty, Mona; Wender, Richard; Smith, Robert. "Promoting Cancer Screening Within the Patient Centered Medical Home." *CA Clinical Journal of Cancer* 61(6):397-408, 2011.

[1015] Mosquer, Ricardo A.; Avritscher, Elenir B. C.; Samuels, Cheryl L.; Harris, Tomika S.; et al. "Effect of an Enhanced Medical Home on Serious Illness and Cost of Care Among High-Risk Children with Chronic Illness – A Randomized Clinical Trial." *Journal of the American Medical Association* 312(24):2640-2648, 2014.

[1016] Marjoua, Youssra; Bozie, Kevin J. "Brief History of Quality Movement in US Healthcare." *Current Reviews in Musculoskeletal Medicine* 5:265–273, 2012.

[1017] Chakravarty, Abhuit; Ranyal, Rk. "Contemporary Issue: Total Quality Management – the New Paradigm in Healthcare Management." *Medical Journal Armed Forces India* 57:226-229, 2001.

[1018] Lohr, Kathleen N. (Editor); Committee to Design a Strategy for Quality Review and Assurance in Medicare, Institute of Medicine. *Medicare: A Strategy for Quality Assurance, Volume II: Sources and Methods.* National Academy Press. Washington, D.C., 1990.

[1019] Norris, Meredeth. "Editor's Message. My Patient-Centered Medical Home." *Osteopathic Family Physician* 6(1):6-7, 2014.

[1020] Jabbarpour, Yalda; DeMarchis, Emilia; Bazemore, Andrew; Grundy, Paul. *The Impact of Primary Care Practice Transformation on Cost, Quality, and Utilization. A Systematic Review of Research Published in 2016.* Prepared By the Patient-Centered Primary Care Collaborative. 601 Thirteenth Street, NW Suite 430, North Washington, DC 20005. July, 2017.

[1021] Diamond, Frank. "'High Quality Saves Money,' Or So the Story Goes." *Managed Care*. May 1, 2011, Page 3.

[1022] The National Health Expenditure Accounts (NHEA). U.S. Centers for Medicare & Medicaid Services. Baltimore, 2018. https://www.cms.gov/Research-Statistics-Data-and-Systems/Statistics-Trends-and-Reports/NationalHealthExpendData/NationalHealthAccountsHistorical.html

[1023] Ibid.

[1024] Ibid.

[1025] Ibid.

[1026] *Webster's New Collegiate Dictionary.* G & C, Merriam Company. Springfield, Massachusetts, P. 507.

[1027] I understand that many in the fields of economics, politics, and sociology scorn the use of GNP and prefer to use other measures of economic performance such as Gross Domestic Product, Gross National Income, and Green National Product. To compare apples with apples, I chose to work with the GNP because it was the economic performance measure used by those measuring and comparing Healthcare Expenditures from country to country.

[1028] Organization for Economic Cooperation and Development (OECD) Health Data, 2017. OECD (2017), Health at a Glance 2017: OECD Indicators, OECD Publishing, Paris, http://dx.doi.org/10.1787/health_glance-2017-en.

[1029] Ibid.

[1030] Ibid.

[1031] King, Diana E; Matheson, Eric, Chirina, Svetlana; et al. "The Status of Baby Boomers' Health in the United States. The Healthiest Generation?" *Journal of the American Medical Association Internal Medicine* 173(5): 385-386, 2013.

[1032] Ginzberg, Eli. "High-Tech Medicine and Rising Health Care Costs." *Journal of the American Medical Association* 263(13):1820-1822, 1990.

[1033] Schwartz, William. From a speech given in Washington. Reported by The Associated Press. May 15, 1993.

[1034] I personally researched these office call numbers by asking area offices what they charge to see patients.

[1035] Anderson, D. R et al. "The Relationship Between Modifiable Risks and Group-Level Health Care Expenditures." *American Journal of Health Promotion* 15(1):45-52, 2000.

[1036] U.S. Department of Health and Human Services. *Healthy People 2010: Understanding and Improving Health.* Government Printing Office. Washington, D.C., 2000.

[1037] Ibid.

[1038] Department of Health and human Services. *Center for Disease Control and Prevention. An Ounce of Prevention . . . What Are the Returns?* 2nd Edition. Atlanta, 1999.

[1039] Herron, R. E.; Cavanaugh, K. "Can the Transcendental Meditation Program Reduce the Medical Expenditures of Older People? Longitudinal Cost Reduction in Canada." *Journal of Social Behavior and Personality* 17:415-442, 2005.

[1040] Ibid.

[1041] Herron, R. E.; Hillis, S. L. "The Impact of the Transcendental Meditation Program on Government Payment to Physicians in Quebec: An Update." *American Journal of Health Promotion* 14(5):284-291, 2000.

[1042] Wammes, Joost Johan Godert; van der Wees, Philip J; Tanke, Marit A C; et al. "Systematic Review of High-Cost Patients' Characteristics and Healthcare Utilization." *British Medical Journal* Open July 2018.

[1043] Herron, R. E. "The Impact of the Transcendental Meditation Program on the Medical Expenses of High-Cost People (In Review.) Herron, R. E.; Hillis, S. L. "The Impact of the Transcendental Meditation Program on Government Payment to Physicians in Quebec: An Update." *American Journal of Health Promotion* 14(5):284-291, 2000.

[1044] Orme-Johnson, David W. "Medical Care Utilization and the Transcendental Meditation Program." *Psychosomatic Medicine* 49(1):493-507, 1987.

[1045] National Health Statistics Group, Office of the Actuary. "National Health Expenditures, 1996." Health Care Financing Review 19(1):345; HCFA Publication Number 03400. Health Care Financing Administration. U.S. Government Printing Office. Washington, D.C., Fall, 1997.

[1046] Orme-Johnson, D. W.; Walton, K. "All Approaches to Preventing and Reversing Effects of Stress Are Not the Same." *American Journal of Health Promotion* 12(5):297-299, 1998.

[1047] Milliman & Robertson, Inc. Table 17. *Colorado Workers Compensation Closed Claim Study 1996.* Tillinghast/Towers Parrin. Denver, 1996, 1995, 1994, 1993, 1992, 1991.

[1048] Pope, Thomas L.; Riddervold, Hans O. "Low-Back Pain: When to Get Spine Films." *Diagnosis.* June 1982. Pp. 71-87.

[1049] Barton, J. E.; Haight, R. O.; Marsland, D. W.; et al. "Low Back Pain in the Primary Care Setting." *Journal of Family Practice* 3(4):363-366, 1976.

[1050] Pope, Thomas L.; Riddervold, Hans O. Op. Cit.

[1051] Blair, Steven N.; Kohl III, Harold W.; Barlow, Carolyn E.; Paffenbarger, Jr., Ralph S.; Gibbons, Larry W.; Macera, Caroline A. "Changes in Physical Fitness and All-Cause Mortality. A Prospective Study of Healthy and Unhealthy Men." *Journal of the American Medical Association* 273(14):1093-1098, 1995.

[1052] Laino, Charlene. "CVD Risk Reduction Stressed." *Medical Tribune* 36(23): 1. December 7, 1995.

[1053] Ornish, Dean. *Dr. Dean Ornish's Program for Reversing Heart Disease.* Ballentine Books. New York, 1990.

[1054] Ibid.

[1055] Ornish, Dean; Scherwitz, Larry W.; Billings, James H.; Gould, K. Lance; Merritt, Terri A.; Sparler, Stephen; Armstron, William T.; Oirts, Thomas A.; Kirkeeide, Richard L.; Hogeboom, Charissa; Brand, Richard J. "Intensive Lifestyle Changes for Reversal of Coronary Disease." *Journal of the American Medical Association* 280(23):2001-2007, 1998.

[1056] Schneider, R. H.; Myers, H. F.; Marwaha, K.; Rainforth, M. A.; Salerno, J. W.; Nidich, S. I.; Norris, K. C. "Stress Reduction in the Prevention of Left Ventricular Hypertrophy: A Randomized Controlled Trial of Transcendental Meditation and Health Education in Hypertensive African Americans." *Ethnicity & Disease* 29(4):577-586, 2019.

[1057] Walton, K. G.; Olshansky, E. H.; Schneider, R. H. "Trials of Maharishi AyurVeda for Cardiovascular Disease: A Pooled Analysis of Outcome Studies with Carotid Intima-Media Thickness." *Journal of Preventive Cardiology* 4(1):615-23, 2014.

[1058] Fuller, R. Buckminster; Farrell, Barry. "Playboy Interview: R. Buckminster Fuller – A Candid Conversation with the Visionary Architect/Inventor/Philosopher." *Playboy Magazine.* January 1971. Pp 199-200.

www.ingramcontent.com/pod-product-compliance
Lightning Source LLC
LaVergne TN
LVHW052016200926
848481LV00005B/1503